Handbook *of*
Equine Emergencies

D1483562

Content Strategist: *Robert Edwards*
Content Development Specialist: *Veronika Watkins*
Project Manager: *Anne Collett*
Designer/Design Direction: *Christian Bilbow*
Illustration Manager: *Jennifer Rose*
Illustrator: *Antbits Ltd*

Handbook *of*
Equine Emergencies

Debra Archer, BVMS PhD CertES DipECVS MRCVS FHEA

Philip Leverhulme Equine Hospital,
School of Veterinary Science,
University of Liverpool, UK

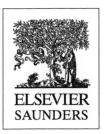

ELSEVIER
SAUNDERS

Edinburgh London New York Oxford Philadelphia St Louis Sydney Toronto 2013

ELSEVIER
SAUNDERS

ISBN 978-0-7020-4545-5

British Library Cataloguing in Publication Data
A catalogue record for this book is available from the British Library

Library of Congress Cataloging in Publication Data
A catalog record for this book is available from the Library of Congress

Notices
Knowledge and best practice in this field are constantly changing. As new research and experience broaden our understanding, changes in research methods, professional practices, or medical treatment may become necessary.

Practitioners and researchers must always rely on their own experience and knowledge in evaluating and using any information, methods, compounds, or experiments described herein. In using such information or methods they should be mindful of their own safety and the safety of others, including parties for whom they have a professional responsibility.

With respect to any drug or pharmaceutical products identified, readers are advised to check the most current information provided (i) on procedures featured or (ii) by the manufacturer of each product to be administered, to verify the recommended dose or formula, the method and duration of administration, and contraindications. It is the responsibility of practitioners, relying on their own experience and knowledge of their patients, to make diagnoses, to determine dosages and the best treatment for each individual patient, and to take all appropriate safety precautions.

To the fullest extent of the law, neither the Publisher nor the authors, contributors, or editors, assume any liability for any injury and/or damage to persons or property as a matter of products liability, negligence or otherwise, or from any use or operation of any methods, products, instructions, or ideas contained in the material herein.

 your source for books, journals and multimedia in the health sciences
www.elsevierhealth.com

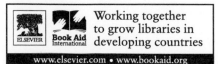
Working together to grow libraries in developing countries

www.elsevier.com • www.bookaid.org

The Publisher's policy is to use paper manufactured from sustainable forests

Contents

Contents

Contents

Contents

Preface

• •

Any emergency situation can be potentially stressful at the best of times and those that occur in equines bring their own unique challenges for the veterinary surgeon. Dealing with the horse, pony, donkey or mule is only part of it; good communication with the client, being aware of legal and safety issues and interacting in a professional manner with other emergency services or members of the public are all key in handling an emergency situation well. It has been a challenge to cover a broad range of equine emergency situations that may be encountered and yet keep this book concise and to a size that can be carried around easily. Varying levels of veterinary expertise and differing opinions, regional variation in diseases and emergency situations that may be encountered, differences in facilities and equipment available and owner economics will play a key part in the approach used and no single approach will necessarily be best. There is also a lack of evidence-based studies regarding the best approach or therapy to use in many situations. I hope that I have managed to provide a practical and concise approach to a variety of emergency situations that will be of use to a wide range of veterinary surgeons. This approach is based on standard or best current practice and relevant evidence-based approaches or outcomes where available. This handbook does not aim to cover a range of diagnostic techniques or referral-level care as this information can be accessed in a number of excellent, more specialist texts and to which readers are referred to. Where relevant, links to useful websites are also provided. It is hoped that the supplementary web-based information will complement the text in this book and provide a quick and easy-to-use summary together with video and audio files. Being prepared for all eventualities can make life much easier and less stressful when that call comes in, and knowing a few handy tips and particular things to avoid or look out for has certainly helped me over the years. I hope that this book will assist in providing this information and will ultimately help to provide the best care for our equine patients.

DA
2013

Acknowledgements

I am extremely grateful to the many knowledgeable, dedicated and kind veterinary colleagues that I have met or worked with and to the many equine patients and their owners who have taught me so much. As a new veterinary graduate working in practice, dealing with an emergency such as an injured horse late at night was much easier to deal with in a supportive environment (thank you to Brian, Martin, Tally, Nina, Alasdair, Alex and team at Scott Veterinary Clinic). I would also like to thank all my colleagues at the Philip Leverhulme Equine Hospital for their help and support. I am very grateful to a number of people who been kind enough to provide feedback on certain areas of the material in this book, including Rachael Conwell, Fernando Malalana, Harry Carslake, Richard Hepburn, David Bardell, Edd Knowles, the Resident team at the hospital, Josh Slater, Derek Knottenbelt, Alex Dugdale, Jonathan Pycock, Nicky Jarvis, Alex Thiemann, Alasdair Foote, David Green, Paul Farrington, Karen Coombe, Peter Green, Nicola Harries, Sarah Gasper, Peter Milner, Peter Clegg, Neil Townsend and Jim Green. Thanks also to Robert Edwards, Veronika Watkins and Anne Collett at Saunders Elsevier for their enthusiasm for this project and for being so patient. And finally, a special thank you to my parents and brother, and to Bruce and Callum.

Acknowledgements

Dedication

· ·

To Professor Barrie Edwards ('Prof')

Abbreviations and symbols

↑	increased
↓	decreased
±	with or without
~	approximately
α2	alpha 2
AAEP	American Association of Equine Practitioners
AHS	African horse sickness
ADR	adverse drug reaction
ALDDFT	accessory ligament of the deep digital flexor tendon
ALP	alkaline phosphatase
AP	auriculopalpebral
ARF	acute renal failure
asap	as soon as possible
ASNB	abaxial sesamoid nerve block
AST	aspartate aminotransferase
AVD	assisted vaginal delivery
BCS	body condition score
BEVA	British Equine Veterinary Association
BGA	blood gas analysis
BMI	body mass index
BS	broad spectrum
BW	body weight
C	cervical vertebra
C&S	culture and sensitivity
Ca^{2+}	calcium
CDET	common digital extensor tendon

CHO	carbohydrate
CK	creatine kinase
Cl⁻	chloride
CN	cranial nerve
CNS	central nervous system
CrCd	cranio-caudal
CRT	capillary refill time
CSF	cerebrospinal fluid
CT	computed tomography
CV	cardiovascular
CVD	controlled vaginal delivery
CVM	cervical vertebral malformation
d	day(s)
DDFT	deep digital flexor tendon
DDSP	dorsal displacement of the soft palate
DDx	differential diagnosis
DE	digestible energy
DFTS	digital flexor tendon sheath
DIC	disseminated intravascular coagulation
DIPJ	distal interphalangeal joint
dL	decilitre(s)
DMI	dry matter intake
DP	dorsopalmar/dorsoplantar
DV	dorsoventral
EDTA	ethylenediaminetetraacetic acid
EEE	Eastern equine encephalitis
EGS	equine grass sickness
EHV	equine herpes virus
EI	equine influenza
EIA	equine infectious anaemia
EIPH	exercise-induced pulmonary haemorrhage
EMS	equine metabolic syndrome
EPM	equine protozoal myeloencephalitis
ERS	exertional rhabdomyolysis syndrome

ERU	equine recurrent uveitis
EVA	equine viral arteritis
FEI	Fédération Equestre Internationale
FNA	fine needle aspirate
g	gram(s)
G	gauge
G –ve	Gram negative
G +ve	Gram positive
GA	general anaesthesia
GFR	glomerular filtration rate
GGT	gamma glutamyltransferase
GIT	gastrointestinal tract
GLDH	glutamate dehydrogenase
GP	guttural pouch
GPM	guttural pouch mycosis
h	hour(s)
Hb	haemoglobin
HIE	hypoxic ischaemic encephalopathy
HQ	hindquarters
HR	heart rate
HYPP	hyperkalaemic periodic paralysis
ICS	intercostal space
IM	intramuscular
IOP	intraocular pressure
IV	intravenous
kg	kilogram(s)
L	litre(s)
LA	local anaesthetic
LCT	large colon torsion
LDH	lactate dehydrogenase
LF	left forelimb
LH	left hindlimb
LM	lateromedial
LMN	lower motor neurone

LN	lymph node(s)
LRS	lactated Ringer's solution
LSN	last seen normal
MC/MT3	third metacarpal/metatarsal bone
MCPJ	metacarpophalangeal joint
MCV	mean corpuscular volume
Mg^{2+}	magnesium
$MgSO_4$	magnesium sulphate
min	minute(s)
mL	millilitre(s)
MM	mucous membranes
MRI	magnetic resonance imaging
MTPJ	metatarsophalangeal joint
Na^+	sodium
NB	navicular bursa
NI	neonatal isoerythrolysis
NMS	neonatal maladjustment syndrome
NSAID	non-steroidal anti-inflammatory drug
O_2	oxygen
OBL	oblique
OP	organophosphate
P3	third (distal) phalanx
PCR	polymerase chain reaction
PCV	packed cell volume
PHF	Potomac horse fever
P1	first phalanx
PIPJ	proximal interphalangeal joint
PLR	pupillary light reflex
PM	post-mortem
PMI	point of maximal intensity
PO	per os
PPID	pituitary pars intermedia dysfunction

psi	pounds per square inch
PSSM	polysaccharide storage myopathy
PU/PD	polyuria/polydipsia
q.	every
RAO	recurrent airway obstruction
RBC	red blood cells
RFM	retained foetal membranes
RHS	right-hand side
RR	respiratory rate
SAA	serum amyloid A
SC	subcutaneous
SDFT	superficial digital flexor tendon
SI	small intestine
SIRS	systemic inflammatory response syndrome
SL	suspensory ligament
SPAOPD	summer-pasture-associated obstructive pulmonary disease
SPL	subpalpebral lavage system
T°	temperature
TBSA	total body surface area
TG	triglycerides
THO	temporohyoid osteoarthropathy
TP	total protein
TPR	temperature, pulse and respiration
UMN	upper motor neurone
URT	upper respiratory tract
US	ultrasonography
VD	ventrodorsal
VEE	Venezuelan equine encephalitis
WBC	white blood cells
WEC	worm egg count
WEE	Western equine encephalitis
WNV	West Nile virus

The basics

General approach to dealing with equine emergencies

Equine emergencies can present a diverse range of challenges. Being prepared to deal with all eventualities (having a plan A, B and sometimes C!) will not only optimise the care that can be given to the patient but also will minimise some of the stress associated with these situations. The key aims are to:

▶ Provide life-saving interventions and ensure human safety is not compromised.

▶ Obtain a full history and perform a full clinical examination.

▶ Perform appropriate and relevant further diagnostic investigations.

▶ Inform the owner/carer of treatment options, enabling them to make informed decisions.

▶ Identify cases where more specialist investigations and/or treatment may be required and initiate discussions with the client at an early stage.

▶ Administer appropriate analgesic, antimicrobial or other medications based upon available clinical evidence – responsible use of antimicrobials is essential (e.g. see British Equine Veterinary Association 'Protect ME' guidelines www.beva.org.uk)

▶ Provide physical protection or support (e.g. bandaging ± splinting) where required.

▶ Interact in a professional manner with other emergency services and veterinary surgeons.

▶ Specify when or in what circumstances re-evaluation should be performed.

▶ Provide advice on prevention where appropriate.

Useful information and paperwork to have

▶ If new to a practice or performing locum work, having some basic information and paperwork to hand can save a lot of stress and hassle.

▶ If new to working in a particular region or country it is important to be aware of equine diseases that are particularly common to that region (including common causes of toxicosis, e.g. poisonous plants or evenomation such as snake bites) and to be aware of any current/recent disease outbreaks.

▶ Useful information and documents to have on hand when dealing with emergencies include:

- contact telephone numbers of practice partners/assistants
- practice consent forms (including euthanasia, general anaesthesia and sedation)
- headed practice paper
- contact telephone numbers for local/regional referral centres and maps/directions (to give to clients)
- names and contact numbers of local horse transporters and equine ambulance services
- names and contact numbers of horse disposal agents/horse cremation companies
- contact details for relevant local/national governmental animal health authorities, e.g. DEFRA.

Equipment

▶ A list of standard and supplementary equipment is given in Table 1.1 – this list is not exhaustive but will provide a guide as to what might be needed when dealing with equine emergencies.

▶ In some situations it may be easier to have specific kits that can be taken to an emergency (e.g. dystocia).

Eye kit – suggested contents
- Ophthalmoscope (if not in standard kit).
- Pen torch.
- Fluorescein stain.
- +/– Rose Bengal stain.
- Mydriatics – tropicamide, atropine.
- Ocular local anaesthetic solutions (e.g. proxymetacaine).
- Local anaesthetic for regional nerve blocks.
- Topical ophthalmic antimicrobial medications (e.g. gentamicin, chloramphenicol).
- Topical ophthalmic steroid medications.
- Small bag of sterile saline.
- Suture material – sizes 2, 3 and 3.5 metric absorbable (3-0, 2-0 and 0 USB), 3.5 metric (0 USB) non-absorbable.
- +/– Subpalpebral lavage kit.

Table 1.1 List of standard and optional equipment that may be required when dealing with equine emergencies

Equipment	Standard	Supplementary
General equipment	Stethoscope Thermometer Direct ophthalmoscope Bowls Clippers Disposable latex gloves (sterile and non-sterile) Rectal gloves Duct tape Chlorhexidine and povidone iodine scrub Surgical spirit Torch/head torch (ideally one that sits at eye level) Penknife Twitch Funnel jug and stirrup pump Hoof knives and hoof testers Shoe removal kit and apron/chaps Stomach tubes (small (foal), medium and large) Lubricant (KY jelly/obstetric lubricant) Haussman gag, dental syringe and mirror Clinical and sharps waste and normal waste bags Paper roll Nylon headcollar and strong lead rope	Refractometer Bucket Small oxygen cylinder, tubing and demand valve Portable lactate measuring device Tracheostomy tube Sterile small and large plastic drapes Plastic bags and labels Urinary catheter
Equipment for administering medications	Syringes (1 mL, 2.5 mL, 5 mL, 10 mL, 20 mL, 35 mL, 50 mL, catheter tipped 60 mL) Needles (14–25G, various lengths) IV catheters (12 and 14G, 8-cm length), extension set, bungs	
Medications (see Table 1.2)	Antimicrobials – IV/IM and oral preparations and in sterile vials (joint medication) Analgesics (NSAIDs/opioids) – IV/oral preparations Sedatives – α2 agonists, butorphanol, acepromazine Tetanus toxoid and antitoxin Topical medications/ wound preparations Oral electrolyte solutions/MgSO4 Steroids (injectable/oral preparations) Antispasmodic medication (butylscopolamine) Oxytocin Clenbuterol and atropine (IV preparations) Sterile fluids (1 L and 5 L bags LRS) and giving sets (small and large animal IV sets) Euthanasia solutions (see p. 389)	

(Continued)

Table 1.1 List of standard and optional equipment that may be required when dealing with equine emergencies (Continued)

Equipment	Standard	Supplementary
Suturing equipment	Scalpel blades (Nos. 10, 11, 15, 22) Scalpel handles (No. 3 and 4) Sterile basic suture pack Sterile cotton swabs Skin stapler / staple remover Suture materials (non-absorbable and absorbable)	
Dressings, bandaging and splints	Cotton wool rolls and poultice material Bandaging material, primary dressings, soft conforming and knitted bandages, cohesive bandages and elastoplast Materials for splinting limbs (p. 383) Foot support – laminitis cases	Nappies (foot dressings)
Laboratory tests/further investigations	Blood tubes – plain/EDTA/lithium heparin/ sodium citrate Formalin in small jars (biopsy specimens) Swabs	Blood culture medium
Biosecurity	Alcohol hand gel Normal moist handwipes Disinfectant Disposable overalls, boot covers Inexpensive stethoscope that can be disposed of	
Clothing/ protective wear	Waterproof coat/trousers Sturdy shoes/boots	Hard hat Reflective tabard/ arm band (vet/ veterinarian)
Extras	Mobile telephone and charging device Veterinary formulary Maps Digital camera	

Emergency field anaesthesia kit (store appropriately when not in use)

- Ketamine/diazepam/α2 agonists.
- Selection of appropriate needles and syringes.
- IV catheters, extension set, bung and suture material.
- Adrenaline 1 mg/mL.
- +/– Endotracheal tubes (pony 20 mm, horses 25 mm, 30 mm).

Foaling/foal resuscitation kit

May be more important where dealing with large numbers of brood mares during foaling season.

- Sterile lubricant, calving ropes, stomach tube and stirrup pump.
- Small oxygen cylinder and demand valve.
- Endotracheal tubes – 8 and 10/12 mm, 55-cm long.
- 5 mL and 2 mL syringes, 20 G, 25mm (1") and 14 G, 25–40 mm (1–1.5") needles.
- Clean towels.
- Large syringe and suction tubing/bulb syringe.
- Self-inflating resuscitation bag (ambubag).
- Adrenaline 1 mg/mL.
- Pen torch.
- 1 L bags LRS × 4.
- Fluid giving set.
- 14G IV catheters and suture material.
- 6F dog urinary catheter.
- ± Foetotomy kit.
- ± Spinal needles (epidural anaesthesia) 19G, 90 mm (3.5").

Horse handling and restraint

▸ Your own personal safety and that of other people around you is critical – emergency situations can sometimes allow little time to consider these factors.

▸ Ensure that you have suitable protective footwear.

▸ When dealing with an unpredictable horse (fractious/trapped/neurological abnormality), wearing protective headgear (e.g. hard hat) may be sensible.

▸ Check that people holding horse/assisting you are competent and are not placed in unnecessary danger.

▸ Be aware of danger zones – kicks, bites, injuries caused by being hit by horse's head, collapse.

▸ Even when horses appear heavily sedated they can be unpredictable and can still kick and bite accurately – ensure handlers are aware of this.

Communication with clients and legal records

▸ Emergency situations can sometimes provide little time to communicate findings and discuss treatment options with the owner/carer and sometimes they may not be present when you arrive – it is important to be aware of the legal issues and national equine veterinary body recommendations regarding treatment of horses (including euthanasia) in these situations (see p. 328).

▸ The priority after human safety is to ensure the welfare of the horse and if in doubt, seek an opinion from a veterinary colleague.

▸ Communication skills will sometimes be put to the test as emergency situations may provoke a variety of emotions in owners, carers, riders and bystanders, ranging from anger, guilt and remorse to grief – remaining calm and professional at all times helps (even if it is sometimes difficult).

▶ Accurate notes should be made at the earliest possible opportunity – as with all medico-legal documents, where written this should be in a legible fashion using black pen (other colours do not photocopy clearly). These details should include:

- Date, time and name of client (and if they are the horse's owner)
- horse name and signalment
- presenting complaint as described by the client
- relevant medical history
- results of clinical examination and any tests performed – a clinical examination checklist is ideal to ensure that normal and abnormal findings are noted
- problem list
- preliminary diagnosis and any differential diagnoses
- definitive diagnosis and when this was made
- treatment administered
- summary of advice provided to the client, including when repeat veterinary examination is recommended
- record details if a second opinion or referral was sought/offered
- signed consent forms (where relevant).

Biosecurity

▶ Infectious and potentially zoonotic conditions (see p. 278) will be encountered in some emergency situations.

▶ Be aware of diseases that are notifiable and their clinical presentations (see Ch. 15).

▶ Veterinary surgeons have the potential to pass infection between premises via infection on their hands/clothing (including footwear)/vehicle (including via tyres) or equipment.

▶ Personal hygiene includes:

- hand washing/use of alcohol-based hand gels
- wearing of gloves if appropriate
- prompt change of contaminated clothing and cleaning/disinfection of footwear
- wearing of protective clothing (e.g. disposable coveralls/gowns and shoe covers) where appropriate.

▶ Cleaning and disinfection of equipment between patients is vital, including:

- rectal thermometers
- nasogastric tubes
- endoscopes / dental equipment.

▶ See p. 387 for details of how to isolate a potentially infectious horse on the premises.

Dealing with other emergency services/rescue authorities

▶ You will be expected to be able to sedate, anaesthetise or euthanase horses, so necessary equipment should be taken with you when dealing with these incidents.

▶ You should also be suitably attired (protective foot and headwear, although some services will provide the latter) and should be identifiable as a vet (e.g. armband, reflective tabard).

▶ On arrival at the scene of an emergency, find out who is in charge and identify yourself to them.

▶ Discuss the plan, including safety issues.

▶ Remember that human life is always a priority over that of an animal.

Referral of horses

▶ Identify cases that may require more intensive care, detailed investigations or surgical intervention and initiate an honest discussion with the owner/carer at an early stage.

▶ If referral is declined, the client should be aware of the potential outcomes.

▶ Contact the referral centre and provide a succinct, clear clinical summary, including presenting signs and treatment administered – these centres are usually very willing to provide advice if you are unsure about referral or treatment options.

▶ Discuss the likely prognosis and range of costs based on the information provided and whether the referral clinic is able to admit the horse for further treatment.

▶ Ask the referral centre whether any specific treatment/procedures (e.g. bandaging and splinting, passage of nasogastric tube) are requested prior to transport.

▶ Ask what the referral centre's payment policy is (e.g. whether a deposit is required on admission).

▶ Inform the client of these discussions – it does not reflect well on the referral hospital or referring veterinary surgeon if the owner arrives at the hospital unprepared for the likely cost of treatment or a hopeless/very poor prognosis.

▶ In insured cases, the policy holder should check that the policy is valid, what conditions and costs are covered, any exclusions in place and the insurance company should be contacted at the earliest possible opportunity.

▶ If transport is not available, transport arrangements should be initiated at an early stage – valuable time can be wasted organising transport in a horse that is sick/deteriorating.

▶ In the case of a sick neonatal foal, it may be more appropriate to send the foal ahead of the mare in a suitable vehicle (see p.230 for referral of sick foals).

▶ Contact the referral centre to confirm whether the horse is being sent to the clinic (or not), let them know an estimated time of arrival and provide them with appropriate contact details for the client/transporter.

▶ Send a written summary of findings of clinical examination (including results of further diagnostic tests), medications given and the time these were administered if possible/ send these details with the client/transporter or by fax/email to the clinic as soon as they are available.

▶ Provide the client/transporter with accurate directions and contact details for the clinic.

▶ If there are any significant delays or problems during transport, ensure that the referral centre is contacted.

Next time....

▶ Emergency situations can sometimes provide little time to think about what to do and treatment may have to be undertaken quickly.

▶ When things do not go to plan, it is worth thinking about what went wrong and what you would do differently next time (including any extra equipment/medications that you would use) – speaking to other colleagues about their experience often yields many useful tips and advice.

▶ Remember to also focus on the good – make a note of what worked well and remember it for next time (forgetting this can be frustrating!).

Normal values and drug dosages (see formulary on http://www. equineemergencieshandbook.com/)

Knottenbelt D C 2006 Equine Formulary 4th edn, Saunders Elsevier.

Corley K, Stephen J 2008 The Equine Hospital Manual, Blackwell Publishing.

Table 1.2 Medications that may be commonly administered in emergency situations in adult horses (see formulary on http://www. equineemergencieshandbook.com/).

Drug name	Dosage and route	Use/comments
Acepromazine	0.02–0.06 mg/kg IV 0.03–0.1 mg/kg IM	Sedative, vasodilator, anxiolytic Rarely may case priapism/paraphimosis in male horses
Adrenaline (epinephrine)	0.01–0.02 mg/kg IV (lowdose)	Asystole, anaphylaxis can be repeated q. 3–5 min
Amikacin	10 mg/kg IV or IM q. 24 h (adults)	Antimicrobial G –ve action – combine with penicillin for BS cover
Atropine	0.005–0.02 mg/kg IV	Bronchodilation – severe exacerbation of RAO/SPAOPD causing respiratory distress. Beware gut stasis/excitement.
Buprenorphine	0.004–0.01 mg/kg IV	Analgesia of 4–8 h duration
Butorphanol	0.01–0.04 mg/kg IV 0.04–0.2 mg/kg IM	Analgesic and sedative – often combined with α2 agonist
Butylscopolamine (hyoscine)/metamizole (Buscopan Compositum®)	5 mL/100 kg BW	Antispasmodic/analgesic – treatment of colic Transient ↑ HR following administration (parasympatholytic activity of butylscopolamine)
Butylscopolamine (hyoscine)	0.3 mg/kg IV	Antispasmodic – colic, assist rectal examination
Carprofen	0.7 mg/kg IV q. 24 h 0.7 mg/kg IM q. 24 h* 0.7 mg/kg PO q. 24 h	NSAID analgesic
Cefquinome**	1–2 mg/kg IV or IM q. 12–24 h	4th generation cephalosporin antimicrobial – BS activity
Ceftiofur**	2.2 mg/kg IV or IM q. 12–24 h* (adults)	3rd generation cephalosporin antimicrobial – BS activity
Clenbuterol	0.8 µg/kg IV q. 12 h 200 µg (total) IV slow or IM (uterine relaxation)	Bronchodilator, tocholytic (uterine relaxation)

Detomidine	0.005–0.02 mg/kg IV 0.02–0.05 mg/kg IM	α2 agonist – sedative/analgesic (usually combined with butorphanol)
Dexamethasone	0.02–0.2 mg/kg IV	Corticosteroid – risk of laminitis low but take care when using in high-risk horses
Diazepam	0.02–0.1 mg/kg IV	Control of seizures; as part of anaesthetic induction
Dimethylsulphoxide (DMSO)	0.5–1.0 g/kg as 10% solution IV q. 12 h	Control of cerebral oedema
Doxycycline	10 mg/kg PO q. 12 h	Tetracycline antimicrobial – BS activity
Enrofloxacin**	7.5 mg/kg PO q. 24 h 5 mg/kg IV q. 24 h	Fluoroquinolone antimicrobial Do not use in young, skeletally immature horses – risk of cartilage damage
Flunixin meglumine	0.25–1.1 mg/kg IV q. 12–24 h	NSAID analgesic/anti-inflammatory/anti-pyretic 'Anti-endotoxic' dose 0.25 mg/kg IV q. 6 h
Frusemide (furosemide)	0.5–2 mg/kg IV q. 6 h	Diuretic – pulmonary oedema, acute renal failure
Gentamicin	6.6 mg/kg IV q. 24 h	Aminoglycoside antimicrobial – predominantly G –ve activity
Ketoprofen	2.2 mg/kg IV q. 24 h	NSAID
Meloxicam	0.6 mg/kg IV or PO	NSAID
Metronidazole	10–25 mg/kg PO q. 12 h 35 mg/kg per rectum q. 12 h	Antimicrobial – predominantly anaerobic activity Oral route – can become anorexic
Morphine	0.12–0.3 mg/kg IV or IM	Opioid analgesic – can see excitatory behaviour if horse is not in severe pain
Omeprazole	1–4 mg/kg PO q. 24 h 0.5 mg/kg IV q. 24 h	Proton pump inhibitor – treatment of gastric ulcers (4 mg/kg PO initial dose, maintenance 1 mg/kg)
Oxytetracycline	5 mg/kg slow IV q. 12 h	Tetracycline antimicrobial – BS activity

(Continued)

Table 1.2 Medications that may be commonly administered in emergency situations in adult horses (see formulary on http://www.equineemergencieshandbook.com/) (Continued)

Drug name	Dosage and route	Use/comments
Oxytocin	10–20 IU/450-kg horse IV (slow) or IM	Various reproductive uses – promotes uterine contraction and milk-letdown (see Ch. 8)
Penicillin G (sodium/potassium)	25 000 IU/kg IV q. 6 h	β-lactam antimicrobial – predominantly G +ve activity, anaerobes
Penicillin G (procaine)	22 000–25 000 IU/kg IM q. 12 h	β-lactam antimicrobial – predominantly G +ve activity, anaerobes
Pentobarbital	2–10 mg/kg IV q. 4 h or as needed	Control of seizures (also euthanasia, see p. 391). Euthanasia solutions are not guaranteed to be sterile
Phenobarbital	5–12 mg/kg IV loading dose	Control of seizures
Phenylbutazone	2.2–4.4 mg/kg IV or PO q. 12 h	NSAID analgesic
Polymyxin B	1000–5000 IU/kg IV q. 8–12 h (dilute in 5% glucose or dextrose)	Binds endotoxin – efficacy questionable if given after initial endotoxic insult
Romifidine	0.04–0.08 mg/kg IV	α2 agonist sedative – usually combined with butorphanol
Suxibuzone	6.25 mg/kg PO q. 12 h initially (reduce dose sequentially after 48 h)	NSAID analgesic; ponies should only receive half the dose rate recommended for horses
Tetanus antitoxin	up to 100 IU/kg (lower for prophylactic use – see manufacturer recommendations)	Prophylactic (SC, IM) and therapeutic use (IV, SC, IM) against C. tetani toxicoinfection
Trimethoprim-sulphonamide	15–24 mg/kg IV q. 8–12 h / 30 mg/kg (combined) PO q. 12–24 h	BS antimicrobial
Xylazine	0.2–1.0 mg/kg IV	α2 agonist sedative – usually combined with butorphanol

*Not licenced for use via this route.
**Protected use recommended by BEVA.
'Protect ME' guidelines www.beva.org.uk

Appendix

GENERAL HISTORY CHECKLIST

- ☐ Signalment – age, breed, gender ± in foal/foaled recently
- ☐ Duration of ownership
- ☐ Use/current level of exercise
- ☐ Current diet
- ☐ Current stabling/management
- ☐ Stereotypic behaviours
- ☐ Parasite and dental prophylaxis
- ☐ Previous medical problems/surgery
- ☐ Ongoing medical problems
- ☐ Current medications
- ☐ Vaccination status
- ☐ Any known drug allergies/reactions
- ☐ Insurance status
- ☐ Current problem
- ☐ When it started/was first noted
- ☐ Signs noted
- ☐ Progression of signs and any in-contacts affected
- ☐ Any treatment already performed

This may be tailored towards individual situations as appropriate.

Vital signs – adult horse/pony

Heart rate	24–40 beats/min
Respiratory rate	12–15 breaths/min
Temperature	37.5–38.4°C

CLINICAL EXAMINATION CHECKLIST

- ☐ General demeanour/mentation
- ☐ Body condition
- ☐ Obvious wounds/scars

Head and neck

- ☐ *MM colour*
- ☐ *Arterial pulse quality*

- [ ] Ears and temperature of extremities
- [ ] Eyes
- [ ] Facial symmetry
- [ ] Nasal airflow/discharge
- [ ] Submandibular LN size
- [ ] Jugular patency/evidence of distension or pulsation

Thorax

- [ ] Heart rate
- [ ] Heart rhythm/murmurs
- [ ] Respiratory rate
- [ ] Abnormal lung sounds – ausculation/percussion
- [ ] Abnormal swelling/wounds

Abdomen

- [ ] GIT sounds in each quadrant
- [ ] Abdominal distension
- [ ] Abnormal swelling/wounds

Perineum/urogenital

- [ ] Rectal temperature
- [ ] Anal tone
- [ ] Penis/prepuce or vulva
- [ ] Mammary glands
- [ ] Urination (if observed)

Limbs

- [ ] Weight-bearing
- [ ] Digital pulses
- [ ] Abnormal swellings/scars/cuts
- [ ] Lameness at walk

Normal values for an equine adult

Check the laboratory's own normal reference ranges for haematology and biochemistry – these will vary between different laboratories. See texts/ contact the laboratory for normal values in non-adult equines.

Haematology

Total erythrocytes (RBC)	$6.8–12.9 \times 10^{12}$/L
Haemoglobin (Hb)	120–145 g/L

Haematology

Packed cell volume (PCV)	0.36–0.42 L/L (36–42%)
Mean cell volume (MCV)	41–49 fL
Total leucocytes (WBC)	6.0–12.0 × 10⁹/L
Neutrophils	2.7–6.7 × 10⁹/L (45–55% of WBC)
Lymphocytes	1.5–5.5 × 10⁹/L (35–50% of WBC)
Eosinophils	0.1–0.6 × 10⁹/L (0–5% of WBC)
Monocytes	0.0–0.2 × 10⁹/L (0–3% of WBC)
Platelets	240–550 × 10⁹/L

Serum biochemistry

Albumin	22–36 g/L
Serum alkaline phosphatase (ALP)	<250 IU/L
Ammonia	<40 mmol/L
Aspartate transaminase (AST)	80–250 IU/L
Bile acids	10–20 μmol/L
Bilirubin (total)	24–50 μmol/L
Creatine kinase (CK)	90–200 IU/L
Gamma glutamyltransferase (γGT)	<40 IU/L
Glucose	4.9–6.2 mmol/L
Total protein (TP)	62.5–70.0 g/L (serum) 65.0–73.0 g/L (plasma)
Globulin	17.0–40.0 g/L
Glutamate dehydrogenase (GLDH)	<6 IU/L
Lactate	<2.0 mmol/L
Lactate dehydrogenase (LDH)	76–400 IU/L
Triglycerides (TG)	0.1–0.8 mmol/L
Urea	3.5–8.0 mmol/L

Electrolytes

Calcium (total)	2.5–4.0 mmol/L
Chloride	90.0–105.0 mmol/L
Potassium	3.5–5.5 mmol/L
Sodium	134.0–143.0 mmol/L

Peritoneal fluid

Appearance	Light yellow, clear
TP	<20 g/L
Lactate	<2.0 mmol/L
WBC	<5 × 10^9/L

Synovial fluid

Appearance	Yellow, clear, viscous
TP	<20 g/L
WBC	<1 × 10^9/L
Neutrophils (%)	<10%

Urine

Appearance	Pale yellow to light brown, often cloudy and contains mucus
Specific gravity	1.012–1.040
pH	7.5–9.5
RBC/Haem	None in normal horses
Glucose	None in normal horses
Protein	None in normal horses (1+ on protein dipstick normal for alkaline urine)
Sediment	Calcium carbonate crystals normal

Conversion factors

Temperature	
°F = 9/5 (°C) + 32	°C = 5/9 (°F) − 32
Length	
1 cm = 0.394 inch	1 inch = 2.54 cm
Weight	
1 kg = 2.2 pounds (lb) 1 lb = 0.454 kg 1 tonne = 2204 lb	
Volume	
1 L = 1.76 UK pint = 2.11 US liquid pints	
1 UK pint = 20 fluid ounces (fl oz) = 0.568 L	
1 US liquid pint = 16 fl oz = 0.473 L	
1 US quart = 0.946 L	
Others	
g/L × 0.1 = g/dL	

2

Wounds and other integumentary emergencies

Wounds 🔊

Wounds are a common emergency encountered in horses and it is important that appropriate first aid, assessment and treatment are performed in order to get the best possible cosmetic and functional outcome.

Advice to owner/agent prior to arrival

▶ If there is profuse haemorrhage, place a clean, ideally sterile dressing (e.g. gamgee) and hold firmly over the site, topping up with sequential layers of cotton wool (or any clean, absorbent material in a dire emergency, e.g. a small towel).
▶ If the horse is unable to weight-bear or is very lame, it should not be moved unless it is in imminent danger.

Initial first aid and history taking

Administer first aid as appropriate

▶ Control any severe external haemorrhage (see p. 186).
▶ If very lame, assess the limb for possible fracture or tendon/ligament injury (see p. 38).
▶ If the horse is distressed, check its cardiovascular and respiratory status to rule out acute internal haemorrhage (see p. 186)/dyspnoea (see p. 85) prior to administering sedation.
▶ Control seizures if present following traumatic injuries to the head (see p. 144).

Obtain a full history

Specific questions that should be asked include:
▶ Any previous/ongoing medical problems and current medication.
▶ Tetanus status.
▶ When the wound was sustained or if unknown when LSN.

- ▶ How it happened/circumstances surrounding injury:
  - bites from other mammals – consider the likelihood of rabies in endemically infected regions (see p. 287)
  - puncture wounds on nose, head and distal limbs – consider the likelihood of snake bite depending on geographic region/season (see p. 304).
- ▶ Whether a penetrating object was involved:
  - obtain details about the type of object and depth of penetration (ideally have a look at it) and description of anything removed from the wound
  - wood is particularly prone to splintering – care should be taken during initial examination to check that no fragments remain (US can be very helpful in locating fragments undetected on palpation).
- ▶ If there was significant haemorrhage.
- ▶ If there was significant blunt trauma, e.g. horse hit a wall.
- ▶ Any initial lameness.
- ▶ If any wound treatment has already been performed and what has been administered.

Perform a full clinical examination

Initial physical examination

- ▶ Assess for evidence of shock – check HR, MM, RR.
- ▶ Assess the horse's mentation and general physical status.
- ▶ Check for any concurrent problems that may have resulted in the horse sustaining the wound, e.g. signs of colic.
- ▶ Make a note of the wound(s) sustained and carefully check for other, less obvious injuries:
  - this is particularly important in horses that have a long hair coat/feathered legs as other small wounds (especially puncture wounds) can be missed
  - dried blood/localised swelling provide useful clues – the haircoat should then be clipped for more detailed evaluation.
- ▶ Assess the horse for signs of concurrent damage to adjacent or underlying structures, e.g. evidence of lameness or ocular trauma.
- ▶ Determine whether the surroundings and facilities are suitable for assessment of the wound(s) or if the horse needs to be moved to a more appropriate site – the area should be clean, dry and well lit.

Perform a detailed examination of the wound(s)

- ▶ ± Administer sedation if required.
- ▶ Assess the likely age of the wound (recent/old) and degree of contamination (relatively clean/dirty/grossly contaminated).
- ▶ Apply sterile gel to any exposed subcutaneous tissues (e.g. hydrogel/unopened tube of KY jelly) to stop any hairs becoming lodged in the wound and acting as a foreign body.
- ▶ Dampen the hair around the wound using water/sterile gel (this helps to clump hairs together, minimising hair contamination of the site) and clip around the site – if the area is grossly contaminated with blood/mud, remove this using water first (ideally warm water).
- ▶ Clean around the site using chlorhexidine/povidone iodine scrub solution in warm water and cotton wool/swabs, but ensure that this fluid does not run into the wound.

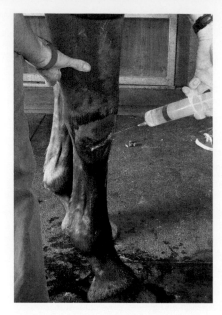

Figure 2.1 Lavage of a wound prior to sterile digital exploration.

▶ Remove the sterile gel and lavage the wound (Fig. 2.1).
▶ The lavage solution must not be cytotoxic (or it will delay wound healing) and ideally fluids should be warmed (to minimise vasoconstriction at the site).
▶ Suitable lavage solutions include:
  ▪ sterile polyionic fluids, e.g. saline, LRS
  ▪ 0.05% chlorhexidine solution (2.5 mL of 2.5% scrub in 100 mL water)
  ▪ 0.1% povidone iodine (1 mL of 10% scrub in 100 mL water).
▶ The ideal pressure is around 10–15 psi. This can be achieved by using:
  ▪ 35- or 60-mL syringe and 18/19G needle
  ▪ clean plastic spray bottle
  ▪ commercial sprays (e.g. Aquaspray®).
▶ Once the site has been thoroughly lavaged, apply sterile gloves and use a finger or sterile probe to determine:
  ▪ the depth and direction of the wound
  ▪ the presence of any foreign material e.g. soil, wood fragments
  ▪ subcutaneous pockets
  ▪ bone/tendon exposure.
▶ Consider the likelihood of communication between the wound and a synovial structure (Table 2.1 and Figs 2.2–2.4) and potential for synovial sepsis (see p. 47).
▶ Determine whether the thoracic (see p. 86) or abdominal cavities (see p. 75) may have been penetrated.

Table 2.1 Key synovial structures to consider when assessing wounds sustained to the limb

Region of limb	Synovial structures
Distal limb (distal to hock/carpus)	Distal interphalangeal joint (coffin joint/DIP) Navicular bursa (NB) Proximal interphalangeal joint (pastern joint/PIP) Metacarpo/tarso phalangeal joint (fetlock joint MCP/MTP) Digital flexor tendon sheath (DFTS)
Proximal forelimb (carpus and above)	Carpometacarpal joint Middle carpal joint Antebrachiocarpal joint Extensor tendon sheaths (common and lateral digital extensor tendons) Carpal sheath Elbow joint Scapulohumeral joint (shoulder joint) Bicipital bursa
Proximal hind limb (hock and above)	Tarsometatarsal joint (TMT) Centrodistal joint; distal intertarsal joint (DIT) Talocalcaneal-centroquartal joint; proximal intertarsal joint (PIT) Talocalcaneal joint Tarsocrural joint Calcaneal bursa Tarsal sheath Extendor tendon sheaths (long and lateral digital extensor tendons) Femoropatellar joint Femorotibial joint Coxofemoral joint (hip joint)

Further assessment and treatment

▸ Knowledge of the regional anatomy and cause of injury is important when assessing wounds affecting different areas (see Figs. 2.5–2.9).

▸ Decide whether further assessment (e.g. radiography, US) or specific treatment (e.g. further exploration under GA) is required and whether you have the facilities/expertise to perform this, or if examination at hospital facilities/referral may be more appropriate.

▸ Decide how the wound would be managed best – primary closure/healing by secondary intention or delayed closure (tertiary) based on:
  ▪ time since injury occurred
  ▪ degree of contamination and infection
  ▪ evidence of tissue defects
  ▪ presence of flaps of tissue and their viability.

▸ In general, wounds that should be sutured include:
  ▪ wounds that are fresh (i.e. <8 h old) with healthy-looking tissue at the wound margins
  ▪ wounds around the eyelid, nostrils and lips

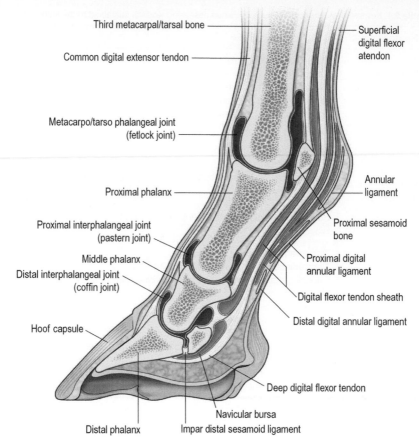

Figure 2.2   Key anatomic structures of the distal limb including synovial structures.

▶ If suturing of the wound is indicated, decide if this can be performed under standing sedation and local anaesthesia or if it would it be easier and safer for this to be performed under GA (at a hospital premises or on site) or at a specialist facility.

▶ Wounds in high-motion areas that are suitable for suturing may require immobilisation, e.g. distal limb casts/cast bandages – in these cases wound closure may be best performed in hospital/referral facilities.

▶ Administer NSAIDs and BS antimicrobials.

▶ Check tetanus status.

HANDY TIP

Owners often expect wounds to be sutured and it is important to explain why this is not necessarily the best option, e.g. grossly contaminated/infected wound that will break down within a few days (negating the time and cost of suturing), or the risk of sealing infection within a wound, which will delay wound healing.

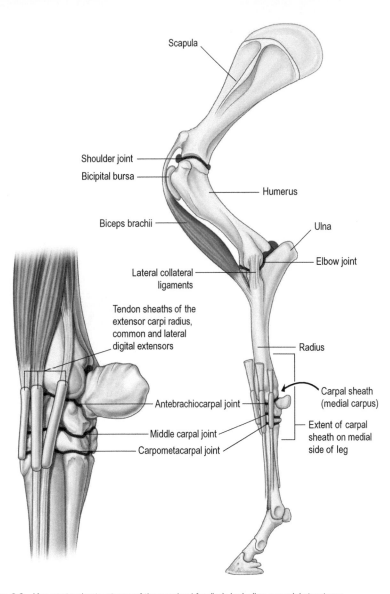

Figure 2.3 Key anatomic structures of the proximal forelimb including synovial structures.

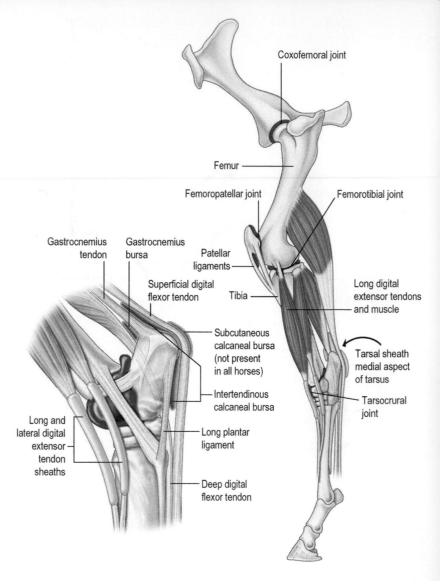

Figure 2.4 Key anatomic structures of the proximal hindlimb including synovial structures.

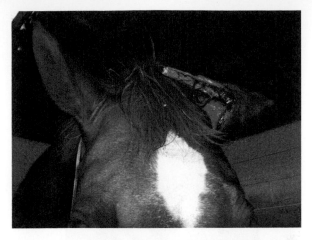

Figure 2.5   Stick injury to the ear of a horse. It is important to try to ensure no wood fragments remain, as splintering frequently occurs and will result in a foreign body reaction and delayed wound healing.

Courtesy of Rachael Conwell.

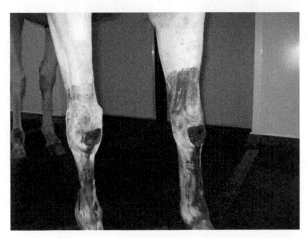

Figure 2.6   Wounds sustained to the dorsal aspect of the carpi after the horse fell onto a road. It is important to determine whether synovial structures have been involved when wounds have been sustained in the region of a joint or tendon sheath.

Prophylaxis against tetanus

- If vaccinated against tetanus in last 12–24 months – no further treatment required.
- Deep/heavily contaminated wound in a horse that has not been vaccinated against tetanus in the last 12 months – administer tetanus toxoid vaccine.
- Unvaccinated horse (or unknown recent vaccination history) with a deep/contaminated wound – administer both tetanus toxoid vaccine and tetanus antitoxin but administer in separate syringes at different body sites to reduce the risk of serum hepatitis developing subsequently.

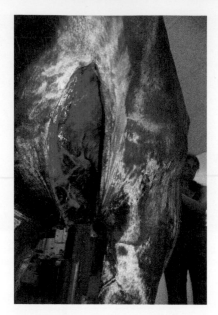

Figure 2.7   Wound sustained to the axilla of a horse. It is important to determine involvement of deeper structures, e.g. thoracic cavity, when assessing wounds in this region and to minimise movement of the horse following wound repair. Subcutaneous emphysema may develop in these cases.

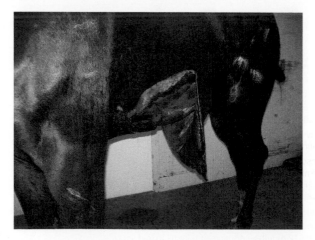

Figure 2.8   Assessment of wounds overlying the thoracic and abdominal cavities should determine whether penetration into these cavities has occurred (see p. 86 and p. 75).

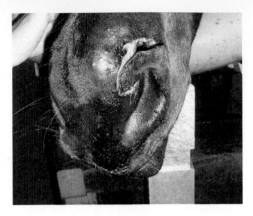

Figure 2.9 Wounds sustained to the nostrils or eyelids must undergo careful repair to ensure a functional and cosmetic result (see p. 102 and p. 109).

Primary closure of wounds

▶ See relevant sections for suturing of eyelids (see p. 109) and lips (see p. 79)/nostrils (see p. 102).

▶ Plan how you are going to suture the site (suture material type and pattern), whether placement of a drain is required and how the site will be protected afterwards.

▶ Check you have all the necessary equipment (including suture materials, stents and drains) and that you are working in an area where you will be undisturbed and sterility will not be compromised.

▶ Decide whether local anaesthetic nerve blocks are appropriate – these are most helpful when suturing wounds around the head (see p. 365) and lower limb.

▶ In other locations, it may be easiest to infiltrate local anaesthetic around the site using a ring block:

    ▪ avoid injecting local anaesthetic solution directly via the wound margins

    ▪ avoid use of anaesthetic solutions that include adrenaline – these will have detrimental effects on wound healing

▶ Decide whether further sedation is required/twitch should be applied before starting.

▶ Remove any necrotic, non-viable tissue and foreign material, as their presence will delay wound healing and may contribute to wound dehiscence.

▶ Preserve tissue flaps wherever possible, especially where involving the eyelid margin, nostrils and distal limbs, as they will act as a biological dressing and will provide some protection.

▶ Gentle scarification of the wound margins using a small (e.g. No. 10/15) scalpel blade to induce a small amount of haemorrhage is useful to remove superficial necrotic material.

KEY TIP

Do not apply antibacterial scrub solutions that would normally be used to prepare the skin prior to surgery to wounds at their normal concentrations as they will cause significant cellular damage, delaying wound healing and contributing to wound dehiscence.

Staples and suture materials

▶ Skin staples are very useful in some situations (e.g. small skin flaps on the head) and can usually be placed relatively easily and quickly.
▶ In general, staples should not be placed where skin edges are under any degree of tension.
▶ See Tables 2.2 and 2.3 for types of suture materials and patterns to use according to tissue type.
▶ Needles:
  ▪ non-cutting (taper point) – fat, muscles and viscera
  ▪ cutting (conventional/reverse/tapered) – fascia and skin.

Table 2.2 Guideline for suture material selection.

Structure being sutured	Suture material type	Suture size	
		USB	Metric
Skin (appositional)	Non-absorbable monofilament	2-0–0	3–3.5
Skin (tension)	Non-absorbable monofilament	0–2	3.5–5
Subcutis	Absorbable monofilament or multifilament	3-0–2-0	2–3
Muscle	Absorbable monofilament or multifilament	2-0–2	3–5
Fascia	Slow absorbable monofilament or multifilament	0–3	3.5–6
Tendon	Slow absorbable monofilament	2	5
Vessel (ligatures)	Absorbable monofilament or multifilament	3-0–0	2–3.5

Adapted from Céleste and Stashak (2008).

Table 2.3 Suture patterns indicated for closure of different tissue types

Suture pattern	Tissue types in which they may be used
Simple interrupted	Skin (appositional), subcutis, fascia
Simple continuous	Skin (appositional), subcutis, fascia
Ford interlocking	Skin (appositional)
Interrupted horizontal mattress	Skin (tension), subcutis, fascia, muscle
Interrupted vertical mattress	Skin (tension), subcutis, fascia, muscle
Cruciate	Fascia, occasionally skin
Continuous intradermal/subcuticular	Intradermal skin closure

- Suture pattern:
  - generally simple interrupted sutures are most suitable for closure of skin, except where there is a degree of tension on the site
  - drip tubing can be used to create stented (quilled) sutures – this helps to ↓ pressure necrosis where mattress sutures are used (Fig. 2.10).

Drains

- If there is a subcutaneous pocket where fluid is likely to accumulate, development of a seroma can be avoided by bandaging the limb and/or and placing a drain.
- This can be done easily with minimal equipment other than a latex (Penrose) drain (see specialist texts for use of more complex drains in larger cavities).
- Drains should never exit the suture line (this will ↑ the risk of dehiscence):
  - place a curved artery forceps into the most dependent portion of the subcutaneous pocket with the instrument curved towards the skin
  - open the jaws of the forceps and make a small incision (depending on the size of the drain) between the jaws, taking care not to incise into any important adjacent structures
  - advance the tips of the forceps through the skin, grasp the drain and pull a 3–5-cm portion into the cavity
  - ± place a single suture to secure the drain to the skin (to prevent it being displaced)
  - enclose the end of the drain within the wound dressing where appropriate (to prevent ascending infection)
  - remove in 48–72h (most serum/blood should have drained from the site by this time).

Wound dressings and bandaging

- In general for all wounds of the distal limb a primary sterile, absorbent, non-adherent dressing should be applied over the site and the limb bandaged to reduce movement, protect the site and reduce contamination (see p. 381).
- Stent bandages can be use to protect other regions where bandaging is difficult (see website or specialist texts).
- Sutured/stapled wounds in other areas may not require dressings/bandaging.

Second intention/delayed primary closure (tertiary healing)

- Apply sterile hydrogel ± non-adherent, absorbent dressing (depending on wound location) to aid debridement.
- Bandaging (± use of splints/cast bandage) of distal limbs is important – ↓ movement and swelling, protects against trauma and contamination.
- See specialist texts/articles for ongoing wound management, including performing skin grafts.

Ongoing care

Analgesia/anti-inflammatory medication

- Generally, administration of NSAIDs IV followed by course administered PO is appropriate (depending on degree of swelling and initial response to medication).
- Care should be taken not to mask potential synovial sepsis – if in any doubt, provide initial analgesia IV and reassess again in 24h.

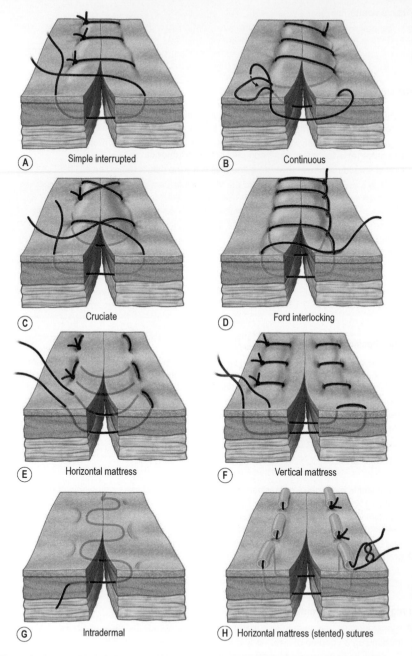

Figure 2.10 Line drawing of suture patterns that may be used in the closure of equine wounds.

(A) Simple interrupted
(B) Continuous
(C) Cruciate
(D) Ford interlocking
(E) Horizontal mattress
(F) Vertical mattress
(G) Intradermal
(H) Horizontal mattress (stented) sutures

Antimicrobial therapy

▶ Depends on the degree of initial contamination, damage to surrounding tissues and ongoing tissue inflammation.
▶ Generally BS antimicrobials administered initially IV or IM followed by administration PO for up to 5–7 d.

General aftercare

▶ Box rest is indicated in wounds at sites of high motion/axillary region:
  ▪ owners should monitor the horses feed intake and faecal output (↑ risk of colon impaction).
▶ Discuss when bandage changes need to be performed:
  ▪ frequent changes (e.g. every 48 h) if very exudative/bandage slips or less frequent (e.g. every 5 d) if minimal exudation and bandage does not slip.
▶ Skin sutures/staples require removal in 10–14 d.
▶ Warn the owner about possible complications that may occur:
  ▪ bone sequestration where periosteal damage has occurred (± radiography required in 4–6 weeks)
  ▪ wound dehiscence
  ▪ foreign material remaining in situ (e.g. wood fragments)
  ▪ sores associated with bandaging

Urticaria

Urticarial reactions are common in the horse and in severe cases may require emergency management.

Clinical signs

▶ Multiple, raised oedematous plaques.
▶ ± Accompanied by pruritus.
▶ ± Anaphylaxis in severe cases.

Assessment and treatment (Fig. 2.11)

▶ Treat anaphylactic reaction if evident (see p. 270).
▶ Nettle stings can result in urticarial reactions and acute ataxia (see p. 306).
▶ Acute onset lesions may resolve spontaneously in 24–48 h.
▶ Dexamethasone 0.02–0.1 mg/kg IV (depending on initial severity) usually results in rapid resolution of the lesions.
▶ Determine if ongoing therapy is required, e.g. persistence of lesions:
  ▪ prednisolone 0.5–1 mg/kg/d – reducing dose
  ▪ ± antihistamines (hydroxyzine hydrochloride 1.0–1.5 mg/kg q. 8–12 h).
▶ Based on the history and clinical examination, determine the most likely cause (often by exclusion of potential causes) and prevent repeat exposure to the inciting antigen:
  ▪ stop drug administration/change to unrelated drug and avoid in the future
  ▪ remove from environment (if environmental cause suspected)

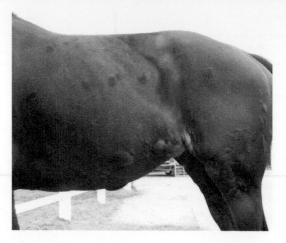

Figure 2.11   Urticaria in a horse evident as multiple raised plaques over the trunk and hindquarters.
Courtesy of Derek Knottenbelt.

▶ Lesions can take 1–2 weeks (and as long as 6–10 weeks to fully resolve).
▶ If lesions persist or >3 episodes occur, further investigations, including biopsy, dietary and environmental restrictions, are warranted.

Possible causes of urticaria

- Drugs (may be carrier/preservative).
- Food/feed additives.
- Insect bites.
- Environmental allergens (contact with irritant plants and chemicals or exposure to inhaled allergens).
- Infectious skin conditions (parasites/bacteria/fungi/viral).
- Systemic disease (e.g. cutaneous vasculitis).
- Physical – exercise/pressure/cold.
- Transfusion reactions.
- Chronic idiopathic.

Cellulitis/lymphangitis

Cellulitis and lymphangitis are common conditions, and affected horses may initially be presented for assessment of severe, acute lameness. Diffuse bacterial infection of the dermis and subcutaneous tissues can dissect through deeper tissue planes, causing severe inflammation in one or more limbs, and it can be difficult to differentiate between the two conditions. Lymphangitis may be associated with particular infectious diseases in certain geographic regions, including ulcerative lymphangitis due to *Corynebacterium pseudotuberculosis* (worldwide) and epizootic lymphangitis due to *Histoplasma farciminosum* (Africa, Middle East).

Clinical signs

▶ Cellulitis – acute painful swelling often in a single limb.
▶ Lymphangitis – diffuse soft tissue swelling affecting an entire limb with prominent superficial lymphatic vessels.
▶ Heat and pain on palpation.
▶ Severe lameness.
▶ ± Pyrexia.
▶ ± ↑ HR.
▶ Skin can become devitalised and suppurates or sloughs.
▶ Lymphangitis – lymphatic vessels become enlarged and thickened ± localised oedema and ulcers along their course.
▶ Can develop laminitis, bacteraemia, osteomyelitis, extensive tissue necrosis, widespread thrombosis, endotoxaemia and extensive skin loss.

Initial assessment

▶ Obtain a thorough history. Specific questions that should be asked include:
  ▪ any history of trauma or recent surgery on the limb
  ▪ recent pastern dermatitis.
▶ Perform a thorough clinical examination:
  ▪ look for any wounds, draining tracts or other underlying cause (e.g. foreign body penetration)
  ▪ determine whether synovial sepsis is possible (wounds in close proximity to a joint/tendon sheath, see p. 47).
▶ Undertake further investigations as required:
  ▪ blood samples for haematology – ↑ fibrinogen, normal/ ↑ systemic WBC
  ▪ radiography/US – rule out other musculoskeletal injury
  ▪ swabs taken from any discharging sites for bacterial C&S
  ▪ US can assist identification of pockets of fluid that may be used to obtain samples for bacterial culture
▶ ± Drainage of sites (depending on location and proximity to other structures).

Treatment and prognosis

▶ Aggressive treatment is required.
▶ Start BS antimicrobials, e.g. penicillin/gentamicin:
  ▪ alter regimen based on results of C&S.
▶ Administer NSAIDs – sufficient analgesia required to encourage weight-bearing.
▶ ± Administer corticosteroids:
  ▪ can be used in severe cases of lymphangitis to reduce fibrosis
  ▪ may be indicated in severe cases of celluliutis, but only once infection is under control.
▶ Bandaging, hydrotherapy, in hand walking.
▶ Place foot support on the contralateral limb (see laminitis, p. 45).
▶ Surgical treatment may be required in severe cases.
▶ Following recovery, horses rarely regain the original contour of limb and are predisposed to recurrence.

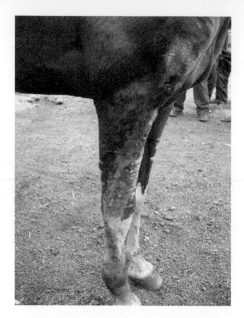

Figure 2.12 Epizootic lymphangitis in a horse in Ethiopia. This is a notifiable disease in the UK (see Ch. 15).
Courtesy of Fernando Malalana.

▶ Consider infectious causes, e.g. ulcerative lymphangitis due to *Corynebacterium pseudotuberculosis* or *Histoplasma farciminosum* (Epizootic lymphangitis – Fig. 2.12) in high-risk regions (refer to texts for further details).

Burn injuries

These are relatively uncommon and usually occur in horses that have become trapped in stable/barn fires. In developing countries, burn injuries may be seen in debilitated horses that have fallen onto domestic outdoor fires. Occasionally, thermal burns may be seen secondary to lightning strikes (see p. 317) or contact with caustic substances. It is important to discuss duration of therapy, likely prognosis and costs at the onset. In severe cases prolonged care will be required (possibly for life) and euthanasia may be a reasonable option in these horses.

Initial first aid and assessment

▶ Provide immediate first aid care and initial assessment, as for fire and smoke injuries (see p. 318).
▶ Administer NSAIDs (if not already performed).
▶ Estimate the extent of the burns using the rule of nines (Table 2.4) – the percentage of total body surface area (TBSA) affected by burn injuries is correlated with mortality.
▶ Evaluate the severity of the burns (Table 2.5) – the depth of burn injuries is correlated with morbidity.

Table 2.4 Estimation of total body surface area (TBSA) affected by burn injuries

Region	Percentage of TBSA
Each FL	9
Each HL	18
Head and neck	9
Thorax	18
Abdomen	18

Table 2.5 Grading of burns according to the depth of the tissues involved

Type of burn	Tissues involved	Clinical signs and sequelae	Prognosis
1st degree	Most superficial layers	Painful, erythema, oedema and sloughing of superficial layers Generally heal without complications	Good
2nd degree (superficial)	Involve stratum corneum, stratum granulosum and a few basal layer cells – tactile and pain receptors intact	Heal rapidly with minimal scarring in 14–17 d	Good
2nd degree (deep)	Involve all layers of the epidermis Germinal cells within sweat glands and hair follicles spared	Erythema, oedema Can heal spontaneously in 3–4 weeks Usually associated with significant scarring unless skin grafting performed	Fair
3rd degree	Loss of epidermal and dermal components, including adnexa	White – black colour, lack of pain Fluid exudation, tissue swelling, eschar formation Shock, wound infection ± septicaemia common	Guarded–poor
4th degree	Involve all layers of skin as well as underlying muscle, fat, ligaments, fascia and bones		Poor–hopeless

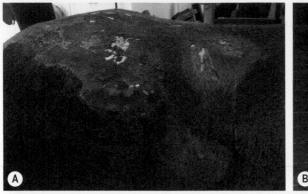
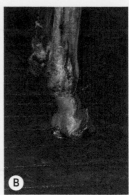

Figure 2.13 (A,B) Burns injury in a horse following a stable fire. First- and second-degree burns were sustained primarily over the head, dorsum of the body and the distal limbs.

▶ Determine whether there is involvement of adjacent/deeper structures, e.g. eyes, blood supply to distal limbs, possible involvement of synovial structures (Fig. 2.13).

▶ Perform a full clinical examination to rule out any concurrent injuries which may alter treatment and prognosis (e.g. other traumatic injuries sustained).

▶ Discuss the likely prognosis and treatment, including euthanasia, where indicated:
  ▪ most burn injuries are superficial, easily managed and heal in a short time
  ▪ euthanasia is indicated in deep partial to full thickness burns (2nd–4th degree) involving 30–50% or more of the total body surface area (TBSA)
  ▪ in severe burns, long-term care can take up to 1–2 years
  ▪ development of infection, pruritus, self-trauma and scarring may prevent the horse from returning to normal function.

Perform wound management

▶ Sedation may be required – check CV status first.
▶ Cool the skin with cold water (4 °C).
▶ Clip the surrounding hair and gently debride any devitalised tissue.
▶ Lavage the site copiously with 0.05% chlorhexidine solution.
▶ Apply a water-based antimicrobial ointment, e.g. silver sulfadiazine, aloe vera, nitrofurazone.

Make a plan for ongoing treatment including wound management

See p. 318 and specialist texts for further details – the key points include:

▶ Intensive care required for treatment of severe burns/burn shock or pulmonary injury – hospitalisation/referral indicated.
▶ Pain management:
  ▪ NSAIDs
  ▪ ± opioids if required (e.g. morphine, butorphanol, CRI lidocaine or ketamine).

▶ Determine how the wound is going to be managed – open/closed:
  ▪ usually open wound management with application of topical antimicrobials – silver sulfadiazine
  ▪ skin grafting may be indicated.
▶ Ensure strict hygiene when performing wound management.
▶ Maintain environmental temperature (28–33 °C) – loss of thermoregulation can occur if large areas are affected.
▶ Optimal nutritional support – humans with burns have a hypermetabolic response requiring 1.4–2 × resting energy requirements:
  ▪ ensure good-quality forage, concentrates and oil supplementation
  ▪ weight loss – nutrition must be addressed.
▶ Monitor for development of anaemia.
▶ Antimicrobials are not indicated unless there evidence of infection:
  ▪ use according to C&S results.

Frostbite

This is relatively uncommon in adult horses but may occur in sick and debilitated individuals and neonates during periods of extremely cold weather.

Clinical signs

▶ Most commonly affected areas: glans penis, ear tips, heels and coronary bands.
▶ Skin initially appears pale.
▶ Followed by erythema, scaling and hair loss.
▶ Can develop severe, dry necrosis and gangrene.

Treatment

▶ Assess for evidence of hypothermia (see p. 216).
▶ Thaw affected regions with warm water (41–44 °C).
▶ Apply antimicrobial ointments that do not contain steroids.
▶ Administer NSAIDs as required.
▶ Surgical debridement, if required, should not be performed until there is obvious demarcation between healthy and non-viable areas.
▶ These sites may be more susceptible to cold injury in the future.

Gunshot injuries

These are relatively uncommon and usually occur at pasture due to horses being accidentally or occasionally deliberately shot. The degree of injury will depend on the type of bullet (high vs low velocity), site of bullet penetration and subsequent anatomic injury. Injuries are most commonly sustained to the skeletal muscles, abdomen and eyes. Secondary infection can occur due to contaminants being drawn into the vacuum created by the bullet.

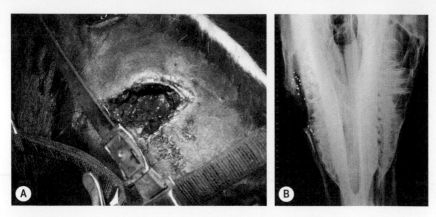

Figure 2.14   (A,B) Gunshot injury to the face of a horse involving the paranasal sinuses and teeth roots – visual assessment, palpation and radiography enabled damage to deeper structures to be assessed.

Initial assessment and treatment

▶ Administer first aid as appropriate, e.g. control any haemorrhage.

▶ Assess the bullet wound(s) in the same way as other wounds.

▶ Determine the likely structures involved, depending on the anatomic location and findings on examination (see Fig. 2.14).

▶ Decide if further diagnostic evaluations are required to evaluate damage to deeper structures, e.g. radiography, US.

▶ Where penetrating injuries of the abdomen have occurred, immediate surgical exploration is warranted:

■ this may be hindered by limited access to some regions of the abdomen and peritoneal contamination may have already occurred.

▶ Debride and lavage the wound and ensure there is adequate drainage – this is more important than removal of the bullet/pellets.

▶ Administer BS antimicrobials.

▶ Administer NSAIDs.

▶ Careful observation following the injury for any secondary effects.

▶ ± Perform delayed wound closure 4–5 d later.

References and further reading

• **Adam, E.N., Southwood, L.L.,** 2006. Surgical and traumatic wound infections, cellulitis and myositis in horses. Vet. Clin. North Am. Equine Pract. 22, 335–361.

• **Céleste, C., Stashak, T.S.,** 2008. Selection of suture materials, suture patterns, and drains for wound closure. In: Stashak, T.S., Theoret, C.L. (Eds.), Equine wound management (second ed.). Wiley Blackwell, Ames, Iowa, pp. 193–224.

• **Fjordbakk, C.T., Arroyo, L.G.,** Hewson, J., 2008. Retrospective study of the clinical features of limb cellulitis in 63 horses. Vet. Rec. 162, 223–236.

- Hanson, R.R., 2005. Management of burn injuries in the horse. Vet. Clin. North Am. Equine Pract. 21, 105–123.

- Hassel, D.M., 2007. Thoracic trauma in horses. Vet. Clin. North Am. Equine Pract. 23, 67–80.

- Marsh, P.S., 2007. Fire and smoke inhalation injury in horses. Vet. Clin. North Am. Equine Pract. 23, 19–30.

- Mellish, M.A., Adreani, C.M., 2008. Management of a gunshot wound in a mare. Can. Vet. J. 49, 180–182.

- Pilsworth, R., Knottenbelt, D., 2007. Urticaria. Equine Vet. Educ. 19, 368–369.

- Scott, D.W., Miller, W.H., 2011. Environmental skin diseases. In: Scott, D.W. (Ed.), Equine Dermatology (second ed.). Elsevier, St. Louis, Missouri, pp. 398–420.

- Vatistas, N.J., Meagher, D.M., Gillis, C.L., et al. 1995. Gunshot injuries in horses: 22 cases (1971–1993). J. Am. Vet. Med. Assoc. 207, 1198–1200.

- Whelchel, D.D., Chaffin, M.K., 2009. Sequelae and complications of *Streptococcus equi* subspecies *equi* infections in the horse. Equine Vet. Educ. 21, 135–141.

Musculoskeletal emergencies are common in horses and it is important to have a good knowledge of the regional anatomy, particularly in relation to the location of synovial structures, tendons and ligaments. Traumatic injuries are common and attending veterinary surgeons should be equipped to provide suitable first aid in these cases, including bandaging and splinting, prior to further assessment at hospital/referral facilities if required.

General approach to acute, severe lameness

Advice over the telephone

▶ Advise the owner/agent not to move the horse until veterinary assessment has been performed, unless it is in imminent danger.

▶ Provide instructions on how to control any haemorrhage if relevant (see p. 187).

▶ If an object such as a nail has been found in the foot and is above the level of the shoe (i.e. it has the potential to be driven further into the foot on weight-bearing), advise the owner to remove the object and keep it, making a careful note as it is removed regarding where it penetrated, how much of the object was embedded into the foot (can mark with a pen) and what direction it headed in.

▶ If the foreign body is embedded within the foot (or is below the level of the shoe and is unlikely to be driven further into the foot), advise the owner to leave it in situ, not to move the horse unless it is in imminent danger and await your arrival – this can make it easier to determine the likely structures involved and radiographs can be taken with the object in situ (provided that this does not unduly delay decision making or treatment).

Initial assessment and first aid

▶ If the horse is distressed, quickly assess MM colour, HR and neurological status and administer sedation (α2 agonist/butorphanol IV).

▶ Obtain a succinct history about the circumstances in which lameness developed:
  - known traumatic event/sudden-onset lameness at exercise
  - if unknown, when LSN and the horse's management at that time (e.g. stabled or out at pasture with other horses)
  - if any wounds have been noted/objects removed from the foot.

▶ If an injury has been sustained on the course during competition or where it is not safe or possible to perform further assessment, it may be more appropriate to transport the horse to a suitable area nearby for further examination following appropriate first aid treatment.

▶ If a fracture or tendon injury is suspected, the limb must be bandaged and splinted appropriately first to prevent exacerbation of the injury (see p. 383).

▶ Occasionally, the injury may be so severe that immediate destruction of the horse is warranted, e.g. open, comminuted long bone fracture – in competition situations/if unsure, get a second veterinary colleague to examine the horse and confirm this decision.

> **KEY TIP**
> Do not be pressured into making any hasty decisions and if immediate humane destruction is not warranted or the diagnosis is uncertain, transport the horse to hospital/referral facilities for further assessment and treatment.

Further assessment

Obtain a full history. Specific questions that should be asked include:

▶ Any history of previous lameness, tendon/ligament injury or myopathy.

▶ When the horse was last shod.

Perform a full clinical examination. Specific assessment that should be performed includes:

▶ Assess the horse visually from the front, back and both sides:
  - assess the horse's posture
  - look for any obvious swelling/deformity/asymmetry of the limbs and pelvis or gluteal musculature (see Fig. 3.1)
  - note any obvious wounds

▶ Determine which leg(s) are affected.

▶ Assess the degree of lameness.

▶ Wash off any mud and palpate all the limbs carefully, noting any:
  - swelling (generalised/focal/evidence of synovial effusion)
  - wounds (do not underestimate small wounds)
  - ↑ digital pulses
  - objects stuck in the foot
  - pain on application of hoof testers/direct application of pressure over the site
  - pain/resentment to flexion and extension of a joint or region of a limb
  - ↓ range of motion of a joint/abnormal motion

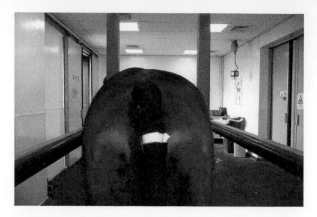

Figure 3.1   Asymmetry of the hindquarters and pelvic region in a racehorse that sustained a fracture of the pelvis during racing competition.

- palpable or audible crepitus (can place a stethoscope over the affected area whilst the limb is manipulated)
- altered tone/heat/pain/swelling or asymmetry in any muscle groups

Common causes of acute severe lameness
- Solar abscess.
- Laminitis.
- Cellulitis (see p. 30).
- Synovial infection.
- Fracture.
- Tendonitis.
- Tendon laceration/rupture.
- Myopathy.

> **HANDY TIP**
> Hoof testers should be applied to the foot of the affected limb to rule in/out foot pain as a cause of lameness, particularly if there is no history of a known traumatic incident.

Further diagnostic evaluation and aftercare

▶ Further diagnostic tests will depend on the suspected problem (Table 3.1).
▶ Consider whether hospitalisation/referral is indicated.
▶ Provide appropriate initial treatment (see relevant sections).
▶ Discuss ongoing management and repeat veterinary evaluation with the owner/carer.
▶ If relevant, provide details of clinical findings, assessment and treatment administered for the horse's usual veterinary surgeon (e.g. injuries sustained and treated during competition).

Table 3.1 Diagnostic tests that may be indicated in the assessment of acute, severe lameness

Diagnostic test	Common indications	Comments
Radiography	Suspected fracture/joint subluxation Assessment of wounds to rule in/out bone pathology Baseline and repeat evaluation of rotation/sinking of P3 in laminitis cases	
US	Diagnosis and assessment of tendon/ligament injury and progression Assessment of wounds Diagnosis of pelvic fractures	Air in the tissues impedes visualisation
Synoviocentesis	Suspected synovial sepsis	Avoid sampling through cellulitic/ contaminated tissues
MRI	Penetrating injuries to the foot Acute/severe lameness of the distal limb where other diagnostic tests are inconclusive	
Scintigraphy	Suspected pelvic/stress fractures	
Serum biochemistry/ urinalysis	Suspected myopathy/ rhabdomyolysis and monitoring of progression	

> **KEY TIP**
> When advising that horses are kept rested in a stable, food intake should be adjusted accordingly and faecal output monitored (↑ risk of colic due to colonic impactions and displacements).

Transport of horses with musculoskeletal injuries

- First aid treatment must have been provided prior to transport including appropriate bandaging and splinting of the limb if required (see p. 383).
- A horse ambulance or a small/low-chassis horsebox is ideal.
- Minimise the distance the horse walks to the vehicle and minimise the ramp incline – use loading ramps if available.

- Confine the horse so that it can lean on vehicle walls/partitions.
- Ensure the horse has sufficient head and neck movement to aid its balance.
- Ideally, transport the horse facing forward (fractures of HL)/backwards (fractures of FL):
  - this may be impractical due to horsebox design
  - horses may travel better in a familiar environment and orientation.
- ± Use slings in an ambulance to support horse if it temporarily wants to reduce the load on its limbs:
  - slings must not be used to partially suspend the horse
  - ensure the sling does not create discomfort/irritation.
- If legal, ideally a handler should travel with the horse to keep it calm.
- Provide a hay net to keep the horse distracted.
- Unload the horse carefully and slowly:
  - make sure it is suitably restrained
  - minimise the slope of the ramp and distance to walk to examination facilities.

Solar abscess and nail bind

These are a common cause of severe lameness. Nail bind is more likely in a horse that has developed progressive lameness in the first 3–5 d after being shod. Solar abscesses should always be ruled out in horses presenting with acute single limb lameness of unknown cause by thorough evaluation, including palpation of the foot and digital pulses, response to hoof testers and paring of the sole.

Clinical signs

▶ Progressive/acute unilateral lameness.
▶ ↑ Digital pulses in the affected limb.
▶ ↑ Heat in the hoof wall.
▶ Pain response to application of hoof testers.
▶ ± Softening around the coronary band/heel bulbs (abscess).
▶ ± Cellulitis of the distal limb (abscess).

Initial assessment and treatment

▶ Obtain a general history. Specific questions that should be asked include:
  - recent farriery
  - duration of lameness and circumstances in which it developed
  - if any objects have been removed from the foot
  - history of laminitis/other medical problems
  - tetanus status.
▶ Perform a general clinical examination and check for evidence of concurrent medical problems, e.g. Cushing disease or evidence of previous laminitis – can develop recurrent solar abscesses.

▶ Apply hoof testers in a systematic fashion to the solar surface – if the horse has recently been shod, application of hoof testers over individual nails may identify the offending one, which can then be removed.

▶ Apart from cases of nail bind, it is usually easiest to remove the shoe – it may be less painful to remove the nails individually rather than levering the shoe off.

▶ Pare the foot and explore any areas of darkened horn.

▶ Abscess formation is confirmed by release of black/brown malodorous fluid.

▶ Pare the area to remove damaged solar tissue and create drainage.

▶ Administer tetanus toxoid/tetanus antitoxin if required (see p. 23).

▶ Antimicrobials are not required unless there is evidence of cellulitis.

▶ ± Short course of NSAIDs if the horse is painful on the limb/evidence of cellulitis.

▶ Apply a dry dressing to the foot daily until the abscess has drained fully (see p. 383).

▶ ± Liaise with a farrier to have a hospital plate fitted if there has been severe under-running of the sole and there is a large solar defect.

If an abscess cannot be found

▶ Pain on percussion of the foot using hoof testers may ↑ suspicion of fracture of P3 (radiography indicated).

▶ Carefully examine the rest of the limb to rule out another cause for lameness.

▶ ± Perform ASNB to confirm the foot as the source of pain.

▶ Apply a wet poultice and dressing over the foot and re-evaluate again after 24 h box rest.

▶ Do not administer antimicrobials.

▶ ± Administration of NSAIDs (may mask lameness, making it difficult to assess progress).

▶ If the horse remains lame, consider further diagnostic examination, including radiography.

Solar penetrations

These are common and are usually due to nails and other sharp objects becoming embedded in the foot. The cause of acute lameness in these cases is usually fairly obvious unless thorough examination of the foot has not been performed. A good knowledge of the regional anatomy of the foot is essential. Involvement of the DDFT, DIP, NB and DFTS may have catastrophic consequences for the horse and surgical treatment should be undertaken promptly. Depending on expertise and facilities available, it may be more appropriate for the horse to be evaluated further at hospital/referral facilities if these structures are suspected to have been involved.

Initial approach

▶ Obtain a history. Specific questions that should be asked include:
  ▪ when the penetration occurred/when the horse was LSN
  ▪ if the object has already been removed, where the object penetrated, to what depth and in which direction
  ▪ tetanus status

▶ Examine the offending object if has already been removed.

▶ If the object remains in situ and radiographs can be obtained without undue delay to further treatment, obtain LM and DP views (± further views as required) with the object in situ prior to removing it – this will provide an immediate assessment of the likely structures involved.

▶ Perform a full clinical examination – rule out other potential cause of lameness in that limb.

▸ Assess the degree of lameness.

▸ Check for effusion of the DIP and DFTS and whether any pain is elicited on pressure over the DDFT over the palmar/plantar area of the pastern (may be indicative of pain related to effusion of the NB).

▸ ± Administer sedation.

▸ ± Perform ASNB if the horse is very painful.

▸ Pare the area around the tract – will usually find an area of haemorrhage that can be followed.

▸ Look for any evidence of synovial fluid leakage from the tract (relatively uncommon as the tract will seal over quickly following removal of the object).

▸ ± Following paring of the region and thorough cleaning, probing of the tract may be undertaken using a sterile malleable probe (taking care not to introduce further material into the tract).

▸ Determine whether the penetration is superficial and unlikely to involve vital structures or whether synovial structures are likely to have been involved (see Fig. 3.2).

Management of superficial foot penetrations

▸ Administer tetanus toxoid/tetanus antitoxin if required (see p. 23).

▸ Administer penicillin IV/IM.

▸ Administer NSAIDs IV.

▸ Do not keep on oral NSAIDs – may mask signs of synovial sepsis.

▸ If there is continued severe lameness/lameness worsens, consider possible synovial structure/DDFT involvement.

Further investigation and treatment of deep foot penetrations

▸ They may be easiest to perform at hospital/referral facilities, depending on expertise/ facilities available – contract referral centre for further advice:

  ▪ MRI examination of the foot may provide vital information in some cases if facilities available/economics allow.

▸ Administer medication prior to transport:

  ▪ BS antimicrobials (penicillin/gentamicin)

  ▪ NSAIDs

  ▪ ± tetanus toxioid or antitoxin if indicated

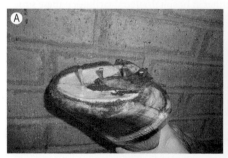
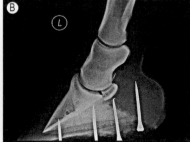

Figure 3.2 (A) Cadaver limb with nails inserted via the solar surface into the foot. (B) A latero-lateral radiograph of the foot demonstrates the relevant anatomical structures that may be involved, depending on the location of the nail.

- Radiograph the foot if not already performed:
  - ± with probe in place
  - ± instillation of contrast agent into a tract (this is difficult and does not confirm lack of communication with a synovial structure).
- Synoviocentesis of DIP, DFTS, NB:
  - assessment of WBC count, TP, cytology and submit for C&S
  - ± instillation of contrast agent into synovial structures to confirm communication with the tract.
- Optimal treatment where synovial structures have been penetrated: arthroscopic lavage of affected synovial structure(s).
- Prognosis – depends on the structures involved and duration of time since the penetration occurred in relation to surgery.

Acute laminitis

This is a common cause of acute-onset bilateral FL lameness which, in the UK, is usually seen in horses at pasture. Laminitis can result in lameness on all four limbs or more uncommonly clinical signs predominate in the HL – the latter cases can be more challenging to diagnose and may be confused with colic, myopathy or neurological disease. Acute laminitis may occur as a one-off episode in high-risk individuals or may be an acute exacerbation of disease in horses with chronic laminitis.

Possible causes of laminitis

- Pasture-associated laminitis – particularly in spring/autumn (Northern Hemisphere) and in individuals with a high BCS
- Endocrinopathies (PPID/EMS)
- Grain (CHO) overload
- Severe, non-weight-bearing lameness in the contralateral limb
- Endotoxaemia/SIRS e.g. retained foetal membranes/metritis, colitis

Clinical signs

- Lameness – classic shuffle-like gait.
- Laminitic stance – weight shifting between feet, loading weight on the caudal part of the feet.
- ↑ Digital pulses.
- ↑ Heat.

Initial assessment and treatment

- Obtain a full history. Specific information that should be obtained includes:
  - duration of clinical signs
  - prior history of laminitis
  - recent medical problems/administration of medication
  - concurrent illness including severe lameness/metritis

Table 3.2 Obel classification of the severity of laminitis

Obel grade	Clinical signs
1	Horse alternately and incessantly lifts its feet Lameness not evident at walk but stilted gait evident at trot
2	Horse exhibits stilted gait at walk but moves willingly A foot may be lifted off the ground without difficulty
3	Horse moves reluctantly and resists attempts to have a foot lifted
4	Horse refuses to move, doing so only if forced

▶ Perform a full clinical examination. Specific assessment should include:
  - assessment of BCS
  - evidence of prior laminitis (laminitic rings)
  - suspicion of EMS/PPID – take relevant diagnostic samples
  - concurrent illness (see relevant sections/texts)
  - palpate the limbs and gluteal muscles – exclude other causes of lameness
  - palpate the coronary bands for evidence of a depression at the site
  - evaluate the solar surface for solar prolapse of P3 (if the horse is willing to lift the foot)
  - apply hoof testers to determine the location of pain (particularly around the toe)
  - determine the Obel grade of laminitis (provides baseline measure, assists determining prognosis/progression – Table 3.2).

▶ Provide analgesia and ↓ inflammation in the laminae:
  - phenylbutazone 4.4 mg/kg IV followed by oral NSAIDs (take care not to overdose in small ponies – obtain an accurate weight).

▶ Alter laminar perfusion:
  - administer acepromazine 0.02 mg/kg IV – will also ↓ anxiety
  - efficacy of other treatments, e.g. pentoxifylline, unproven.

▶ Provide mechanical support:
  - if shod, remove the shoe unless the horse finds it too painful to do so
  - it is often less painful for the horse if the clenches are rasped down and each nail is removed individually, with the horse stood on a soft conforming surface (e.g. in a stable with deep bedding)
  - ± facilitated by performing an ASNB
  - if the shoe is left on, pack the mid/caudal ⅓ of the solar surface
  - if unshod/following shoe removal apply commercial foot support products (e.g. Styrofoam pads, solar support systems using silicon-based materials)
  - if these are not available, basic support can be providing by placing padding over the caudal ⅓ of the hoof, e.g. rolled-up bandage taped in place (unlikely to be sufficient in larger horses) or by keeping them on a deep, conforming surface (see below).

▶ Minimise further structural changes:
  - keep confined to a stable (or enclosed in a field shelter) on a deep (>20 cm) bed – ideally sand/peat moss bed (unless Styrofoam pads have been placed)

- if these facilities are not available, fence off a stable-sized area in a paddock (not lush grass/extremely bare).
▶ Remove/treat the initiating cause (see relevant sections/texts).
▶ Where laminitis has developed at pasture:
  - remove from pasture (see above)
  - record BCS and body weight (weigh tape)
  - initiate immediate dietary changes, including removal of treats (carrots, apples) and any concentrate feed
  - work out the quantity of forage needed (approx. 1.5–2.0% of BW/d), get the owner/carer to weigh this and soak it in cold water for 8–16h before feeding
  - do not starve affected individuals – high risk of hyperlipaemia developing (especially obese ponies/donkeys).
▶ Determine if radiographs are required immediately (e.g. severe lameness/suspicion of rotation or sinking of P3 on palpation of the coronary band/response to hoof tester application over the toe):
  - determine rotation/sinking
  - baseline measurement if progression occurs
  - LM views of all four feet – markers on dorsal hoof wall and point of frog (see texts/website).
▶ Reassess again in 24–48h (depending on severity and initiating cause).
▶ Liaise with the horse's usual farrier and communicate what ongoing veterinary/farriery care is required with the owner/carer.

Prognosis

▶ Survey of first-opinion pasture-associated laminitis cases in the UK (Menzies-Gow et al. 2010b):
  - 95% survival at 8 weeks following laminitis episode
  - clinical outcome good in 72% cases
  - better prognosis associated with lower body weight, lower BMI, Obel grades 1 and 2.

Synovial sepsis

This is a commonly encountered emergency situation that can have catastrophic consequences for the horse if not identified and treated early. In adult horses, sepsis usually develops subsequent to a skin laceration or puncture that has penetrated a joint or tendon sheath. Less commonly it may be iatrogenic following synovial anaesthesia or medication (see p. 272). A good knowledge of the regional anatomy of the limb is essential and the possibility of synovial sepsis should be considered in any horse that has sustained a wound in close proximity to a joint or tendon sheath (see p. 19–22).

Clinical signs

▶ Acute-onset/progressive severe lameness.
▶ If open and draining, evidence of synovial fluid leakage and variable lameness.
▶ ± Wound (laceration/puncture) close to/directly communicating with a synovial structure.
▶ Heat, pain and swelling.

Obtain a general history. Specific questions that should be asked include:

▶ When the wound occurred or if unknown when the horse was LSN.

▶ If any objects (e.g. thorns) have been removed from the limb.

▶ Tetanus status.

▶ Degree and progression of lameness.

Perform a full clinical examination and more specific evaluation of the limb(s).

▶ Evaluate any other concurrent traumatic injuries (see relevant sections).

▶ Assess the degree of lameness – severe non-weight-bearing lameness is uncommon in the acute stage and the possibility of a fracture should be ruled out.

▶ Apply hoof testers to the foot – rule out a subsolar abscess.

▶ Perform a detailed evaluation of the limb to assess the location and depth of each wound and proximity to any synovial structures (see p. 19).

▶ Ensure small puncture wounds are not missed – clip hair away from areas with matted blood/localised swelling.

▶ Remember that if the wound was sustained during flexion/extension of the limb, the wound may be distant to the site of trauma.

▶ Determine whether there is effusion of any synovial structures or evidence of cellulitis:

  ▪ it can be difficult to differentiate between primary cellulitis and synovial sepsis as the cause of lameness – cellulitis that occurs secondary to synovial sepsis will usually be more focal around the synovial structure area (rather than more diffuse swelling that occurs in generalised cellulitis unrelated to synovial sepsis p. 30)

  ▪ the degree and location of any cellulitic reaction may influence whether synoviocentesis should be performed (see p. 346).

▶ Determine if there is evidence of synovial fluid leakage from any wounds (this may be more obvious when the limb is flexed and extended):

  ▪ this fluid is yellow and sticky and forms a 'string'

  ▪ do not confuse with serum exudating from the site.

▶ Following aseptic preparation of the site, evaluate the wound further using a sterile gloved finger or a sterile probe (see p. 16).

If involvement of a synovial structure is considered highly unlikely

▶ Administer BS antimicrobials.

▶ ± Administer tetanus toxoid/antitoxin if required (see p. 23).

▶ If the horse is in pain, administer NSAIDs IV:

  ▪ if the diagnosis is uncertain, ongoing administration of NSAIDs should be avoided (risk of masking signs of deteriorating lameness if synovial sepsis is present).

If synovial sepsis is obvious or highly likely (Fig. 3.3)

▶ Consider further assessment at hospital/referral facilities.

▶ Confirm the diagnosis by synoviocentesis (see p. 346 & Fig. 3.4):

  ▪ ± perform US and radiography first if the risk of performing synoviocentesis may outweigh the benefits (e.g. iatrogenic introduction of infection into a non-septic synovial structure).

▶ Confirm that damage has not occurred to adjacent soft tissue structures or bone:

  ▪ radiography/US if not already performed.

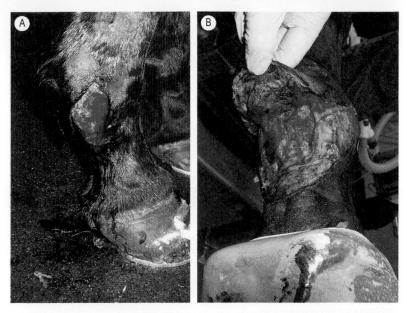

Figure 3.3 (A,B) Wounds to the distal palmar/plantar pastern region are common and may involve the DFTS/DDFT. In this case a small puncture wound resulted in sepsis of the DFTS.

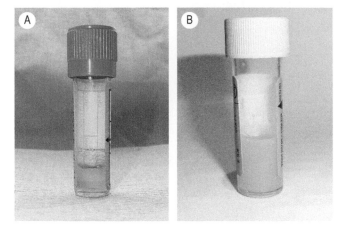

Figure 3.4 Samples of synovial fluid obtained from a normal (A) and septic (B) synovial structure. The septic sample is grossly turbid in appearance and had elevated TP and WBC counts (see p. 346).

▸ Optimal treatment of confirmed synovial sepsis: arthroscopic assessment and lavage under GA (contact referral centre/seek specialist advice).
▸ If this is not an option, needle flushing can be performed under heavy sedation/GA: (see texts)
  ▪ regional nerve block/instil LA into joint
  ▪ place 16G needles into affected synovial structure(s)
  ▪ lavage 3–5-L sterile LRS through the joint/tendon sheath using a giving set.

Prognosis

▸ Depends on a number of factors, including other structures involved, and treatment performed (see texts/seek specialist advice).

Acute tendonitis

Tendon injuries are most commonly sustained during intense exercise (including training and during competition) and usually involve the flexor tendons/suspensory ligaments of the forelimbs. The injury may be uni- or bilateral and may involve re-injury of previously injured tendon(s).

Clinical signs

▸ Localised swelling and heat (Fig. 3.5).
▸ Lameness – may not be obvious immediately following injury but will worsen over subsequent hours.

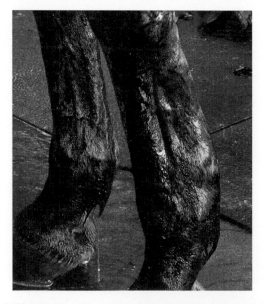

Figure 3.5　Acute SDFT tendonitis – 30 min after sustaining the injury, marked soft tissue swelling is evident over palmar aspect of the metacarpal region of the left forelimb.

Initial assessment and treatment

▶ Obtain a full history. Specific information that should be obtained includes:
  ▪ the circumstances surrounding injury – when and how
  ▪ previous history of tendonitis – which limb and tendon, how long ago.
▶ Perform a full clinical examination and further evaluation of the affected limb(s):
  ▪ less severe tendon injuries might present with mild pain/swelling at the site only
  ▪ assess any wounds and rule in/out the possibility of tendon laceration (see below)
  ▪ look for any postural changes that may ↑ suspicion of tendon rupture (see Table 3.3)
  ▪ palpate each tendon individually with the limb weight-bearing and non-weight-bearing
  ▪ determine the size and shape of each tendon (SDFT, DDFT, ALDDFT, SL) and whether pain is elicited when digital pressure is applied over each.
  ▪ determine which tendon(s) are most likely to be affected (may not be possible in some cases where there is diffuse, severe swelling).
▶ Immediately following injury, apply ice/ice water to the site for 30 min, stop for 30 min and place a temporary support bandage – repeat × 3.
▶ Administer NSAIDs IV, e.g. phenylbutazone 4.4 mg/kg IV.
▶ Administer dexamethasone 0.1 mg/kg IV.
▶ Bandage the limb:
  ▪ placement of a support bandage can help to reduce the degree of swelling and inflammation at the site
  ▪ place a Robert Jones bandage plus dorsal splint/proprietary splint for severe injuries.

Table 3.3 Postural changes that may indicate the tendons affected in cases of rupture/complete laceration or displacement.

Postural abnormality	Likely injury
Reduced ability to extend digit – rapid dorsal flip of hoof at walk	Rupture/laceration extensor tendons
Hyperextension of fetlock, normal foot placement	Rupture/laceration SDFT
Hyperextension of fetlock and elevation of toe	Rupture/laceration both SDFT/DDFT
Elevation of toe, normal fetlock position	Rupture/laceration DDFT 🎥
Marked hyperextension of the fetlock	SL rupture ± flexor tendons 🎥
Distress, reluctant to bear weight/walk on HL	Displacement of the SDFT off the tuber calcis 🖼
Hock can be extended when the stifle is flexed (loss of reciprocal apparatus)	Laceration/rupture of the peroneus tertius tendon

▶ Stable rest, NSAIDs & bandaging.
▶ US assessment in 24–48h and again 3–4 weeks later, discuss exercise regime based on the results of these (see texts/ seek specialist advice).
▶ Prognosis depends on a variety of factors:
  ▪ the location and extent of the tendon injury
  ▪ whether one or both limbs are affected
  ▪ use of the horse
  ▪ whether this is a repeat injury.

Tendon lacerations, ruptures or displacements

They are usually traumatic in nature and are frequently associated with a wound. Injuries may be sustained by wire/other sharp objects or after being struck by a limb (overreach injury or from another horse). Such injuries should always be considered in any horse that has sustained a wound over the palmar/plantar aspect of the pastern or over the dorsal, plantar or palmar metacarpus/tarsus.

Clinical signs

▶ Lameness – depends on the degree of damage and structures affected.
▶ Extensor tendons – may not be lame.
▶ Flexor tendons and SL – will be lame.
▶ ± Distress – evident where the SDFT has luxated over the tuber calcis.
▶ Obvious postural abnormality – depends on structure(s) affected (Table 3.3).

Initial assessment and first aid

Obtain a full history. Specific information that should be obtained includes:
▶ When and how the injury was sustained or, if unknown, when the horse was LSN.
▶ The degree of lameness evident.

Perform a full clinical examination.
▶ Assess any concurrent injuries and provide treatment as appropriate.
▶ Assess the horse's posture.
▶ Assess any wounds (see p. 16):
  ▪ these may be distant to the site of tendon injury depending on the position of the limb at the time the injury occurred
  ▪ the size of the wound does not correlate with degree of tendon damage – do not underestimate small wounds
  ▪ extensor tendons and the SDFT/DDFT are directly underneath the skin and may be completely or partially transected (look for tendon fibres).
▶ ± Perform US evaluation.
▶ Determine which structures are involved and the extent of contamination.
▶ Assess whether concurrent synovial sepsis is possible/likely.
▶ Discuss the options with the owner/carer.
▶ Optimal treatment of tendon lacerations and ruptures involves surgical exploration and treatment in hospital/referral facilities (depending on the structures involved – contact referral centre).

▸ SDFT luxation – surgical management (for return to function)/conservative management.
▸ Immediate euthanasia may be indicated in certain tendon ruptures/lacerations (see p. 329):
  ▪ if unsure seek a second opinion.
▸ Administer NSAIDs IV, phenylbutazone 4.4 mg/kg or flunixin 1.1 mg/kg.
▸ Administer BS antimicrobials, e.g. penicillin/gentamicin.
▸ ± Administer acepromazine if the horse is distressed (e.g. SDFT luxation).
▸ Apply a dressing to the wound – hydrogel and absorbent, non-adherent dressing.
▸ Provide limb support prior to transport (see p. 383).
▸ Distal limb injuries:
  ▪ flexor tendons – alignment of dorsal cortices Robert-Jones bandage (RJB) plus splint or cast bandage
  ▪ extensor tendons – RJB.
▸ SDFT luxation – full limb RJB.

Prognosis with surgical management

▸ Extensor tendons – good.
▸ Flexor tendons – fair.
▸ Reduced where there is concurrent involvement of synovial structures.

Fractures/joint luxations

These usually occur during high-speed exercise (training or competition) but can occur as a result of traumatic injury sustained at pasture. Fractures may be immediately obvious or suspected based on the degree of lameness.

Clinical signs

▸ Usually acute, severe lameness.
▸ Competition situations (effects of adrenaline) – may have initial mild lameness that progressively worsens.
▸ Localised heat, pain and swelling.
▸ ± Abnormal limb contour/posture.
▸ ± Resentment of flexion/extension of the limb.
▸ ± Abnormal range of joint motion.
▸ ± Crepitus.
▸ ± Severe distress.
▸ ± Wounds and other soft tissue injuries.
▸ ± Severe haemorrhage.

Initial first aid and assessment

▸ Provide emergency treatment – e.g. control haemorrhage, assess CNS signs.
▸ ± Sedation (α2 agonist/butorphanol IV):
  ▪ often need to administer a high/increased dose if the horse is distressed and under the influence of adrenaline to achieve a suitable level of sedation.
▸ Perform a rapid but careful visual assessment and palpate the entire limb to determine the likelihood of a fracture/luxation and its location (see Fig. 3.6).
▸ Assess any concurrent traumatic injuries.

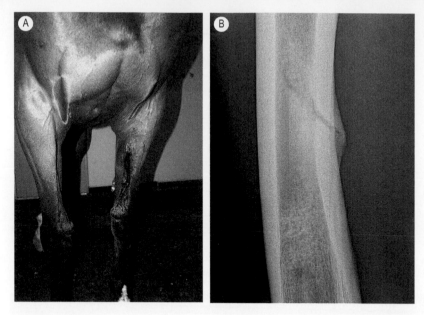

Figure 3.6 (A) Severe lameness and swelling of the medial radius in a horse that has sustained a radial fracture. (B) These fractures may not be evident radiographically for several days/weeks and various views may be required to demonstrate the fracture line. Where suspected, these cases should be kept box rested and a full limb Robert Jones bandage together with a lateral splint applied (see p. 383).

▶ Administer analgesia IV – phenylbutazone 2.2–4.4 mg/kg or flunixin/ketoprofen.
▶ Administer BS antimicrobials if wounds have been sustained.
▶ Perform initial wound management (see p. 16).
▶ Immobilise the limb as appropriate – bandaging ± splinting (see p. 383) or application of bandage casts / commercial splints (see texts/website):
  ▪ if unsure of the location of injury, random bandaging and splinting can do more harm than good.
▶ Decide what further diagnostic evaluation is required and how, where and when this will be performed:
  ▪ at a suitable adjacent area/nearby hospital
  ▪ at a referral centre (contact centre for further advice).
▶ Organise transport if necessary (see p. 41).
▶ Immediate euthanasia may be indicated in certain circumstances (see p. 328).
▶ If unsure, seek an opinion from a second veterinary surgeon or make a decision only once further diagnostic evaluation has been performed.

KEY TIP

If a horse with a fractured limb is to be transported, the limb must be appropriately immobilised where required – failure to do so may result in closed, simple fracture becoming open and comminuted with potential catastrophic consequences.

Further assessment

▸ Radiographic assessment:
   ▪ minimum of 4 views – DP/CrCd, Lat, Obl × 2 (may not be possible in proximal limb)
   ▪ ± additional specific views
   ▪ if an unstable fracture is suspected, can obtain initial radiographs with the bandage still in place
   ▪ may need stressed views if joint subluxation suspected
   ▪ not all fractures may be immediately evident radiographically.
▸ ± US.
▸ ± MRI if indicated.

Treatment and prognosis

Treatment options and prognosis depend on multiple factors, including fracture location and configuration, size of horse, economics and treatment facilities/equipment available – seek specialist advice if unsure.

Exertional rhabdomyolysis syndrome (ERS)
. . . .

This is a common muscular disease syndrome in horses. The sporadic form is usually related to overexertion beyond a horse's level of fitness but may occur in horses undergoing intensive exercise following a period of rest for a few days during which time nutrition has remained unchanged. The recurrent form (more common) can be associated with underlying genetic and metabolic causes. This is not usually associated with overexertion, often occurring during warm-up or early in the exercise period.

Clinical signs

▸ Lameness/stiffness during or immediately following exercise.
▸ Mild–severe lameness.
▸ ± Myoglobinuria (see p. 176).

Initial assessment and treatment

▸ Obtain a full history. Specific questions that should be asked include:
   ▪ level of fitness and current exercise programme
   ▪ recent changes to exercise programme or diet
   ▪ previous history of ER
   ▪ any history of recent trauma.
▸ Perform a full clinical examination:
   ▪ rule out other potential causes of a stiff gait, including laminitis or pelvic injuries
   ▪ palpate the muscles to identify abnormal spasm/pain.
▸ Take blood and urine samples.
▸ Confirm the diagnosis by serum biochemistry and assess renal function:
   ▪ creatine kinase (CK) – peaks at 2–12 h, can reach 100,000,000 IU/L or more, returns to near normal in 24–36 h
   ▪ aspartate transaminase (AST) – peaks at 24 h, can reach 10,000 or more IU/L, can remain elevated for 21 d.

▶ Obtain a urine sample and assess for evidence of myoglobinuria (see p. 177):
  ▪ peaks 12–24 h, remains elevated for 5 d, increased levels may persist for 14–21 d.

Ongoing management

▶ Fluid therapy (oral/IV) is essential in severe cases even if myoglobinuria is not evident to minimise the risk of renal failure developing subsequently (see Ch. 9).
▶ Administer NSAIDs, IV flunixin 1.1 mg/kg or phenylbutazone 4.4 mg/kg (in severe cases, administer only after fluid therapy has been initiated – reduce risk of renal damage).
▶ ± Sedation if distressed (α2 agonist/butorphanol).
▶ ± Administer acepromazone 0.02 mg/kg IV –↓anxiety.
▶ Monitor urination and evidence of discoloration of urine (see p. 176).
▶ Repeat assessment based on severity and response to initial treatment.
▶ In acute, sporadic cases, keep the horse box rested until they are able to move freely.
▶ In recurrent cases, implement dietary changes and do not box rest them.

Prognosis

▶ Good in mild, sporadic cases; depends on clinical progression of more severe cases (see texts/seek specialist advice).
▶ Recurrent cases – further investigations include muscle biopsy/generic testing, assessment of nutrition and exercise programmes to determine if there is an underlying cause.

Atypical myopathy

This is a severe, non-exertional rhabdomyolysis that occurs in horses at pasture (particularly young horses) and is associated with high mortality. It occurs sporadically worldwide but has been increasingly recognised in Europe. Outbreaks may occur with multiple horses affected in certain geographic locations within a few weeks of each other. Other horses on the premises where a confirmed/suspected case has been identified should also be examined for evidence of atypical myopathy.

Clinical signs

▶ Depression.
▶ Congested MM.
▶ ↑ HR.
▶ ↑ RR, dyspnoea.
▶ Weakness/stiff gait.
▶ Myoglobinuria (Fig. 3.7).
▶ Muscle fasciculations.
▶ Recumbency.
▶ ± Death.

Initial assessment and first aid

▶ Obtain a detailed history. Specific questions that should be asked include:
  ▪ duration of clinical signs or when LSN
  ▪ recent illness
  ▪ known traumatic incident preceding recumbency

- whether other horses on the premises are affected
- vaccination status.

▶ Perform a full clinical examination:
  - rule out other causes of weakness/recumbency, including colic and neurological disease (see p. 313).

▶ Obtain a blood sample for haematology and serum biochemistry to confirm the diagnosis and assess hydration/other organ dysfunction.

▶ Obtain a urine sample (may require catheterisation) and assess for the presence of myoglobin (see p. 177).

Further evaluation

▶ Cases often require intensive care – consider hospitalisation/referral.
▶ General treatment as for a recumbent horse (see p. 315):
  - monitor urination ± repeated catheterisation.
▶ Fluid therapy – see p. 179 acute renal failure.
▶ Analgesia: NSAIDs.
▶ Nutrition:
  - CHO-based feeds (fat metabolism deranged in these cases)
  - can administer as gruel by stomach tube (see Ch. 11)
  - ± IV glucose.
▶ ± Metronidazole 15 mg/kg q. 8 h PO (clostridial infection implicated in some cases – evidence lacking).
▶ ± Antioxidants – vitamin E (3000–5000 IU/d) and selenium (10 mg/d).
▶ ± Oxygen supplementation.

Prognosis

▶ Mortality in 70–90% cases within 3–5 d.

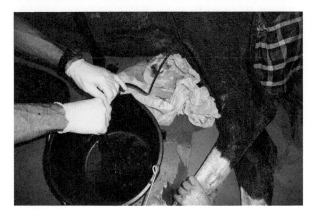

Figure 3.7 Recombent horse with atypical myopathy; myoglobinuria was evident upon catheterisation of the bladder.

References and further reading

- Cripps, P.J., Eustace, R.A., 1999. Factors involved in the prognosis of equine laminitis in the UK. Equine Vet. J. 31, 433–442.

- Dyson, S., 1996. Emergency management of tendon and ligament injuries. In: Guide, A. (Ed.), To the Management of Equine Emergencies. Equine Veterinary Journal Ltd, Newmarket, pp. 29–36.

- Dyson, S.J., Bertone, A.L., 2011. Tendon lacerations. In: Ross, M.W., Dyson, S.J. (Eds.), Diagnosis and Management of Lameness in the Horse (second ed.). Elsevier, St. Louis, Missouri, pp. 806–810.

- Keen, J., 2011. Diagnosis and management of equine rhabdomyolysis. In Pract. 33, 68–77.

- Menzies-Gow, N.J., Stevens, K.B., Sepulveda, M.F., Jarvis, N., Marr, C.M., 2010a. Repeatability and reproducibility of the Obel grading system for equine laminitis. Vet. Rec. 167, 52–55.

- Menzies-Gow, N.J., Stevens, K., Barr, A., et al. 2010b. Severity and outcome of equine pasture-associated laminitis managed in first opinion practice in the UK. Vet. Rec. 167, 364–369.

- Mudge, M.C., Bramlage, L.R., 2007. Field fracture management. Vet. Clin. North Am. Equine Pract. 23, 117–133.

- Parks, A.H., 2003. Treatment of acute laminitis. Equine Vet. Educ. 15, 273–280.

- Richardson, D.W., Ahern, B.J., 2012. Synovial and osseous infections. In: Auer, J.A., Stick, J.A. (Eds.), Equine Surgery (fourth ed.). Elsevier, St. Louis, Missouri, pp. 1189–1201.

- Smith, M.R.W., 2010. Management of joint instability. Equine Vet. Educ. 22, 112–114.

- Smith, R., Schramme, M., 2003. Tendon injury in the horse: current theories and therapies. In Pract. 25, 529–539.

- Wright, I.M., 2011. Racetrack fracture management and emergency care. Racecourse Casualty Management Seminar, 2011 Association of Racecourse Veterinary Surgeons.

- van Galen, G., Serteyn, D., Amory, H., Votion, D.M., 2008. Atypical myopathy: new insights into the pathophysiology, prevention and management of the condition. Equine Vet. J. 20, 234–238.

Oral and gastrointestinal emergencies

Colic

Colic is one of the most common equine emergencies encountered. In many cases the exact cause is unknown and the majority (around 90%) of colic cases seen in first opinion practice resolve with medical treatment. Early recognition of horses that may require surgical management and referral at an early stage, prior to the development of marked alterations in horses' cardiovascular parameters, is critical. This will have a major bearing on a horse's survival following surgery, both in the short and long term. Colic in the foal is dealt with in Ch. 12.

Epidemiology

▶ There are numerous reasons why colic develops, most of these being related to the GIT, but pathological conditions of other organs/systems may result in signs of abdominal pain (Table 4.1).
▶ Certain horse- and management-level factors ↑ the likelihood of particular types of colic (Table 4.2).

Advice to the owner/carer

▶ If the horse is in pain and wants to lie down and roll, it is safer to put the horse in a well-bedded stable with no objects that it can harm itself on until you arrive rather than try to keep the horse walking around.
▶ Owners are often keen to exercise horses with colic – a short period (around 10 min) of walking exercise is acceptable if the horse is not violently painful.

Table 4.1 Non-gastrointestinal causes of abdominal pain ('false colic')

Body system	Lesions that may be mistaken for GIT-related colic
Musculoskeletal	Laminitis Rhabdomyolysis/Atypical myopathy Ruptured pre-pubic tendon/body wall rupture HYPP
Cardiovascular	Haemothorax/haemoperitoneum Ruptured abdominal/thoracic artery Dysrrhythmias/pericarditis Aortoiliac thrombosis Splenic rupture/haematoma Splenic abscess/tumour
Reproductive	Uterine torsion Rupture of uterine/ovarian artery Ovarian haematoma Abortion/premature foaling/dystocia Spermatic cord torsion
Respiratory	Pleuropneumonia/pleuritis
Urinary	Urethral/ureteral obstruction Uroperitoneum
Hepatic/metabolic/endocrine	Exhausted horse syndrome Hyperlipaemia Acute hepatic necrosis (serum hepatitis) Cholangiohepatitis Pancreatitis
Neurological	Hypocalcaemia Tetanus Botulism Seizures Encephalitides
Other	Intra-abdominal abscess/neoplasia Peritonitis

▶ Excessive walking exercise must not be undertaken, nor should horse's be exercised at trot or canter until veterinary assessment has been performed.

Initial assessment

▶ If the horse is violently painful, obtain a brief history, evaluate the horse's MM and HR then administer 0.3–0.4 mg/kg xylazine IV (150–200 mg for a 500-kg horse):
  ▪ this will provide around 10–15 min analgesia, enabling a full clinical examination to be performed prior to making further decisions regarding ongoing analgesia and management (other α2 agonist can be used if xylazine is not available).

Table 4.2 Horse- and management-related factors that may increase suspicion of particular causes of colic in adult horses (see p. 235 for colic in foals)

Horse/management factors	Causes of colic that are more commonly seen in these groups
Pregnant mares	Uterine torsion Bruising/rupture of a viscus or tearing of the mesenteric attachment
Mares that have recently foaled	LCT Uterine/vaginal artery tear Bruising/rupture of a viscus or tearing of the mesenteric attachment Impactions Entrapment of viscus in torn mesentery/broad ligament
Stallions/colts	Inguinal herniation (common) Spermatic cord torsion (rare)
Horses that display crib-biting/windsucking behaviour	Large colon displacements Large colon impactions Epiploic foramen entrapment
Age >7 years old, particularly older ponies	Pedunculated lipoma
Poor dentition	Large colon displacements, impaction and torsion Gastric impaction
Recent stable rest	Pelvic flexure impaction Large colon displacement/torsion
Seasonal factors	EGS more likely in April/May Large colon displacements/torsion – more common in spring and autumn months Large colon impactions – winter months
Geographic region	Sand impaction/enteroliths EGS

▶ Obtain a full history. Specific questions that should be asked include:
- when signs of colic were first seen or, if unknown, when LSN
- recent change in routine, including diet, stabling or premises
- pregnant/recent foaling (mares)
- previous history of colic
- current medical problems/medication
- history of previous/recent EGS on the premises (in relevant geographic regions)
- faecal output over last 24 h – normal/reduced
- evidence of diarrhoea

- routine parasite and dental prophylaxis
- recent administration of an anthelmintic
- whether the horse displays stereotypic behaviours, including crib-biting/windsucking behaviour.

▸ Observe the horse briefly before entering the stable. Take note of:
  - the horse's general demeanour and whether it is exhibiting signs of colic – rule out possible causes of colic unrelated to the GIT ('false colic', see Table 4.1)
  - any signs of disturbance in the stable and evidence of faeces
  - abrasions around the head or other extremities may indicate that the horse was violently painful at some stage prior to being found with colic
  - note any abdominal distension.

▸ Perform a full clinical examination. Specific information that should be obtained includes:
  - MM colour, pulse quality and temperature of extremities
  - HR – take prior to administering any medication
  - RR and effort
  - T°
  - gastrointestinal borborygmi (gut sounds; normal/absent/increased)
  - presence of digital pulses
  - palpate the scrotum and inguinal region in stallions/colts – rule out inguinal herniation.

▸ Determine whether further tests are indicated:
  - if the horse is not exhibiting overt signs of colic and the cardiovascular parameters are within normal limits these may not be indicated at this stage
  - in horses exhibiting moderate/severe signs of abdominal pain or recurrent signs of mild colic despite initial treatment, rectal examination and passage of a nasogastric tube should be performed.

▸ Rectal examination (see p. 344).
▸ Passage of a nasogastric tube (see p. 339).
▸ Abdominocentesis (see p. 341).
▸ Haematology/biochemistry:
  - PCV/TP
  - systemic lactate
▸ abdominal US 3.5–5 MHz linear/curvilinear transducer (see website)
  - basic assessment – evaluation of inguinal regions and ventral midline for small intestinal distension/motility, large colon distension and thickness, excess peritoneal fluid.

Initial treatment and management

▸ Decide whether the horse can be treated medically, where surgical intervention is potentially required (Table 4.3) or where euthanasia is indicated (see p. 66).
▸ Where signs of moderate or severe colic are evident, discuss potential referral for surgery at an early stage and start planning transport – this is a common cause of delay in getting horses to referral centres.
▸ Decide on appropriate analgesia/antispasmodic medication. As a general guide:
  - phenylbutazone or butylscopolamine/metimazole (Buscopan compositum®) are good initial choices in cases of mild colic
  - where more moderate signs of colic are evident, consider α2 agonist (romifidine/detomidine)/butorphanol combinations.

Table 4.3 Criteria that can help to determine whether medical or potential surgical management is indicated (NB this should be based on a combination of several criteria)

	Medical management indicated	Surgical management may be required
Heart rate	<50 beats/min	>50 beats/min
Degree of pain	Mild/moderate	Moderate/severe
Response to analgesia	Good response to mild/moderate analgesia	Poor/partial response to potent analgesia
GIT sounds	Normal/increased	Reduced/absent
Abdominal distension	None	Moderate/marked
PCV	<40%	>40%
TP	55–70g/L	>70g/L
Systemic lactate	<2.0mmol/L	>3mmol/L
Nasogastric reflux	<2L	>2L
Peritoneal fluid appearance	Clear, straw-yellow coloured	Orange/red or turbid
Peritoneal TP	<20g/L	>25g/L
Peritoneal lactate	<1mmol/L	Any increase in serial samples/>2.5mmol/L
US examination of the small intestine	Small intestinal motile and normal wall thickness	Distended, amotile loops ± oedema of the wall
US examination of the large intestine	Normal wall thickness and position	Increased colon wall thickness

▸ **Use of flunixin should be considered carefully due to its potent analgesic and particularly endotoxic properties which can delay identification of the need for surgery** (or failure for owners to seek further veterinary advice if the horse is still showing colic signs, even if they are less severe than initially). As a guide:

  ▪ in horses with severe signs of abdominal pain where surgery is not an option, flunixin is a good choice of analgesic – if there is no response to this, together with α2 agonist/butorphanol combinations, euthanasia is indicated

  ▪ where a decision has been made to refer a horse with colic for potential surgery and the horse is painful, flunixin can be administered in these cases (check with the referral centre first or let them know it has been administered)

  ▪ consider other analgesics in the case of mild/moderate signs of colic of unknown aetiology where surgery is an option – administration of flunixin in the early stages of intestinal strangulation (particularly of the small intestine) will mask increases in HR and PCV that would indicate progressive endotoxic shock until severe gastrointestinal compromise becomes evident (Figs 4.1, 4.2).

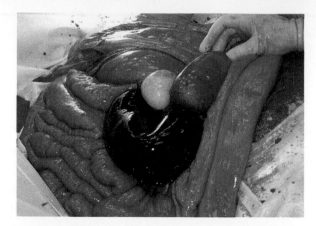

Figure 4.1 Pedunculated lipoma causing small intestinal strangulation. Administration of flunixin in the initial stages in such cases can mask early signs of ischaemic pain and the development of endotoxaemia, delaying the decision to refer for surgery.

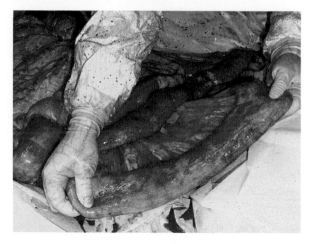

Figure 4.2 Small intestine that had been entrapped in the epiploic foramen. Early surgical intervention avoided the need to resect the affected small intestine, improving the horse's chance of survival.

▶ Decide whether other medical therapies are required if a specific diagnosis can be made (see p. 65).

KEY TIP

In general, avoid use of flunixin in horses with mild/moderate signs of colic of unknown aetiology where referral for surgery is an option – identification of the need for surgery may only be obvious once severe GIT compromise has occurred (with a subsequent ↓ prognosis despite surgery).

Ongoing management

▶ Discuss your initial assessment with the owner/carer and leave a record of your findings with them in case the horse needs to be reassessed (possibly by a different colleague):

  ▪ increasing HR, PCV and lactate can assist identification of horses that require potential surgical management/more intensive medical therapy.

▶ In general, water should be left with the horse but feed removed until faeces have been passed, and the horse should be monitored by the owner/carer every 30 min until signs of colic have resolved.

▶ Reassess the horse again in around 2 h, sooner if signs of colic recur.

▶ In the case of horses with signs of mild colic that respond to treatment, reassessment may not be indicated and it may be more appropriate to call the owner in 2 h/ask them to contact you to confirm that the horse is back to normal.

▶ Gastrointestinal rupture should be suspected in horses that have been acutely painful but then exhibit profuse sweating and a sudden reduction in pain:

  ▪ confirm by abdominocentesis (see p. 343) – euthanasia is indicated if this is confirmed (check this diagnosis is consistent with clinical signs – they will have severe CV compromise).

▶ In medically treated cases of colic, if a likely cause has been established (e.g. poor dentition/poor parasite prophylaxis), ways in which the risk of colic can be minimised in future should be discussed.

> **KEY TIP**
>
> Owners should be informed of the importance of early referral for potential surgical management and should be aware of the potential consequences if this option is declined.

Medical therapy for specific types of colic

Pelvic flexure impaction

▶ Administer 5–6 L water/oral electrolyte solutions by stomach tube q. 2–4 h (this may be easier to perform in hospital facilities); there is no evidence of any benefit in using liquid paraffin (mineral oil) in these cases.

▶ ± Administer an osmotic laxative as a one-off treatment – 0.5–1.0 g/kg of magnesium sulphate (Epsom salts) added to fluids administered by stomach tube.

▶ Withhold feed but allow access to water.

▶ If there is no softening of the impaction and passage of faeces within 24–36 h or if there is progressive deterioration in clinical parameters/increased level of pain, referral for potential surgery should be considered.

Large colon displacement

▶ Medical management is indicated if affected horses have normal CV parameters, signs of only mild/moderate pain and if gross large intestinal distension is absent.

▶ Oral ± IV fluids.

▶ Gentle exercise.

▶ Monitor carefully (q. 2–4 h) – may be more practical in hospital facilities; horses can occasionally deteriorate quickly if vascular occlusion develops.

▶ Nephrosplenic entrapment:

  ▪ can try phenylephrine treatment to ↓ splenic size and assist repositioning of the large colon (risk of haemorrhage in horses >15 years old)

- confirm by rectal examination ± US of the left paralumbar fossa
- administer phenylephrine 3 μg/kg/min given as an IV infusion in 500 mL or 1 L sterile saline/LRS over 15 min (22.5 mg total dose for 500-kg horse) followed by lunging exercise for 15 min
- repeat assessment to determine if successful or not – if not, potential surgical management may be indicated.

Referral of horses with colic

▶ If in doubt, referral centres are usually very happy to discuss management of colic cases.
▶ Time should not be wasted administering IV fluids unless there is a significant delay in obtaining transport or if the referral centre is some distance away.
▶ A nasogastric tube should always be passed prior to transport in a horse with severe pain or where a distended small intestine has been palpated on rectal examination/identified on abdominal US.
▶ Owners should be aware of the need to get the horse to the clinic as soon as possible and should be provided with good directions and the contact telephone number of the referral centre if there are any delays or if they get lost (see Referral of horses, p. 7).

Indications for euthanasia
- Uncontrollable pain despite potent analgesia where surgery is not an option.
- Severe CV compromise:
  - HR >90 beats/min
  - PCV >60%
  - purple MM.
- Gastrointestinal rupture:
  - brown/red ingesta-contaminated peritoneal fluid (see p. 343).

Grain (carbohydrate) overload

Ingestion of large quantities of grain/concentrate feed can have potentially fatal consequences and early and aggressive treatment is essential. Intestinal bacterial fermentation results in systemic absorption of massive quantities of endotoxin. This can result in the development of colic and severe abdominal distension in the early stages, followed by laminitis and diarrhoea.

Initial information to obtain

▶ How much and what type of feed has been ingested.
▶ When this occurred (if known).
▶ Whether any other horses could have also accessed this feed.
▶ If the feed could potentially contain additives such as growth promoters that may have potential additional toxic effects (e.g. poultry feed) – check the label on the feedbag.

Assessment and treatment immediately after carbohydrate ingestion

▶ Assess HR, RR, MM colour, and digital pulses.
▶ Check for evidence of colic/abdominal distension.
▶ Pass a stomach tube to check for any gastric reflux.

▸ If ingestion of large quantities of carbohydrate (CHO) has occurred <1–2h previously it is worth trying to lavage the stomach with repeated administration and removal of 1–2L fluid, particularly if feed can be siphoned off:

  ▪ continue lavage until retrieved fluid contains no further feed material.

▸ Administer activated charcoal 1–3g/kg as a slurry via the stomach tube (PO).

▸ Administer 0.25mg/kg flunixin IV q. 8h.

▸ ± Administer polymyxin B (1000–5000IU/kg diluted in 5% glucose solution IV q. 8–12h).

▸ Initiate treatment as for acute laminitis (see p. 45).

▸ Start cryotherapy of the feet (to try to prevent development of laminitis):

  ▪ cut the top off 4 × 5L fluid drip bags (or a suitable thick, plastic bag/container)

  ▪ place these over the feet and distal limbs

  ▪ fill each bag with crushed ice – replenish as necessary

  ▪ gently tape the bags in place (see website).

▸ Reassess again in 4h, sooner if signs of colic develop.

Assessment and treatment of clinical signs that develop as a consequence of ingestion of large quantities of carbohydrate

▸ Assess MM colour – congestion/cyanosis (severe cases).

▸ Assess HR, RR, GIT sounds and degree of abdominal distension.

▸ Assess digital pulses/evidence of laminitic stance or mild lameness.

▸ Assess degree of dehydration if diarrhoea is evident (see p. 72).

▸ Perform a rectal examination – assess degree of colon distension.

▸ Pass a stomach tube to check for reflux.

▸ ± Administer activated charcoal (contraindicated if >2L reflux obtained).

▸ Intensive medical management is required – consider hospitalisation/referral.

▸ Surgery may be indicated if there is evidence of massive abdominal distension/severe signs of colic:

  ▪ if this is not an option, as a last resort caecal trocharisation can be performed (see texts).

▸ Take blood samples for haematology ± BGA (if available).

▸ Administer flunixin 1.1mg/kg IV.

▸ Start IV fluid therapy (see p. 374).

▸ Administer 2–4L plasma concurrently – ideally hyperimmune plasma if available.

▸ ± Administer polymyxin B (see above).

▸ Initiate treatment for acute laminitis (see p. 45).

Prognosis

▸ Generally poor if signs of colic or laminitis develop.

Equine grass sickness (equine dysautonomia)

Equine grass sickness (EGS) occurs as a result of degeneration of neurones predominantly in the gastrointestinal system. It is more common in certain geographic regions (UK and other parts of Europe, 'Mal Seco' in South America) and there is strong evidence that it is a result of toxicoinfection with *Clostridum botulinim* types C and D. Subacute and acute forms usually present as cases of acute colic, whereas the chronic form may be primarily associated with weight loss, dysphagia and mild colic. In the Northern Hemisphere, cases most commonly occur in the spring (April/May) and young horses (2–7 years old) are at greatest risk.

Clinical signs

▶ Mild/moderate signs of colic.
▶ ↓ Faecal output.
▶ Muscle fasciculations.
▶ Ptosis.
▶ ↑ HR.
▶ Patchy sweating.

Assessment and diagnosis

▶ Presumptive based on clinical signs – rule out other causes of colic, dysphagia or weight loss.
▶ ± Administer topical 0.5% phenylephrine to one eye to determine whether ptosis is reversed in 30 min (this may support the diagnosis in horses with clinical signs consistent with EGS but false +ve and -ve results can be obtained).
▶ Ante-mortem diagnosis can only be confirmed by histological evaluation of an ileal biopsy obtained at laparotomy.
▶ PM confirmation – histopathology of autonomic/enteric ganglia and ileal biopsy.

Treatment

▶ Generally hopeless in acute/subacute cases.
▶ Chronic cases can survive with intensive nursing care.
▶ Useful sources of information include:
  ▪ Equine Grass Sickness Surveillance Scheme (http://www.equinegrasssickness.co.uk)
  ▪ Equine Grass Sickness Fund (http://www.grasssickness.org.uk).

Advice regarding prevention/reducing the risk of EGS in other horses on the premises

  • It is likely that any co-grazers on that pasture may have been exposed to the aetiologic agent and they should be monitored closely (particularly young horses/recent arrivals on the premises).
  • Move the horses to a different pasture if possible (but be aware that the risk increases over a radius of several kilometres for several days following a case).
  • Provide supplementary hay/haylage to horses at pasture for the following 2–3 weeks.
  • Avoid turning young horses or new arrivals onto the affected pasture during high-risk months.

Traumatic abdominal injuries

These may be a result of penetrating injuries into the abdominal cavity, including stake wounds/other penetrating foreign bodies or gunshot injuries (see p. 36). Blunt trauma can also result in traumatic injury, either to the body wall (often sustained by horses hitting their flanks on gates as they pass through a gateway) or to the abdominal viscera.

Potential sequelae following abdominal trauma

▶ Rupture of an abdominal viscus (including the uterus in pregnant mares – see p. 166).
▶ Diaphragmatic or body wall tears.
▶ GIT herniation through abdominal wall/diaphragmatic tears.
▶ Haemorrhage – haematoma/haemoperitoneum.
▶ Peritonitis.

Initial assessment

▶ Obtain a full history. Specific information that should be obtained includes:
  ▪ details about the type of trauma and where on the abdomen it was sustained
  ▪ when the injury happened and any abnormal signs noted since that time.
▶ Perform a full clinical examination. Specific evaluation should include:
  ▪ assessment of CV status
  ▪ check for other traumatic injuries and concurrent thoracic involvement
  ▪ careful examination of the body wall for wounds or alterations in the contour of the abdominal wall.
▶ ± Perform abdominocentesis (see p. 341):
  ▪ confirm peritonitis/haemorrhage/perforation of a viscus.
▶ Further assessment and treatment as required (see relevant sections/texts).

Oesophageal obstruction (choke)

This most commonly occurs when forage/concentrate feed becomes impacted within the oesophageal lumen, usually in the proximal or distal cervical (thoracic inlet) regions. Occasionally it may be a consequence of impaction by carrots, apples, foreign bodies or may be secondary to extraluminal masses or functional abnormalities of the oesophagus.

Clinical signs

▶ Dysphagia.
▶ Coughing.
▶ Ptyalism.
▶ Repeated flexion and extension of the neck.

Initial advice to the owner/carer

▶ Remove any food and water and observe for the next 10–15 min – if the obstruction resolves spontaneously offer the horse water and withhold feed for around 1–2 h.
▶ If signs of choke do not resolve after 15 min or if signs recur, veterinary assessment should be performed.

Initial evaluation

▶ Obtain a full history. Specific details that should be obtained include:
  ▪ duration of signs observed/if unknown when LSN
  ▪ type of feed being ingested at the onset of clinical signs.

‣ Perform a full clinical examination. Specific assessment should include:
  ▪ evaluation of HR, RR and respiratory effort, MM colour, T°
  ▪ assess hydration status (particularly if obstruction of more than a few hours duration)
  ▪ palpate left cervical region – assess for swelling/pain/crepitus
  ▪ perform auscultation of the thorax – check for crackles/harsh respiratory sounds (inhalation pneumonia)
  ▪ rule out other potential causes of dysphagia, e.g. neurological abnormalities.

Initial treatment

‣ Administer sedation IV (α2 agonist/butophanol):
  ▪ sufficient to lower the horse's head and ↓ anxiety.
‣ ± Administration of butylscopolamine IV.
‣ Pass a nasogastric tube (see p. 339):
  ▪ confirm the diagnosis – stomach tube cannot be advanced into the stomach
  ▪ identify the level at which obstruction has occurred (assess visually/measure stomach tube)
  ▪ do not force the tube – risk of perforation of the oesophagus
  ▪ perform initial lavage of the oesophagus. Use (warm) water to remove impacted material.
‣ ± Oxytocin 11–22 IU/kg IV (unproven efficacy – contraindicated in pregnant mares).
‣ If the obstruction cannot be cleared after 10–20 min of trying and the horse is otherwise clinically normal (i.e. no evidence of dehydration/pneumonia), withdraw food and water and repeat evaluation and initial treatment in 4–8 h.

> **HANDY TIP**
>
> Use a stomach tube with a single opening at the end rather than one with multiple fenestrations on the side to perform oesophageal lavage (more effective flushing of luminal contents).

Subsequent management of uncomplicated cases

‣ Once the obstruction has been cleared, provide water only initially (around 12–24 h).
‣ Administer BS antimicrobials if the horse has aspirated significant quantities of food/has ↑ respiratory rate. e.g. Trimethoprim sulphonamides.
‣ Assess the oral cavity for dental problems ± soft tissue lesions as a possible cause.
‣ ± Administer NSAIDs if a painful oral lesion has been identified.
‣ Reintroduce feed gradually (over 24–48 h) – grass and soaked pellet feed, avoid long-fibre forage initially.
‣ Further assessment and investigations are required if the horse subsequently becomes dull and anorexic/recurrent episodes of choke occur

> **KEY TIP**
>
> Never force the stomach tube down the oesophagus to clear the impaction – oesophageal perforation usually has grave consequences.

▶ Conservative treatment can be continued for around 12–24 h provided the horse is cardiovascularly stable and does not have ↑ RR/respiratory effort:
   ▪ monitor HR and RR ± PCV/TP during this time
   ▪ administer BS antimicrobials IV/IM.
▶ Longer duration of obstruction will result in clinically apparent systemic dehydration requiring IV fluids (see p. 374) and ↑ risk of inhalational pneumonia.
▶ Advanced assessment and treatment is recommended in cases of oesophageal obstruction >12–24 h in duration – consider hospitalisation/referral.

Advanced assessment and treatment of refractory cases

▶ Endoscopic evaluation of the oesophagus – identify cause of obstruction and location.
▶ Endoscopic examination of the trachea – assess degree of tracheal contamination.
▶ ± US of cervical oesophageal region.
▶ ± Radiography of pharynx and oesophagus (± contrast study).
▶ Lavage of the oesophagus using a cuffed endotracheal tube – sedation/under GA.
▶ Where foreign bodies are identified, removal using specialist forceps or via surgical oesophagostomy.
▶ Treatment of mucosal ulceration with sucralfate.

▶ Good in primary feed impactions that clear in <24 h.
▶ Inhalation pneumonia may complicate management and prognosis.
▶ Strictures may form secondarily to severe mucosal damage/surgical site.
▶ Where secondary to a predisposing cause, prognosis depends on individual inciting lesion.

Oesophageal perforation/tears

These are relatively uncommon and can be iatrogenic (e.g. after forcing a stomach tube) or traumatic in nature. These should be suspected where swelling and crepitus develops over the cervical oesophageal region, particularly following known trauma to the region. This is usually followed by acute deterioration in the horse's systemic parameters due to development of SIRS/endotoxic shock.

▶ Hospitalisation/referral.
▶ Endoscopy – identify tear/perforation, location and depth of tear.
▶ ± Radiography/contrast studies (Fig. 4.3).
▶ ± US assessment of cervical oesophagus.
▶ Surgical management may be possible in cervical injuries (seek specialist advice).

▶ Generally very poor.
▶ Grave where the intrathoracic oesophagus is involved.

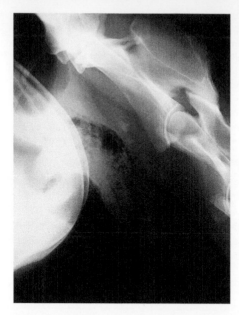

Figure 4.3 Lateral radiograph of the proximal cervical region in a horse that had sustained an oesophageal perforation. Mottled areas of variable radiolucency are indicative of gas and ingesta in the peri-oesophageal tissues.

Acute diarrhoea

Most cases of diarrhoea in the adult horse are mild, transient and self-limiting. However, severe, acute diarrhoea results in massive fluid loss, altered electrolytes, increased absorption of bacterial products and toxins and can be fatal if not treated early and aggressively. Some causes of diarrhoea may be infectious and potentially zoonotic, and good biosecurity is essential in these cases.

Assessment and initial treatment

▶ Obtain a thorough history. Specific information that should be obtained includes:
- when diarrhoea was first observed
- recent illness/weight loss
- parasite prophylaxis – consider larval cyathostominosis in young horses with poor/no parasite prophylaxis, or history of using only adulticides/ fenbendazole (resistance)
- diet and recent diet change
- if other horses are affected (consider salmonellosis, clostridiosis, PHF)
- recent administration of antimicrobials – most antimicrobials have been implicated in cases of colitis (consider salmonellosis, clostridiosis)
- geographical region – consider PHF in endemic regions, sand-related colic in areas with sandy soil)
- vaccination history (PHF if relevant)
- recent/ongoing NSAID administration.

Table 4.4 Possible causes of acute diarrhoea in the adult horse

Salmonellosis (*Salmonella* spp.)
Clostridiosis (*Clostridium* spp.)
Cyathostome nematodes (cyathostominosis)
NSAID (phenylbutazone) toxicity
Dietary change
Grain overload
Sand
Toxins (cantharidin, heavy metals)
Potomac horse fever (PHF)
Peritonitis
Antimicrobial associated (altered intestinal microbiota)
Idiopathic
Infiltrative bowel disease
Liver disease
Stress (following illness/surgery)

▶ Perform a clinical examination. Specific assessment should include:
  ▪ assess hydration status (see p. 375)
  ▪ assess HR and MM
  ▪ palpate digital pulses – evidence of laminitis
  ▪ assess GIT sounds
  ▪ check T°.
▶ ± Rectal examination (if signs of colic evident).
▶ ± Abdominocentesis (if peritonitis suspected).

Take samples for further investigations (see Table 4.4 for possible causes of diarrhoea)

▶ Haematology – assess WBC/differential count, PCV/TP.
▶ Serum biochemistry – creatinine, albumin:globulin, protein electrophoresis.
▶ Faecal samples – parasite larvae / eggs
▶ Presence of sand - suspend faecal sample in water (rectal glove ideal)
▶ Rule in/out Salmonellosis / Clostridiosis if suspected:
  ▪ samples from subsequent 5 piles of faeces (at least 5–10 g or put in selenite broth)
  ▪ culture/serology/PCR/*C. difficile* toxin assay (A) (discuss with laboratory).

Biosecurity

Any horse with 2 of the following 3 criteria should be placed in isolation (see p. 387) until the results of 5 faecal cultures are known:

▶ Diarrhoea.

▶ Pyrexia.

▶ Low systemic WBC.

Initial treatment

▶ Determine appropriate fluid therapy based on hydration status and other clinical parameters.

▶ Oral fluid therapy is indicated if no/only mild signs of dehydration are evident:
- commercial/home-made electrolyte solutions administered by stomach tube
- home-made electrolyte solution – add the following to 4 L water (Hillyer, 2004):
  » 15 g sodium chloride
  » 5 g sodium bicarbonate
  » 4 g dextrose
  » 10 g potassium bicarbonate
  » 10 g potassium chloride.
- check there is no reflux and administer around 8 L/500 kg q. 1–2 h (replace estimated deficits).

▶ IV fluids are indicated where there is evidence of moderate/severe dehydration (see p. 375).

▶ Administer flunixin 0.25 mg/kg IV q. 8 h.

▶ ± Polymyxin B (see Grain overload, p. 66).

▶ ± Administer intestinal protectants:
- di-tri-octahedral smectite (Bio-Sponge™) – see manufacturer instructions.

▶ Use of antimicrobials in these cases is controversial:
- metronidazole 15 mg/kg PO q. 8 h if clostridial colitis suspected/confirmed
- tetracyclines 6.6 mg/kg IV q. 24 h for 5 d in PHF cases.

▶ Nursing care:
- place a rectal sleeve over the tail and secure with sticky tape or Elastoplast (ensure this is not put on too tightly)
- clean perineum regularly, dry the skin and apply barrier cream if evidence of skin scalding
- bandage the distal limbs if limb oedema has developed
- maintain horse's appetite and forage intake – always ensure palatable fresh water is available, together with electrolyte solutions (may not drink these)/fresh forage.

▶ Treatment for cyathostominosis following initial stabilisation:
- administer moxidectin 0.4 mg/kg PO (dose accurately)
- alternatively, administer fenbendazole 7.5 mg/kg PO for 5 d (provided no evidence of resistance to this/previous use), followed by ivermectin 0.2 mg/kg PO on day 6
- concurrent corticosteroid administration (IV dexamethasone followed by oral prednisolone).

Advanced treatment of severe cases

▶ Indications for hospitalisation/referral of horses for intensive care (as a guide):
- tachycardia >60 beats/min
- congested/cyanotic MM
- PCV >50%, TP <50 g/L.

▶ Hospitalisation/referral may be difficult if suitable isolation facilities are not available and infectious colitis is suspected:
  ▪ depends on hospital policy regarding these cases – contact referral centre for advice.
▶ Critical care overview (see texts):
  ▪ hypertonic saline 2–4 mL/kg IV initially
  ▪ plasma/colloid administration
  ▪ supplement potassium and bicarbonate
  ▪ laminitis prophylaxis
  ▪ other symptomatic treatment as required.

Peritonitis

Affected horses may be presented with subtle and relatively non-specific signs of disease or this may be suspected following a penetrating injury to the abdomen. Peritonitis may be defined as primary (idiopathic), secondary and tertiary (recurrence following apparent resolution).

Clinical signs

▶ Depression, lethargy.
▶ Anorexia.
▶ Colic.
▶ ↑ HR.
▶ Pyrexia.
▶ ± Ileus.
▶ ± Weight loss.
▶ ± Diarrhoea.

Diagnosis

▶ Peritoneal fluid:
  ▪ yellow–orange, opaque (Fig. 4.4)
  ▪ ↑ WBC (may be as high as $100–140 \times 10^9/L$), predominantly neutrophils
  ▪ TP >25 g/L
  ▪ cytology – smear and Gram stain
  ▪ C&S – place sample into blood culture system.
▶ Abdominal US (see website/texts).

Treatment and prognosis

▶ Medical management is indicated in most primary cases.
  ▪ BS antimicrobials – penicillin, gentamicin ± metronidazole (reassess based on results of C&S)
  ▪ administer NSAIDs
  ▪ ± IV fluids.
▶ Surgical exploration of the abdomen is indicated in horses with suspected involvement of a viscus or where there is no response to medical therapy (exploratory laparotomy and abdominal lavage or laparoscopy).

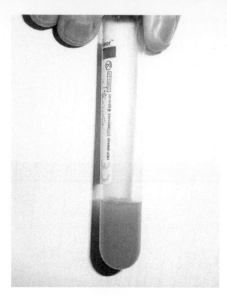

Figure 4.4   Turbid peritoneal fluid obtained from a horse with peritonitis.

Prognosis

▶ 40–70% survival reported.
▶ Around 84% for uncomplicated idiopathic peritonitis.

Dysphagia

Strictly, this is defined as difficulty swallowing but it is usually expanded to include difficulty eating. The underlying cause is broadly defined into three categories: obstructive, neurogenic and pain related (see Table 4.5)

> **KEY TIP**
> Rule out rabies as a cause of dysphagia in endemic areas and do not perform intraoral examination in suspected cases (see p. 287).

Initial assessment

▶ Obtain a full history. Specific information that should be obtained includes:
  ▪ duration of signs observed
  ▪ whether gradual or sudden in onset
  ▪ current management and any recent changes in this

Table 4.5 Possible causes of dysphagia

Pain	Neurogenic	Obstructive
Buccal/lingual abscess Retropharyngeal or intraoral foreign body Dental pathology Trauma to the mouth Retropharyngeal abscess (*Strep. equi* var. *equi*) Masseter myositis Atypical myopathy	Head trauma Guttural pouch disease Pharyngeal paralysis Lead poisoning Botulism Hepatoencephalopathy Equine grass sickness (dysautonomia) Viral encephalomyelitis EPM	Oesophageal obstruction/ stricture Neoplasia

- recent dental prophylaxis/treatment and who performed this
- whether the horse is able to chew or appears to have difficulty swallowing.
▶ Perform a full clinical examination. Specific assessment should include:
  - assess mentation (rabies is an important DDx in affected areas)
  - determine whether there is any swelling around the pharyngeal/neck region
  - assess CV parameters and hydration status
  - auscultation of chest (check for evidence of aspiration pneumonia)
  - assess whether the horse can drink water
  - observe the horse eating if appropriate to try to determine whether the dysphagia is oral, pharyngeal or oesophageal
    » oral – the horse is unable to prehend food/is reluctant to chew food and displays dropping/quidding of food or may exhibit excessive salivation
    » pharyngeal – food is masticated but the horse seems physically unable to swallow it and may exhibit head shaking behaviour
    » oesophageal – food cannot move down the oesophagus into the stomach and the horse may exhibit signs of distress, coughing, nasal discharge, and neck extension when attempting to swallow.
▶ Perform a full neurological examination (particularly evaluation of the cranial nerves – see p. 129).
▶ Perform a detailed intraoral examination:
  - ± sedation (if flexible endoscope available, may choose to perform endoscopic examination of the pharynx and oesophagus first)
  - Haussmann gag and light source
  - ± rigid intraoral endoscope
  - evaluate the oral soft tissues for evidence of inflammation (may be secondary to dental disorders such as fractured teeth/diastemata) or foreign bodies.
▶ Endoscopic evaluation of pharynx, larynx, guttural pouches, oesophagus and trachea:
  - ideally perform without sedation to rule out sedation-induced artefacts as the cause of any abnormalities seen (e.g. oesophageal dilation).
▶ Obtain blood samples for haematology and serum biochemistry:
  - PCV, TP, electrolytes ± ammonia (if available).

▶ Depends on the underlying cause: see relevant sections/texts.
▶ Administer NSAIDs – ↓ inflammation.
▶ ± BS antimicrobial cover – if likely aspiration of food.
▶ If able to swallow water, see if the horse can ingest sloppy food (slurry).
▶ ± Administration of slurry by nasogastric tube.
▶ ± IV fluid therapy.
▶ Check urination and defecation.
▶ Ongoing care, including hospitalisation/referral, will depend on the severity of clinical signs and diagnosis (if established).

▶ Lateral radiographs of the head and neck ± contrast studies.
▶ US – retropharyngeal area/larynx, oesophagus.
▶ ± CT if available.
▶ ± Obtain CSF sample.
▶ ± Viral isolation/serology/PCR.

Mandibular and maxillary fractures

These may be a result of direct trauma or the horse pulling back suddenly whilst grasping a fixed object. Fractures can occur in a variety of different locations and various configurations may be seen. Fractures of the incisive region of the mandible are most common.

▶ Intraoral haemorrhage +/− wound over the mandible or maxilla.
▶ ± Obvious displacement of the incisors.
▶ Unwilling/unable to eat.

▶ ± Administer sedation.
▶ Perform a careful examination of the mouth – fractures of the incisors/incisive plate can be assessed easily by elevating the horse's lips (Fig. 4.5).
▶ Be careful when assessing the mouth – it may be sensible to obtain radiographs first to avoid displacing a fracture if a gag is placed.
▶ Administer NSAIDs and BS antimicrobials.

▶ Confirm the diagnosis and determine the fracture location and configuration (consider referral):
▶ Radiography:
  ▪ lateral, DV, oblique views (Fig. 4.6)
  ▪ intraoral VD view, which is useful for assessing rostral mandibular fractures.

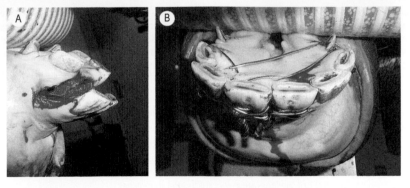

Figure 4.5 (A,B) Fracture of the rostral mandible involving teeth 402 and 403 that underwent repair under standing sedation using cerclage wires (see website for further details).

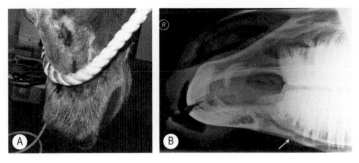

Figure 4.6 (A) A wound sustained to the horizontal ramus of the mandible following a kick from another horse. (B) A unilateral, displaced, oblique fracture (arrow) of the interdental space (arrow) was confirmed on radiography.

▶ ± US of mandible.

▶ ± CT if available.

▶ Options for treatment depends on the fracture location and configuration:

  ▪ simple fractures of the rostral mandible can be treated easily in the sedated horse using cerclage wires (see texts/website) 📖

  ▪ conservative treatment may be indicated in some non-displaced fractures, e.g. vertical ramus of the mandible

  ▪ other fractures frequently require surgical fixation (seek specialist advice).

Lip and tongue lacerations

As with other injuries to the soft tissues of the head, the lips and tongue have a good vascular supply and generally heal well. Lip injuries are relatively common and are usually sustained after horses have been chewing or mouthing on fixed objects on which they have become caught, with resultant tearing of the tissues when they pull back. Tongue injuries are less common and may occur when the horse has accidentally bitten its tongue or subsequent to use of inappropriate bits or use of ropes around the mouth. It is important to try to get the best functional and cosmetic result when performing repair of these injuries.

Lip

Assessment

▶ Perform a full clinical examination and check for other injuries to the head.
▶ Check the mouth for any evidence of intraoral injuries (use a gag and light source to assess the mouth fully if these are suspected).
▶ Determine the extent of the laceration (i.e. full/partial thickness).

Treatment

▶ If partial thickness, conservative management (cleaning, ± antimicrobials and NSAIDs) is often appropriate.
▶ If they are full thickness – best to suture to get the best possible cosmetic and functional result (although dehiscence of the repair can often occur):
  ▪ debride and lavage (see p. 22)
  ▪ suture in 2 or 3 layers – oral mucosa, muscle layer, skin (see website)
▶ If dehiscence/poor cosmetic or functional outcome – further surgery can be performed once any infection and swelling has resolved (seek specialist advice).

Tongue

Assessment

▶ Sedate the horse.
▶ Perform a thorough evaluation of the mouth using a good light source:
  ▪ palpation ± use of an intraoral rigid endoscope
  ▪ check for any other injuries to the mouth/evidence of any foreign bodies.
▶ Can use a gauze bandage tied temporarily around the caudal part of the tongue as a tourniquet and to apply gentle traction in order to examine the more caudal parts of the tongue.
▶ Palpate the tongue for evidence of pain and swelling – if so, suspect a foreign body:
  ▪ ± further assessment with US/radiography.
▶ Assess the location and depth of the laceration and viability of the tissues.

Treatment

▶ Superficial injuries usually heal well without suturing.
▶ May need to amputate the tip of the tongue if it is not viable – horses can cope with removal of tissue to the level of the rostral aspect of the lingual frenulum (Fig. 4.7).
▶ Suturing of deeper lacerations/amputated stump (consider referral):
  ▪ usually best under GA but can do standing with sedation and LA infiltration
  ▪ debride and suture (0 or 1 size absorbable suture)
  ▪ deeper injuries – use mattress sutures and perform in several layers.

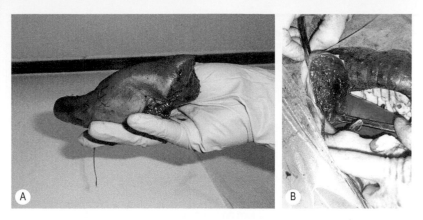

Figure 4.7 (A,B) Tongue laceration sustained in a horse at pasture at the level of the rostral aspect of the lingual frenulum. The horse suffered no long-term effects following the loss of the rostral portion of the tongue.

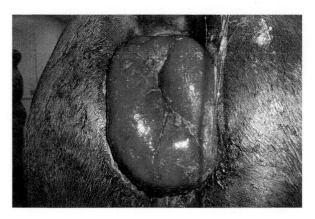

Figure 4.8 Type I rectal prolapse in a horse with severe diarrhoea. It is important to investigate and treat the underlying cause (consider biosecurity measures if potential infectious aetiology).

Rectal prolapse

This usually occurs following periods of prolonged straining; types I and II are most common.

Possible causes of straining and rectal prolapse

▸ Diarrhoea (Fig. 4.8).
▸ Colic.
▸ Intestinal parasites.
▸ Proctitis.

Table 4.6 Classification of rectal prolapse

Classification of rectal prolapse	Definition	Clinical signs
Type I	Prolapse of rectal mucosa through the anus	Mucosa-covered mass at the anus
Type II	Full-thickness prolapse of all/part of the rectal ampulla	Mucosa-covered mass at the anus
Type III	Type II + variable length of small colon intussuscepted into the rectum (but not through the anus)	Mucosa-covered mass at the anus
Type IV	Peritoneal rectum and a variable length of small colon intussuscepted through the anus	Tube-like structure protruding from the anus

▸ Rectal foreign body/mass.
▸ Dystocia.
▸ Retained foetal membranes.

Assessment and treatment

▸ Obtain a full history. Specific information that should be obtained includes:
  ▪ details of any abnormal clinical signs prior to rectal prolapse, e.g. diarrhoea, signs of colic.
▸ Perform a full clinical examination to determine the underlying cause of straining.
▸ Treat any underlying problem as appropriate (see relevant sections/ texts).
▸ ± Administer sedation/butylscopolamine to ↓ straining.
▸ Assess the prolapsed tissue and determine the grade of prolapse and the degree of tissue compromise (Table 4.6).
▸ ± Perform proctoscopy if there is no obvious predisposing cause on initial examination to rule in/out a rectal foreign body/mass.
▸ Obtain peritoneal fluid in types III and IV to determine whether there is evidence of intestinal compromise (see p. 341).

Treatment of types I, II and III rectal prolapse

▸ Reduction of prolapsed tissue under standing sedation:
  ▪ can apply topical local anaesthetic solution/mix with lubricant (e.g. mepivacaine/ lidocaine) and instil into the rectum to reduce straining
  ▪ ± apply sugar/magnesium sulphate solution to reduce mucosal oedema
  ▪ ± caudal epidural anaesthesia (see p. 362) – assist replacement/prevent re-prolapse.
▸ Place a purse-string suture to prevent repeat prolapse:
  ▪ heavy-duty suture/umbilical tape

- take 4 wide bites in the anus
- tie in a bow and loosen q. 2–4h for defecation/manual removal of faeces from the rectum.
▸ Administer oral fluids by stomach tube (soften faeces).
▸ Feed a laxative diet.
▸ Other ongoing treatment as for primary problem (see relevant sections/texts).
▸ Repeat abdominocentesis q. 24h initially in type III prolapses – early detection of peritonitis.
▸ Submucosal resection is indicated if evidence of tissue necrosis/severe swelling precludes reduction or if prolapse recurs:
- can be performed under sedation + epidural anaesthesia/GA – consider referral.

Treatment of type IV rectal prolapse

▸ Seek specialist advice/referral.
▸ If referral is undertaken, it is usually better to leave the prolapse as it is, to enable more accurate assessment by the surgeon:
- conservative treatment – reduction of prolapsed intestine, prevention of re-prolapse (including treatment of underlying cause) and monitoring for intestinal necrosis (peritonitis, colic)
- surgical management – resection and anastomosis.

Prognosis

▸ Good for types I and II (depending on underlying cause).
▸ More guarded in types III and IV – depends on vascular compromise/damage to mesenteric attachments.

Rectal tears

These are most commonly iatrogenic in nature, and diagnosis and management are covered in Ch. 14 (see p. 262). Other possible causes include:
▸ Direct trauma.
▸ Dystocia.
▸ Neurogenic faecal retention.
▸ Secondary to tissue devitalisation (vascular compromise).
▸ Impactions secondary to:
- mural haematoma
- abscess
- neoplasia
- stricture.
▸ Spontaneous.

References and further reading

• **Aleman, M.,** 2009. Dysphagia of neurogenic origin. In: Robinson, N.E., Sprayberry, K.A. (Eds.), Current Therapy in Equine Medicine (sixth ed.). Elsevier, St. Louis, Missouri, pp. 354–357.

- Archer, D.C., 2004. Decision making in the management of the colicky horse. In Pract. 26, 378–385.

- Beard, W., 2009. Fracture repair techniques for the equine mandible and maxilla. Equine Vet. Educ. 21, 352–357.

- Chiavaccini, L., Hassel, D.M., 2010. Clinical features and prognostic variables in 109 horses with esophageal obstruction (1992–2009). J. Vet. Intern. Med. 24, 1147–1152.

- Elce, Y., 2009. Esophageal obstruction. In: Robinson, N.E., Sprayberry, K.A. (Eds.), Current Therapy in Equine Medicine (sixth ed.). Elsevier, St. Louis, Missouri, pp. p351–353.

- Freeman, D.E., 2012. Rectum and anus. In: Auer, J.A., Stick, J.A. (Eds.), Equine Surgery (fourth ed.). Elsevier, Philadelphia, Pennsylvania, pp. p494–505.

- Greet, T., Ramzan, P.H.L., 2011. Head and dental trauma. In: Easley, J., Dixon, P.M., Schumacher, J. (Eds.), Equine Dentistry (third ed.). Elsevier, Edinburgh, pp. 115–127.

- Henderson, I.S.F., Mair, T.S., Keen, J.A., et al. 2008. Study of the short- and long-term outcomes of 65 horses with peritonitis. Vet. Rec. 163, 293–297.

- Hewetson, M., 2006. Investigation of false colic in the horse. In Pract. 28, 326–338.

- Hillyer, M., 2004. A practical approach to diarrhoea in the adult horse. In Pract. 26, 2–11.

- Hudson, N.P.H., McGorum, B.C., Dixon, P.M., 2006. A review of 4 cases of dysphagia in the horse: buccal abscess, lingual abscess, retropharyngeal foreign body and oesophageal obstruction. Equine Vet. Educ. 18, 199–204.

- Lyle, C., Pirie, S., 2009. Equine grass sickness. In Pract. 31, 26–32.

- Naylor, R.J., Dunkel, B., 2009. The treatment of diarrhoea in the adult horse. Equine Vet. Educ. 21, 494–504.

Respiratory emergencies

Respiratory emergencies are relatively common in adult horses, and are usually associated with traumatic, infectious and inflammatory conditions. The most common presentations relate to respiratory distress (dyspnoea) and epistaxis.

Respiratory distress (dyspnoea)

This can be life-threatening and it is essential to be prepared to perform a tracheotomy and place a temporary tracheostomy tube (see p. 356) in the case of severe URT obstructions.

Advice to the owner/carer

▶ Do not move the horse unless it is in imminent danger.
▶ Minimise any stress to the horse, e.g. do not move companions.

Table 5.1 Causes of inspiratory and expiratory dyspnoea

Inspiratory dyspnoea	Expiratory dyspnoea	Mixed inspiratory and expiratory dyspnoea
Obstruction of extrathoracic airways Restrictive lung disorders Space-occupying lesions of the thorax	Obstruction of intrathoracic airways	Fixed obstruction of the airways

Adapted from McGorum and Dixon (2007).

Initial assessment and first aid

▶ If the horse is exhibiting severe respiratory distress, obtain a succinct history about the circumstances leading to the event and perform a rapid assessment.

▶ Check MM for evidence of cyanosis.

▶ Determine if dyspnoea is inspiratory/expiratory or a combination of both (Table 5.1).

▶ Examine the head, neck and thorax for any evidence of wounds or swellings and check for any gross abdominal distension.

- If there is obvious nasal swelling/oedema (e.g. snake bite/severe trauma):
  - place a nasal tube/tubing of suitable diameter and length into the nasal passages or perform a tracheotomy.
- If there is evidence of severe inspiratory dyspnoea and respiratory noise, a URT obstruction is highly likely:
  - perform a tracheotomy (see p. 356).
- If there is a wound over the thorax and air movement can be heard, suspect pneumothorax:
  - cover the wound immediately – cling-film wrapped around the thorax is ideal
  - further evaluation and treatment of the wound can be performed once the horse's condition has stabilised.
- If there is evidence of severe expiratory dyspnoea, a history of RAO/SPAOPD and known exposure to a potential inciting cause:
  - administer atropine 0.02 mg/kg IV (slow) to relieve acute bronchoconstriction.
- If oxygen is available, administer by nasal insufflation 10–15 L/min.
- Administer NSAIDs if required – analgesia/anti-inflammatory effects.
- Do not transport the horse (if required) until their condition has stabilised.

Further assessment following stabilisation

Obtain a full history. Specific questions that should be asked include:

▶ Duration of clinical signs – if unknown when the horse was LSN.

▶ History of prior respiratory disease, e.g. RAO/SPAOPD.

▶ Speed of progression.

▸ If signs have developed following known/suspected trauma or recent change of management (e.g. recent stabling).
▸ Any recent/concurrent illness.
▸ ↓ Performance at exercise noted.
▸ Current/recent administration of medication.
▸ Illness in any in-contact horses.
▸ Vaccination status.
▸ Potential exposure to ragwort or other sources of toxins.
▸ Recent long distance transport.
▸ Recent importation.

Perform a general examination to rule out concurrent disease. Specific assessment should include:

▸ Check for other non-respiratory causes of respiratory distress, e.g. colic, hydrops conditions (pregnant mare).
▸ Check T° – if pyrexic, consider infectious disease aetiology.
▸ Assess MM colour and CV status.
▸ Assess RR, depth and degree of abdominal effort, respiratory pattern:
  ▪ rapid/normal
  ▪ shallow/deep
  ▪ regular/irregular.
▸ Check for evidence of any respiratory noise and determine its location.
▸ Examine the nasal region for:
  ▪ evidence of any nasal discharge – unilateral/bilateral, type of discharge (mucoid/purulent/haemorrhagic/containing particulate feed material)
  ▪ overt swelling of the region (e.g. acute swelling following trauma/insect sting/snake bite)
  ▪ bilateral nasal airflow
  ▪ evidence of a malodorous smell from the nares/mouth.
▸ Examine the head:
  ▪ look for signs of external trauma/palpate for swelling/crepitus
  ▪ palpate the submandibular and parotid region – evidence of enlarged LN or guttural pouch(es).
▸ Examine the cervical region:
  ▪ palpate the trachea
  ▪ check for emphysema/crepitus
  ▪ auscultate the trachea.
▸ Examine the thorax:
  ▪ perform auscultation and percussion over the lung fields
  ▪ palpate the ribs
  ▪ auscultate the heart
  ▪ NB do not perform re-breathing examination.

Treatment and further evaluation

▸ Specific treatment and further diagnostic tests will depend on the provisional diagnosis made (Table 5.2).

Table 5.2 Possible causes of respiratory distress in the adult horse

Common respiratory causes	Uncommon respiratory causes	Non-respiratory causes
Retropharyngeal abscess (*Strep. equi* var *equi*)	Arytenoid chondritis	Hyperthermia/exhaustion
Recurrent airway obstruction	Progressive ethmoidal haematoma	Proximal oesophageal obstruction
Pneumonia/pleuropneumonia	Severe pharyngeal lymphoid hyperplasia	Severe anaemia/ haemolysis
Diaphragmatic hernia	Tracheal collapse	Severe abdominal distension (e.g. colonic distension, hydrops conditions)
Guttural pouch empyema	Laryngeal oedema	
Pneumothorax/fractured ribs		
Bilateral laryngeal paralysis		Pain
Severe nasal oedema (post GA/acute jugular vein obstruction/anaphylaxis)		Endotoxic shock
		Cardiac failure
Severe nasal swelling (trauma/snake bite)		Botulism
		Poisoning
		Altitude

▶ Further diagnostic tests may include:
  ▪ endoscopy
  ▪ ± tracheal wash
  ▪ radiography
  ▪ US
  ▪ haematology/serum biochemistry
  ▪ ± CT
  ▪ ± BGA.

Pneumonia/pleuropneumonia

This can be challenging to diagnose in the early stages and pleurodynia (pleural pain) that is evident can be mistakenly attributed to pain associated with colic or laminitis. It occurs most commonly in competition horses or those who have undergone recent long distance travel and it can be career and life-threatening if not diagnosed and treated early.

Predisposing factors

▶ Long distance transport (>500 miles).
▶ Strenuous exercise.
▶ General anaesthesia.
▶ Oesophageal obstruction.

▸ Viral respiratory infection.
▸ Dysphagia.
▸ Inhaled foreign bodies.
▸ External thoracic injury.

Clinical signs

▸ Pyrexia.
▸ ↓ Appetite, depression and lethargy.
▸ ↑ HR.
▸ ↑ RR.
▸ Dependent oedema of the sternal region.
▸ Reluctance to move/abduction of elbows.
▸ ± Soft productive cough.
▸ ± Nasal discharge.

Diagnosis

▸ Presumptive diagnosis based on history (predisposing factors) and findings on clinical examination:
  ▪ auscultation and percussion of thorax
  ▪ other causes of pleural effusion should also be considered – in the UK this is more commonly associated with neoplasia, e.g. lymphoma, mesothelioma.
▸ Confirmation of diagnosis – consider hospitalisation/referral if this is an option:
  ▪ US – assess if unilateral/bilateral, severity
  ▪ thoracocentesis – US guidance, assess WBC, TP and submit for C&S
  ▪ endoscopy trans-tracheal wash for cytology and C&S (aerobic and anaerobic)
  ▪ radiography (once pleural drainage performed)
  ▪ haematology and serum biochemistry.

Treatment and prognosis

Ongoing treatment includes (see specialist texts):
▸ BS antimicrobials (penicillin and gentamicin IV ± metronidazole):
  ▪ may need to change if no response to therapy – antimicrobial choice based on C&S results.
▸ NSAIDs – flunixin 1.1 mg/kg IV.
▸ Pleural drainage (Fig. 5.1):
  ▪ perform via catheter/teat cannula or ideally a commercial thoracic cannula
  ▪ 7th ICS – determine optimal site using US
  ▪ repeat daily/maintain in situ (chest drain and one-way valve, e.g. Heimlich valve/cut end of latex glove or condom).
▸ ± IV fluids.
▸ ± Preventive therapy vs laminitis (e.g. ice therapy of feet, see p. 67).
▸ US monitoring of progression, abscess formation).

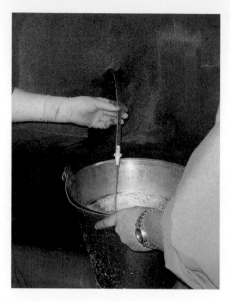

Figure 5.1 Drainage of sanguinous, malodorous fluid from the thorax of a horse with pleuropneumonia.

▸ Depends on duration of disease prior to diagnosis, severity, types of bacteria involved and complications that may develop.
▸ Good/fair prognosis for survival if treated early and appropriately (43–98% survival reported).
▸ Reasonable prognosis for return to previous athletic function.

Inhalational pneumonia

Horses have a relatively poor cough response compared to other species and this may contribute to development of inhalational pneumonia in certain conditions/situations, including:

▸ Oesophageal obstruction (especially >24 h in duration).
▸ Dysphagia.
▸ Aspiration of gastric contents, e.g. under GA.
▸ Iatrogenic – during stomach tubing of fluids (see p. 264).

▸ ± Suction of inhaled material from the lungs (if possible).
▸ Treatment for pulmonary oedema in acute/severe cases (see next section).
▸ Identify and treat concurrent/initiating problem.
▸ Administer NSAIDs IV.

Table 5.3 Potential causes of pulmonary oedema in adult horses

URT obstruction	Severe nasal oedema
	Severe bilateral laryngeal paralysis
	Severe laryngeal/pharyngeal swelling
Acute pulmonary injury	Acute alveolitis/interstitial disease
	Aspiration
	Smoke inhalation
	Anaphylaxis
	Adverse drug reactions
	Infectious diseases (e.g. AHS, Hendra)
	Endotoxaemia/SIRS
	Embolism
	Transfusion reaction
Cardiac	Cardiac failure

▸ Administer BS antimicrobials.
▸ Decide if hospitalisation/referral is warranted for further assessment and intensive treatment.
▸ Supportive therapy as required, e.g. IV fluids.
▸ Monitor closely for development of pleuropneumonia, e.g. US monitoring to identify pleural effusion/lung pathology.

Aspiration of liquid paraffin (mineral oil)

▸ This is usually iatrogenic and can result in development of a severe, potentially life-threatening lipoid pneumonia (see specialist texts/seek specialist advice).
▸ Severity of clinical signs and prognosis depends on the amount aspirated.
▸ Consider hospitalisation/referral for intensive treatment.

Prognosis

▸ Depends on severity and duration; generally poor following aspiration of liquid paraffin in severe cases (successful treatment using corticosteroids has been reported).

Pulmonary oedema

This is an immediate, life-threatening condition that requires rapid and aggressive treatment. It can develop subsequent to acute pulmonary injury or secondary to URT obstruction or cardiac failure (Table 5.3).

Clinical signs

▸ Pink/white frothy material from the nares (see Fig. 10.2, p. 194).
▸ Inspiratory stridor.

- ▶ Respiratory distress.
- ▶ ↑ HR.
- ▶ ↑ RR.
- ▶ Severe – marked distress (can react violently).
- ▶ ± Collapse and death.

Initial treatment

- ▶ If distressed, administer acepromazine 0.02 mg/kg IV or xylazine 0.2–0.4 mg/kg IV.
- ▶ Perform nasal intubation/tracheotomy if an URT obstruction is suspected.
- ▶ Administer furosemide 1 mg/kg IV.
- ▶ Nasal insufflation of O_2 (if available) 10–15 L/min:
  - ± administration directly into the trachea using a 14G needle/catheter inserted between the tracheal rings (to ↑ speed of O_2 absorption).
- ▶ Administer dexamethasone 0.1 mg/kg IV.
- ▶ ± Administer clenbuterol 0.8 μg/kg IV (sweating, tachycardia, ↓ BP) or inhaled salbutamol (2 μg/kg).
- ▶ ± Administer NSAIDs (↓ inflammation/pain).
- ▶ ± Reduce volume of fluid in the airways (if suction is available).

Further investigation and treatment

- ▶ Take a full history and perform a full clinical examination to determine the underlying cause.
- ▶ Consider hospitalisation/referral if appropriate once stabilised.
- ▶ Rule out the possibility of infectious disease, e.g. AHS/Hendra virus in high-risk horses (see Ch. 15).
- ▶ Prognosis – dependent on underlying cause and whether it can be treated.

Acute exacerbation of RAO/SPAOPD

Acute exacerbation of clinical signs can occur in horses previously diagnosed with recurrent airway obstruction (RAO)/summer-pasture-associated obstructive pulmonary disease (SPAOPD). This may occur following accidental exposure to known allergens and, in severe cases, can result in marked expiratory dyspnoea.

Initial treatment

- ▶ If the horse is in severe respiratory distress, administer atropine 0.02 mg/kg IV (slow) - bronchodilation takes 15 min:
  - side effects – ↑ HR, mydriasis, ileus ± colic.
- ▶ Dexamethasone 0.1 mg/kg IV. (can take 4–6 h to have any effect)
- ▶ ± Intranasal oxygen if available.
- ▶ Administer furosemide 1 mg/kg IV.
- ▶ Remove inciting cause/from environment in which the horse had been placed.
- ▶ Discuss ongoing medical therapy (see texts).

Pneumothorax

This is rare but may be suspected in horses that have developed respiratory distress following penetrating trauma to the thorax (open pneumothorax). Less commonly it may develop following URT surgery or in horses with pleuropneumonia (closed pneumothorax) and, rarely, tension pneumothorax can occur (air can enter but not exit the thorax). Haemothorax can occur concurrently and affected horses may have clinical signs consistent with haemorrhagic shock (see p. 186).

First aid and assessment

▸ Check carefully for any wounds over the thorax and palpate the region to check for evidence of crepitus over the ribs.

▸ If there is wound, cover it immediately – cling film wrapped around the thorax is ideal (the wound can be evaluated and treated once the horse is stabilised).

▸ Auscultate and percuss the thorax:
  ▪ ± lack of lung sounds dorsally on auscultation
  ▪ ↑ resonance on percussion.

▸ If severe respiratory distress/cyanosis, administer intranasal oxygen (if available) ± administer directly into the trachea (see Pulmonary oedema, p. 91).

▸ Evacuate air from the thorax:
  ▪ clip and aseptically prepare a site between the 12th and 15th ICS just below the epaxial muscles (± place a few mL of local anaesthetic at the site)
  ▪ keeping close to the cranial part of the rib (avoid blood vessels on caudal aspect), insert a 14G IV catheter/incise through the skin and insert a teat cannula
  ▪ connect to a 3-way tap and syringe
  ▪ aspirate air
  ▪ do this slowly – rapid expansion can cause pulmonary oedema.

Further assessment and treatment

▸ Check that the patient has stabilised (improved MM colour, ↓ RR).

▸ Determine if hospitalisation/referral is required:
  ▪ further investigation of the underlying cause, e.g. radiography/US of the thorax
  ▪ assessment and treatment of wounds, concurrent rib fractures or haemothorax
  ▪ placement of an indwelling catheter if ongoing pneumothorax.

Acute viral respiratory disease

▸ This may be suspected where respiratory disease occurs in a number of in-contact horses.

▸ These uncommonly present as emergencies except in horses that have developed severe pulmonary oedema/pneumonia (see p. 88–92).

Treatment

▸ Symptomatic (see relevant sections).

▸ It is Important to confirm the diagnosis and implement appropriate biosecurity measures until the cause of clinical signs is confirmed (see p. 292):
  ▪ consider EI/EHV-1/AHS (Fig. 5.2)/Hendra where recent outbreaks have occurred/disease occurs in high-risk areas (see Ch. 15).

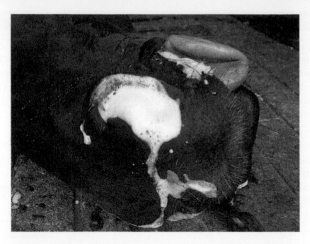

Figure 5.2 Pulmonary oedema evident as a frothy discharge from the nares following collapse and death of a horse with African horse sickness (see Ch. 15).

Courtesy of Derek Knottenbelt.

Retropharyngeal abscess

This is usually caused by infection with *Streptococcus equi* var *equi* (strangles). Immediate isolation of the affected horse(s) and implementation of other biosecurity measures to prevent disease spread is essential (see p. 292 and HBLB codes of practice http://codes.hblb.org.uk).

Clinical signs

▸ Respiratory distress (URT obstruction).
▸ Dysphagia.
▸ ± External swelling caudal to the vertical rami of the mandible.

Initial treatment

▸ Perform a tracheotomy if there are signs of severe respiratory distress (see p. 356).
▸ ± Assess the degree of respiratory tract obstruction (severe cases):
  ▪ endoscopy
  ▪ radiography.
▸ Take pharyngeal swabs/guttural pouch wash and send to appropriate laboratory (confirm diagnosis).
▸ Administer NSAIDs – flunixin 1.1 mg/kg IV initially.
▸ Antimicrobials are usually not recommended if there is evidence of overt abscess formation (may delay eventual abscess maturation and drainage) but penicillin administration may be required in cases of airway obstruction.
▸ ± Surgical drainage of abscess (be aware of anatomical structures in the immediate vicinity).

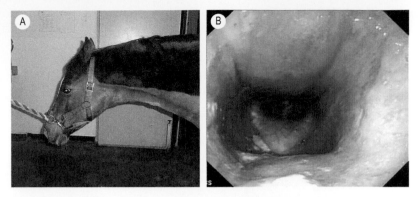

Figure 5.3 (A) Extended head position and swelling behind the vertical ramus of the mandible in a pony with guttural pouch empyema that presented in respiratory distress. (B) The endoscopic image demonstrates the degree of pharyngeal compression due to large quantities of inspissated material that have accumulated in the affected guttural pouch.

Guttural pouch empyema

This is an occasional cause of respiratory distress. Horses usually have a history of *Streptococcus equi* var *equi* infection, sometimes followed by intermittent purulent nasal discharge.

Clinical signs

▶ Head and neck held extended (Fig. 5.3).
▶ Swelling behind the vertical ramus of the mandible.
▶ ± Respiratory distress.

Initial first aid

▶ Perform a tracheotomy if respiratory distress is evident (see p. 356).
▶ Administer NSAIDs IV.
▶ Perform further assessment and treatment following stabilisation:
  ▪ lateral/oblique radiographs
  ▪ endoscopy
  ▪ endoscopic/surgical removal of guttural pouch contents.

Bilateral laryngeal paralysis

This is uncommon and, unlike cases of unilateral laryngeal paralysis, affected horses can present with signs of severe respiratory distress at rest. Concurrent neurological signs may also be evident in horses that have a history of possible exposure to ragwort (or other pyrrolizidine alkaloid-containing plants), lead or organophosphates. Bilateral laryngeal paralysis has been reported more commonly in ponies and is usually associated with hepatic disease secondary to ingestion of pyrrolizidine alkaloid-containing plants.

▶ Severe respiratory distress.
▶ Respiratory stertor.
▶ ± Cyanotic MM.

Assessment and treatment

▶ Perform a tracheotomy (see p. 356).
▶ Endoscopy – confirm diagnosis and rule out other causes of respiratory distress.
▶ Investigate and treat the underlying cause (Ch. 16/specialist texts)
  ▪ hepatic encephalopathy
  ▪ OP/lead poisoning
  ▪ following general anaesthesia
  ▪ idiopathic (uncommon).

Tracheal collapse

This is uncommon and is usually seen in middle-aged, small ponies (Shetlands, miniature horses) and aged donkeys. Collapse usually occurs in the distal portion of the cervical trachea/rostral portion of the intrathoracic trachea. Due to these individuals undergoing low levels of exercise, subclinical disease may have existed previously with acute exacerbation occurring at times of hot/humid weather or due to a concurrent disorder causing respiratory compromise.

Clinical signs

▶ Respiratory distress and stridor.
▶ Severe – can develop pulmonary haemorrhage and epistaxis.

Diagnosis

▶ Palpation of the trachea – a distinct, sharp edge may be felt on the lateral aspect of the cervical trachea (it will not be possible to palpate the affected intrathoracic portion).
▶ Endoscopy – confirm the diagnosis and identify the region affected.
▶ Radiography – rule out external compression/other lesions.

Treatment

▶ Administer oxygen (if available) – see Pulmonary oedema (p. 91).
▶ Check for evidence of hyperthermia – if present, initiate cooling (see p. 214).
▶ Administer NSAIDs.
▶ Keep in a quiet and cool environment.
▶ Most cases can be managed conservatively in the long term:
  ▪ ± surgical management (tracheal stenting).

Tracheal ruptures/tears

These injuries are relatively uncommon and are usually a result of blunt trauma, e.g. kicks, or occasionally due to injury on sharp objects.

Clinical signs

▶ Subcutaneous swelling and emphysema at the site.
▶ Emphysema can spread over rest of the head, trunk and upper limbs.
▶ ± Epistaxis and coughing.
▶ ± External wound present.

Assessment and treatment

▶ Endoscopy of the trachea and oesophagus:
  ▪ determine the location and extent of the injury
  ▪ rule out concurrent injury to the oesophagus.
▶ Radiography of the neck and thorax:
  ▪ rule in/out concurrent injuries.
▶ Small tears – conservative management indicated:
  ▪ usually heal spontaneously
  ▪ NSAIDs
  ▪ BS antimicrobials
  ▪ rest and careful monitoring.
▶ Larger tears – require surgical repair (seek referral/specialist advice).

Prognosis

▶ Good with appropriate management.
▶ Poor if there is concurrent oesophageal rupture (see p. 71).

Epistaxis

Most cases of epistaxis are iatrogenic as a result of nasogastric intubation or endoscopy (see p. 264). Where epistaxis occurs spontaneously, it is usually mild and self-limiting and the underlying cause may not be found, even with extensive investigations. Where epistaxis is severe or multiple episodes occur (particularly over a period of a few days or weeks), the possibility of guttural pouch mycosis (GPM) must be investigated promptly.

Initial assessment and treatment

▶ Advise that the horse is kept quiet and undisturbed in a stable until you arrive – warn of the possibility of collapse if haemorrhage is severe (consider human safety too).
▶ On arrival, obtain a brief history of the circumstances in which epistaxis has happened (see Table 5.4 for common causes of epistaxis) and determine:
  ▪ if epistaxis occurred following trauma to the head or immediately after intense exercise
  ▪ whether any recent episodes of epistaxis have occurred prior to this (↑ suspicion of GPM)
  ▪ how much blood has been lost.

Table 5.4 Common causes of moderate–severe epistaxis and historical/clinical factors that may increase suspicion of each

Possible aetiology	Factors that may increase suspicion
GPM	Several episodes of epistaxis within the previous 1–2 weeks not associated with trauma/exercise
Rupture of longus capitis muscle	Epistaxis following trauma to the head (e.g. rearing over backwards)
Trauma to paranasal sinuses	Epistaxis following trauma to the head
Progressive ethmoidal haematoma	Multiple episodes of epistaxis over several weeks – usually dark (altered) blood
EIPH	Epistaxis immediately following exercise
Iatrogenic	Following nasogastric intubation/other trauma to the nasal passages (e.g. endoscopy)

▸ Assess MM colour, pulse quality and HR.
▸ If there is no history of traumatic injury to the head, and the horse is not tachycardic (HR <60 beats/min) or showing evidence of haemorrhagic shock, administer acepromazine 0.02 mg/kg IV.
▸ If there is continued, profuse arterial haemorrhage and the history is strongly suggestive of GPM, in reality there is little that can be done outside hospital facilities (where immediate general anaesthesia, administration of blood and ligation/occlusion of the internal carotid artery can be attempted).

Further assessment

▸ Obtain a full history. Specific questions that should be asked include:
- when signs of epistaxis were noted or if unknown when LSN
- if epistaxis was associated with known traumatic event (e.g. kick/rearing backwards/fall) or was evident immediately following intense exercise
- whether this was unilateral (and which side) or bilateral
- if the blood was arterial (bright red), venous (darker red), altered (brown/black)
- how much blood was lost
- whether there has been an associated with a mucoid/purulent nasal discharge or evidence of feed material from nasal passages (dysphagia)
- if recent episodes of epistaxis have occurred (particularly in the previous 2–3 weeks)
- recent illness, including respiratory tract infection
- recent long distance transport.

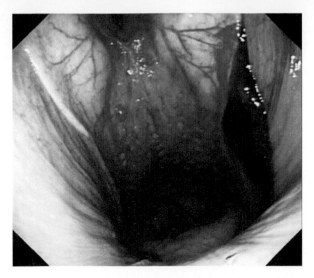

Figure 5.4   Endoscopic image of the pharynx demonstrating a blood clot emanating from the left guttural pouch ostium in a horse in which guttural pouch mycosis was confirmed.

▶ Perform a full clinical examination. Specific assessment should include examination of:
  ▪ other body systems, to rule out concurrent, underlying disease
  ▪ the head – traumatic injuries, evidence of neurological signs, e.g. facial nerve paralysis (see p. 128).

Further management

▶ If expistaxis was mild and self-limiting and there are no significant clues from the history or abnormal findings on clinical examination suggestive of an underlying cause, no further treatment may be indicated at this stage.
▶ Further investigations should be performed if haemorrhage was profuse or if more than one episode of epistaxis occured to determine the source and perform relevant treatment (see texts/seek specialist advice):
  ▪ endoscopy (Fig. 5.4)
  ▪ radiography
  ▪ ± sinoscopy
  ▪ ± CT
  ▪ haematology and clotting profiles.

Guttural pouch mycosis

Fungal infection of the guttural pouch is not uncommon in horses and plaques usually localise over the internal carotid artery or occasionally over the external carotid/maxillary artery. Subsequent erosion of the arterial wall results in epistaxis, and irritation to adjacent cranial nerves that traverse through the guttural pouch can result in concurrent dysphagia. The first few episodes of epistaxis are usually mild in nature but severe, potentially fatal haemorrhage can occur over the following 2–3 weeks unless surgical treatment is performed. Occasionally cases may present with neurological signs only.

Clinical signs

▶ Epistaxis – mild/severe.
▶ ± Coughing (due to pharyngeal/laryngeal neurological dysfunction).
▶ ± Nasal discharge (mucopurulent, contains feed material).
▶ ± Evidence of facial nerve deficits.

Initial assessment

▶ As for epistaxis.
▶ Endoscopic assessment of the larynx and pharynx:
  ▪ confirm evidence of haemorrhage from guttural pouch ostium/ostia (Fig. 5.4)
  ▪ assessment of the internal structures of the GP (only if no evidence of haemorrhage from the GP ostium/ostia)
  ▪ assess laryngeal/pharyngeal function (may have a bearing on prognosis, particularly in the equine athlete) and the degree of aspiration of any food material if there is evidence of dysphagia.

KEY TIP

If there is evidence of a blood clot emanating from the guttural pouch ostium/ostia and the history is highly suggestive of GPM, endoscopic assessment of the guttural pouches outside referral facilities is not advisable in case this results in dislodgement of the clot and recurrence of severe (potentially fatal) epistaxis.

Treatment

▶ Refer for further evaluation and treatment if surgery is an option – discuss timing of referral and patient stabilisation with the referral centre.
▶ Surgical treatment –placement of coils/balloon catheter occlusion/ligation.
▶ If surgery is not an option, conservative management can be attempted (topical antifungal medication – see texts):
  ▪ there is a >50% risk of mortality and owners must be counselled carefully when taking this option due to the risk of acute, fatal haemorrhage occurring.

Rupture of the longus capitis muscles

This is an uncommon cause of epistaxis seen following trauma to the head (usually as a result of the horse rearing over backwards), which is generally self-limiting.

Initial assessment

▶ As for epistaxis (see p. 97).
▶ Perform a full clinical examination to rule out other traumatic injuries.
▶ Perform a detailed evaluation of the head:
   ▪ determine if there are any neurological abnormalities – see CNS trauma (see p. 128)
   ▪ check for concurrent depressions in the contour of the head/wounds.
▶ Perform endoscopic assessment of the URT, including guttural pouches, to confirm the diagnosis.
▶ If skull fractures are suspected consider:
   ▪ radiography
   ▪ ± CT (if available)
   ▪ ± scintigraphy if radiography inconclusive/CT not available.

Treatment

▶ Symptomatic, including treatment of concurrent injuries as appropriate.
▶ Treatment as for acute haemorrhage if severe blood loss (see p. 186).
▶ Keep quiet and monitor carefully for the development of any CNS abnormalities.

Paranasal sinus trauma/skull fractures

Trauma to the skull overlying the paranasal sinuses can result in haemorrhage into the paranasal sinuses, with subsequent development of epistaxis and sinusitis. Fractures may also occur and should be suspected where there is evidence of a wound/swelling together with palpable crepitus or obvious visual deformity at the site.

Assessment and treatment

▶ Check for other concurrent traumatic injuries and evidence of neurological signs.
▶ Perform careful palpation and visual assessment of the head.
▶ Where there is evidence of severe/extensive injury, consider hospitalisation/referral.

Further assessment

▶ Endoscopy to confirm that haemorrhage is emanating from the nasomaxillary aperture.
▶ Radiography.
▶ US – often very helpful in determining the location and size of skull fractures.
▶ ± CT (if available).
▶ Perform sinoscopy via a small trephine portal to assess the paranasal sinuses further and lavage to remove blood (see texts).
▶ Administer NSAIDs, BS antimicrobials and check tetanus status.
▶ ± Surgical management (see Fig. 5.5) (seek referral/specialist advice):
   ▪ elevation and fixation/removal of fragments where there is a palpable/visual depression or where cosmesis is important
   ▪ removal of sequestered bone.

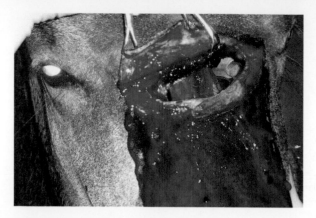

Figure 5.5 Open, displaced fracture of the frontal bone overlying the paranasal sinuses in a horse that had collided with a fixed object in the field.

Lacerations of the nares

These are relatively common and usually occur when a horse rubs its head on wire or gets an object caught on the nares and pulls back. Full-thickness lacerations that are not dealt with properly can result in poor cosmesis and can potentially compromise athletic function if the function of the nares is disrupted.

Assessment and treatment

▶ Determine if the laceration is full/partial thickness.
▶ Partial-thickness lacerations may not require suturing – the head has a good blood supply and they often heal quickly.
▶ Full-thickness lacerations, especially those that involve the margins of the nares must be sutured.

Suture repair

▶ Sedate the horse and, if possible, rest the head on a temporary head stand, e.g. bales of hay or straw covered by a rug.
▶ Ensure there is good lighting.
▶ Perform an infraorbital nerve block (see p. 368)/infiltrate local anaesthetic around the site.
▶ Lavage the wound (see p. 22) and remove as little tissue as possible (even if of questionable viability).
▶ Close the defect in 2 or 3 layers (mucosa ± muscular layer and skin) using 2-0–0 absorbable suture (can use non-absorbable suture in the skin).
▶ Ensure good anatomic reconstruction – work from the margin of the nares:
  ▪ ± place protective stent (see following page).
▶ Administer NSAIDs and BS antimicrobials.
▶ Consider referral/repair under GA for extensive injuries/where good reconstruction cannot be achieved or if dehiscence occurs.

> **HANDY TIP**
>
> It can be difficult to prevent a horse from rubbing the sutures out – a protective stent
> can be fashioned by cutting a suitably sized and shaped small animal buster collar to
> fit over the affected area, creating holes with a 16G needle (make sure the side with the
> roughened surface is outmost) for sutures to be placed through and securing this to the
> outside of the nares with mattress sutures (see website for further details).

Exercise-induced pulmonary haemorrhage

Exercise induced pulmonary haemorrhage (EIPH) is the most common cause of epistaxis.
It is associated with intense exercise and rarely necessitates emergency treatment.
Occasionally severe haemorrhage can occur, resulting in respiratory distress or, rarely, sudden death may occur, due to rupture of a large pulmonary vessel.

Diagnosis and initial treatment

▶ Confirm the diagnosis by endoscopy (haemorrhage originating from bronchi).
▶ ± Radiography (if severe haemorrhage has occurred).
▶ Administer furosemide 1 mg/kg IV.
▶ Administer BS antimicrobials.
▶ Maintain on dust-free management (see texts for ongoing management).

Foreign bodies

These may occasionally become lodged in the respiratory tract anywhere from the nasal
passages down to the bronchi. The most common offending objects are plant materials
such as twigs or brambles.

Clinical signs

▶ Sudden-onset severe snorting, coughing.
▶ ± Epistaxis.
▶ ± Malodorous breath.
▶ ± Haematochezia (coughing up blood).

Diagnosis and treatment

▶ Endoscopic identification of the type and size of the foreign body and its location.
▶ Objects usually become lodged in the oropharynx or laryngopharynx, rarely in the nasal
  passages and occasionally in the trachea or bronchi.
▶ Removal can be undertaken using endoscopic instruments (e.g. endoscopic snares):
  ▪ complications include iatrogenic epistaxis, trauma to the tissues (due to thorns or other
    sharp protrusions) or breakage.

▶ Pharyngeal foreign bodies can occasionally be retrieved manually under GA or heavy sedation following placement of a gag.

▶ Occasionally distal cervical tracheotomy and retrieval is required (see specialist texts/ seek specialist advice).

▶ Ongoing treatment following removal:
  ▪ BS antimicrobials
  ▪ NSAIDs
  ▪ monitor closely – occasionally can develop pleuropneumonia.

References and further reading

• Borer, K., 2009. Management of pulmonary oedema. In: Robinson, N.E., Sprayberry, K.A. (Eds.), Current Therapy in Equine Medicine (sixth ed.). Elsevier, St. Louis, Missouri, pp. 317–319.

• Collins, N.M., Dixon, P.M., 2009. Disorders of the trachea. In: Robinson, N.E., Sprayberry, K.A. (Eds.), Current Therapy in Equine Medicine (sixth ed.). Elsevier, St. Louis, Missouri, pp. 261–263.

• Copas, V., 2011. Diagnosis and treatment of equine pleuropneumonia. In Pract. 33, 155–162.

• Dixon, P.M., McGorum, B.C., Railton, D.I., et al. 2001. Laryngeal paralysis: a study of 375 cases in a mixed-breed population of horses. Equine Vet. J. 33, 452–458.

• Greet, T.R.C., 2010. Endoscopic retrieval of foreign bodies. Equine Vet. Educ. 15, 232.

• Hassel, D.M., 2007. Thoracic trauma in horses. Vet. Clin. N. Am. Equine Pract. 23, 67–80.

• Henninger, R.W., Hass, G.F., Freshwater, A., 2006. Corticosteroid management of lipoid pneumonia in a horse. Equine Vet. Educ. 18, 205–209.

• Lugo, J., 2009. Pneumothorax. In: Robinson, N.E., Sprayberry, K.A. (Eds.), Current Therapy in Equine Medicine (sixth ed.). Elsevier, St. Louis, Missouri, pp. 313–314.

• McGorum, B., Dixon, P.M., 2007. Clinical examination of the respiratory tract. In: McGorum, B.C., Dixon, P.M., Robinson, N.E., Schumacher, J. (Eds.), Equine Respiratory Medicine and Surgery (sixth ed.). Elsevier, Philadelphia, Pennsylvania, pp. 103–117.

• Marsh, P.S., 2007. Fire and smoke inhalation injury in horses. Vet. Clin. N. Am. Equine Pract. 23, 19–30.

• Miskovic, M., Couëtil, 2009. Pleuropneumonia. In: Robinson, N.E., Sprayberry, K.A. (Eds.), Current Therapy in Equine Medicine (sixth ed.). Elsevier, St. Louis, Missouri, pp. 292–296.

• Scarratt, W.K., Moon, M.L., Sponenberg, D.P., et al. 1998. Inappropriate administration of mineral oil resulting in lipoid pneumonia in three horses. Equine Vet. J. 30, 85–88.

• Tremaine, H., 2004. Management of skull fractures in the horse. In Pract. 26, 214–222.

Ophthalmic emergencies

General approach

Ophthalmic emergencies are common and swollen, painful, traumatised or acutely discoloured eyes are an emergency. It is also important to determine whether concurrent injury/illness is evident in other body systems where ophthalmic conditions have occurred secondary to trauma or as a consequence of systemic disease (e.g. infectious disease conditions) (Fig. 6.1).

▶ Attend promptly and take the necessary equipment with you (see p. 2).
▶ Assess and treat any life-threatening injuries first.
▶ Aim to save the eye wherever possible.
▶ Do not cause additional damage to the eye during examination or by administering inappropriate medications.
▶ Refer/seek advice at an early stage.
▶ Revisit at appropriate intervals – do not rely on updates from the owner.

First aid

▶ Get the owner/carer to place the horse in a clean, darkened stable until it is examined.
▶ Tell them not to wipe away any ocular discharges.

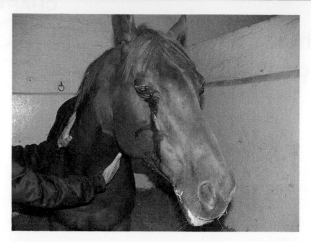

Figure 6.1 Oedema of the supraorbital fossae and oedema/petechial haemorrhage of the conjunctivae in a horse with African horse sickness (see Ch. 15).

Courtesy of Derek Knottenbelt.

▶ Medication must not be dispensed without seeing the horse – there is no 'safe' medication for these cases.

Assessment

▶ Examine in a darkened area – relatively little equipment is required

OPHTHALMIC EXAMINATION CHECKLIST

- ☐ Facial symmetry.
- ☐ Eyelid position and symmetry/blepharospasm.
- ☐ Size, and position of eye.
- ☐ Ocular discharges.
- ☐ Menace response.

Using a transiluminator or a good pen torch.

- ☐ Dazzle reflex.
- ☐ Direct PLR.
- ☐ Consensual PLR.
- ☐ Conjunctiva and sclera.
- ☐ Surface of cornea.
- ☐ Fluorescein uptake and aqueous leakage (Seidel test, see Fig. 6.2).
- ☐ ± Rose Bengal stain.
- ☐ Patency of nasolacrimal duct.
- ☐ Anterior chamber clarity.

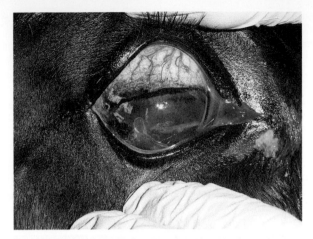

Figure 6.2 Seidel test. After saturating the tear film with fluorescein stain, leakage of aqueous humour from a corneal perforation results in a change in colour due to dilution of the stain.

Courtesy of Fernando Malalana.

- ☐ Size of pupil (miosis/mydriasis).
- ☐ Iris colour and mobility.

Using an ophthalmoscope.

- ☐ Lens.
- ☐ Vitreous.
- ☐ Retina (tapetal and non-tapetal fundus) and optic papilla (optic disc).

KEY TIP

Never press on the eye or force the eyelids open – sedate the horse and perform an auriculopalpebral (AP) nerve block (see p. 367).

HANDY TIP

Supporting the horse's head on a solid table or constructing one using straw/hay bales covered with a rug/blanket can significantly facilitate ocular examination following sedation.

Treatment

▸ Determine at an early stage whether specialist advice should be sought.

▸ Failure to deliver medications into the eye properly is a major cause of therapeutic failure – if there are doubts about an owner/carer's ability or if the horse is non-compliant a subpalpebral lavage (SPL) system can be placed (see p. 379).

▶ Ensure medications are stored appropriately and that the owner/carer is able to administer them (demonstrate this if necessary).
▶ In severe cases, the horse should ideally be hospitalised to enable regular examination and ensure medication compliance; frequent medication may be needed.

> **KEY TIP**
>
> Steroid medications are absolutely contraindicated where there is any evidence of corneal ulceration; if in doubt do not use any corticosteroid medications either topically or systemically.

> **HANDY TIP**
>
> Offering the horse a treat after medicating the eye can improve patient compliance.

Ocular and periocular trauma

These injuries are common and can vary from relatively minor superficial injuries to more severe life- or vision-threatening injuries. Penetrating injuries are usually immediately obvious but injuries to the eye caused by blunt trauma may not be – these can cause significant intraocular damage. Traumatic ocular injuries may also occur in horses with colic or those who have been recumbent for prolonged periods.

Initial approach

▶ Obtain a full history. Specific questions to ask include:
  - the circumstances of injury if the incident was observed
  - when the injury occurred (if known).
▶ Perform a full clinical examination. Specific examination that should be performed includes:
  - check general mentation/neurological status in the case of severe trauma to head – rule out potential brain injury (especially important prior to sedating the horse) and obtain baseline information if subsequent neurological signs develop or deteriorate
  - rule out colic as a potential cause (if circumstances surrounding injury unknown)
  - check for other traumatic injuries
  - assess facial symmetry, including positioning of the eye within the orbit
  - palpate around the orbit for swelling/crepitus.
▶ Perform a full ophthalmic examination:
  - perform menace, dazzle and PLR prior to sedation
  - sedate the horse if neurological status normal ± place AP nerve block (see p. 367)
  - check for any foreign bodies that may be lodged in or around the eye or any concurrent damage to the nasolacrimal duct.
▶ If periocular swelling makes it difficult to open the eyelids (even after sedation and placement of nerve blocks), US examination of the eye and the orbit is very useful – never force the eyelids open or put pressure on the eye (see website).

▶ Common injuries that may be encountered include:
- eyelid laceration
- corneal laceration
- orbital fractures
- damage to the nasolacrimal duct
- lodgement of foreign bodies in or around the globe
- orbital cellulitis/abscess formation
- panophthalmitis
- retinal detachment
- globe rupture.

> **KEY TIP**
>
> Shining a very bright light into the damaged eye and observing for a consensual pupil reflex constriction in the contralateral (normal) eye is a good way of establishing whether a severely damaged eye is still functional.

Eyelid lacerations

There are common injuries in both upper and lower eyelids. The upper eyelid is more commonly affected and is more significant since it is responsible for most of the blink reflex. Injuries to the medial canthus can also involve the nasolacrimal duct.

General points

▶ The eyelids have a good blood supply and, whilst they usually swell significantly following injury, they generally heal very well.

▶ Eyelid lacerations should be repaired as soon and as accurately as possible – repair usually carries an excellent functional and cosmetic outcome.

▶ If these injuries are neglected or if repair is not performed properly, the horse may be left with a long-term, painful eye due to exposure keratitis and corneal ulceration.

> **KEY TIP**
>
> Pieces of tissue from the eyelid margin should never be removed, even if they appear to be of questionable viability.

Initial assessment

▶ Obtain a full history. Specific information that should be obtained includes:
- when and how the injury was sustained
- if unknown, if the horse was in the stable/field at the time (this might indicate how the injury was sustained)
- tetanus status.

▶ Perform a full clinical examination. Specific assessment should include:
- assessment of neurologic status (particularly prior to administration of sedatives)
- examine for other traumatic injuries

- assess for evidence of other systemic disease – eliminate colic/other systemic conditions causing pain that may have been the cause of trauma.
▶ Administer sedation.
▶ Perform a full ocular examination.
  - stain the cornea with fluorescein to rule out corneal injury
  - check for other traumatic injuries to the eye and periocular structures.

Treatment

▶ Decide if the laceration can be sutured under standing sedation following placement of appropriate nerve blocks (see p. 365) or if a GA is required:
  - indications for GA include:
    » complicated injuries
    » uncooperative patient
    » additional trauma to other structures.
▶ Consider hospitalisation/referral in complicated lacerations or where there are inadequate facilities or equipment for assessment and repair.
▶ Injuries should be repaired as soon as possible.
▶ Perform initial wound management:
  - lavage the site with sterile saline
  - keep the cornea moist – apply topical antimicrobial ophthalmic lubricant.
▶ Administer systemic NSAIDs.
▶ Administer BS antimicrobials.

KEY TIP

Scrub formulations, alcohol and chlorhexidine are toxic to the corneal epithelium. Use a 1:50 dilution of 10% povidone iodine solution when performing aseptic preparation directly around the eye.

Suturing of lacerations

▶ If the laceration is partial thickness through the eyelid and there is no involvement of the eyelid margin, suture as for skin lacerations (see Ch. 2).
▶ Where lacerations involve the eyelid margin or are full thickness in nature, ensure that suitable instruments and suture materials are available:
  - suture material used in eyelid repair should ideally be 4-0 (1.5 metric) in size or thinner with a cutting/taper-cut needle.
▶ Administer/top up sedation as indicated to ensure the patient is adequately sedated.
▶ Support the head, e.g. rest on hay bales or other appropriate means of head support.
▶ Good lighting is essential.
▶ Ensure the horse is not stimulated during the procedure.
▶ Perform minimal debridement – tissue should be preserved if at all possible.
▶ In injuries >6h old, use a No. 15 scalpel blade to carefully and gently debride the exposed tissues.
▶ Close full-thickness eyelid lacerations with a minimum of 2 layers (3 layers may be required in some cases).

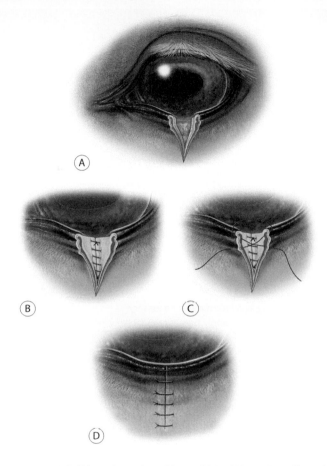

Figure 6.3 Suturing of full-thickness lacerations of the eyelid should be performed in two layers. Use of a figure-of-eight suture to close the eyelid margin prevents the knot or suture ends from rubbing on the cornea.

▶ Deep layer – place sutures in the tarsal plate (white, fibrous tissue) – do not suture the conjunctiva or place sutures through the conjunctiva.

▶ Skin/subcuticular layer – interrupted sutures.

▶ Start at the eyelid margin – where healthy tissue is present, place a figure-of-eight suture (Fig. 6.3) to avoid knots/suture material rubbing on the cornea:
  ▪ this suture can be tied first or pre-placed so it can be tied once the other sutures have been placed.

▶ The golden rules are:
  ▪ make sure the eyelid margin is in as perfect apposition as possible
  ▪ ensure that no suture material is in contact with the cornea
  ▪ if not – remove the suture and start again (Fig. 6.4).

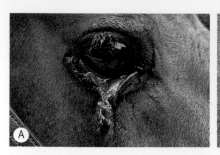 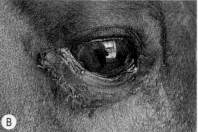

Figure 6.4 (A) Before and (B) following repair of a laceration sustained to the lower eyelid.
Courtesy of Fernando Malalana.

Aftercare

▸ Systemic NSAIDs.

▸ Systemic antimicrobials (3–5 d).

▸ Topical antimicrobial therapy if there has been superficial damage to cornea (see Corneal lacerations below).

▸ Check tetanus status (see p. 23).

▸ Prevent self-trauma – apply a face mask if necessary.

▸ Clean away any discharge and apply barrier cream below the eye if required to prevent skin scalding.

▸ The eye must be checked carefully several times a day by the carer – the eye should remain comfortable (i.e. no suture material rubbing cornea) and the eyelid functional.

Corneal lacerations

These are relatively uncommon but should be ruled out following any trauma to the eye and periocular region.

Initial assessment

▸ As for general eye trauma.

▸ These injuries require careful evaluation – sedate the horse and place an AP nerve block (see p. 367).

▸ Do not force the eyelids open or apply any pressure to the globe.

▸ Check for any evidence of a FB (especially plant material) within cornea and conjunctiva.

▸ Stain the corneal surface with fluorescein:

  ▪ note any uptake and areas within this that have no stain uptake (possible area of corneal perforation/exposure of Descemet's membrane)

  ▪ check for evidence of leakage of aqueous (Seidel test, see Fig. 6.2).

▸ Examine the anterior chamber.

▸ Check the position of the lens.

▸ Assess the fundus.

Table 6.1 Factors associated with prognosis in cases of corneal lacerations

Poor prognosis	Fair prognosis with surgery
≥50% hyphaema	Simple laceration with minimal contamination and iris prolapse
>24 h duration and flat anterior chamber	Formed anterior chamber
Lens rupture/dislocation	Small amount of haemorrhage/fibrin
Detached retina	Iris prolapse with minimal distortion of ocular contents
Extensive laceration with prolapse of ocular contents other than aqueous humour/iris tissue (e.g. vitreous leakage)	
Involvement of sclera and prolapse of uveal tissue	
Proptosis	

Treatment

▶ Partial-thickness, non-penetrating corneal lacerations:
- small loose flaps of cornea can be removed with fine scissors after application of topical local anaesthetic solution
- treat as for corneal ulcers.
▶ Other injuries – seek specialist advice/referral:
- prompt specialist surgical treatment, possibly under GA, is usually required.
- do not cut off any protruding iris or administer topical atropine prior to referral if prolapsed iris is plugging the corneal laceration prior to transport
- for prognosis see Table 6.1.
▶ Enucleation may need to be considered if referral is not an option

> **KEY TIP**
> Only use ophthalmic solutions where there is suspected perforation of the eye – never administer ophthalmic ointments in these situations.

Orbital fractures

These can occur following kicks from other horses or blows to the head, including collisions with fixed objects, and may be missed if a thorough assessment is not performed. Knowledge of the normal regional anatomy is helpful when assessing these injuries (Fig. 6.5).

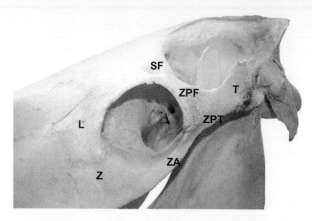

Figure 6.5 Anatomic landmarks in the orbital region. L = lacrimal bone, SF = supraorbital foramen, T = temporal bone, Z = zygomatic bone, ZA = zygomatic arch, ZPF = zygomatic process of frontal bone, ZPT = zygomatic process of temporal bone.

Initial approach

▶ Obtain a detailed history. Specific information to obtain includes:
  - how and when the injury was sustained
  - if unknown, where the horse was at the time of injury.
▶ After a thorough clinical examination, specific assessment should include:
  - check neurological status for concurrent CNS injury
  - check for evidence of epistaxis – this may indicate involvement of the paranasal sinuses (see p. 101)
  - visual assessment of facial symmetry/asymmetry
  - palpation of orbital region for swelling/crepitus/differences in contour compared to the normal side.
▶ Perform a thorough ophthalmic examination – blunt trauma can cause severe intraocular damage:
  - check that the eye is in a normal position and has a normal range of movement – fragments of bone can entrap the eye, causing it to be fixed in an abnormal position
  - check for other clinical abnormalities, including hyphaema
  - stain the cornea with fluorescein and check that the nasolacrimal duct is patent.
▶ Perform US evaluation of the orbit and eye – use the normal side for comparison (see website).
▶ Perform radiography if a fracture is suspected:
  - lateral, DV, DV oblique views of the region
  - VD view (radiographic plate placed on the horse's forehead) can be very useful in these injuries
  - can be difficult to interpret the images obtained due to superimposition – radiograph the other side for comparison if unsure.
▶ ± CT assessment (if facilities available).

Treatment

▸ Minor fractures (i.e. fragments not impinging on the globe/perfect cosmetic result not required):

- conservative management – systemic NSAIDs and BS antimicrobials for 5 d initially
- treatment of concurrent ocular injuries
- reassess frequently (q. 48 h initially).

▸ Fractures that impinge on ocular/adnexal structures or where cosmesis is important:

- surgical management required as soon as the patient has been stabilised
- fractures are easier to elevate/realign <5 d post-injury (suitable surgical skills and equipment are also required).

▸ ± Lavage of the paranasal sinuses if these have been involved (see p. 101).

Acute retinal detachment

▸ There will usually be no vision in the affected eye.

▸ Usually secondary to trauma or ERU.

▸ Can be uni- or bilateral and partial/complete.

▸ Identified during ophthalmic examination – there is evidence of free-floating, undulating grey opaque veils of tissue in the vitreous overlying the optic disc running towards the lens and the tapetum is hyperreflective.

▸ US – classic 'seagull' signs (see specialist texts website).

▸ This diagnosis carries a grave prognosis for vision.

Hyphaema

Blood in the anterior chamber of the eye can be secondary to:

▸ Blunt/penetrating trauma.

▸ Uveitis.

▸ Glaucoma.

▸ Retinal detachment.

▸ Intraocular neoplasia.

▸ Blood dyscrasias.

Initial investigation

▸ Obtain a full history, including:

- duration of clinical signs/when LSN
- any known trauma
- any previous/recent ophthalmic condition(s)
- recent illness
- current/recent medications.

▸ Perform a full clinical examination, specifically checking for:

- traumatic injuries
- clotting disorders – assess MM, whole blood clotting time (see p. 190)
- concurrent systemic disease.

▸ Perform an ophthalmic examination – this may be difficult depending on the quantity of blood present.

▸ ± Perform US assessment of the eye – assess len's position, retina.

▸ If there is no history of trauma/ongoing ocular problems, take blood for serum biochemistry, haematology and clotting profiles to be performed.

Treatment

▸ Treat or investigate any underlying cause (see relevant sections/texts) – hospitalise/refer if necessary.

▸ Initiate therapy with:
  ▪ topical atropine
  ▪ systemic NSAIDs.

▸ Re-evaluate daily until the quantity of blood within the anterior chamber starts to reduce:
  ▪ can take 5–30 d to resolve, depending on quantity of blood and underlying cause

▸ Hyphaema involving >50% of the eye is associated with a poor prognosis for vision.

▸ Sequelae include synechiae, cataracts, glaucoma, blindness or phthisis bulbi.

Corneal foreign bodies

Plant material is the most common foreign body. It is essential to assess the eye thoroughly and carefully and to also assess the iris and anterior chamber.

Clinical signs

▸ May be obvious in the case of large foreign body (FB).

▸ A small FB may only be visualised during detailed examination.

▸ A black speck on the cornea may be a portion of iris sealing a corneal defect.

Treatment

Superficial foreign bodies

▸ Optimal treatment – hospitalise/refer for removal under GA (ideally by a specialist).

▸ If this is not an option, removal can be performed using a 23G needle or 2-mm biopsy punch under heavy sedation with nerve blocks (see p.365) and topical anaesthesia.

▸ Treat as for a corneal ulcer following removal (check FB removal is complete and that perforation of the cornea has not occurred).

Deep/large or penetrating foreign bodies (Fig. 6.6)

▸ To try to save the eye – referral to a specialist with microsurgical expertise and the ability to manage potential perforation of the eye is essential.

▸ Enucleation may be considered if this is not an option.

Corneal ulceration (ulcerative keratitis)

This occurs where there has been loss of the corneal epithelium and exposure of the underlying corneal stroma. Ulcers may be traumatic or non-traumatic and may be sterile or infected (bacterial or occasionally fungal in nature). This is a vision-threatening condition requiring prompt, appropriate treatment.

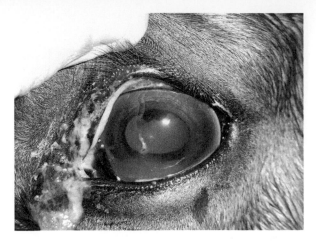

Figure 6.6 Corneal foreign body – a small portion of a thorn was removed surgically.
Courtesy of Fernando Malalana.

> **KEY TIP**
> Florescein staining must be performed in any painful/inflamed eye to ensure that corneal ulceration is recognised and treated at an early stage

Clinical signs

▸ Lacrimation and epiphora.
▸ Blepharospasm.
▸ Photophobia.
▸ Corneal oedema.
▸ ± Miosis.
▸ ± Aqueous opacification (flare).

Initial diagnosis and assessment

▸ Obtain a full history. Specific information to obtain includes:
  ▪ duration of clinical signs or when the eye was LSN
  ▪ whether a traumatic incident was observed/suspected
  ▪ any treatments administered so far.
▸ Perform a full clinical examination with particular attention to:
  ▪ assessment of any traumatic injuries
  ▪ check for and investigate any concurrent systemic illness (e.g. in the case of the recumbent horse or one with neurological abnormalities).
▸ Perform a full ophthalmic examination and check:
  ▪ fluorescein uptake (Fig. 6.7)
  ▪ whether there is evidence of keratomalacia (Fig 6.8), a descemetocele, stromal abscess, corneal laceration/perforation or iris prolapse

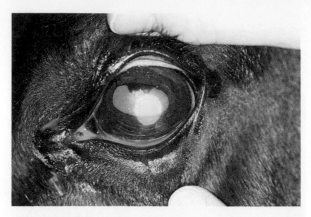

Figure 6.7   Uptake of fluorescein stain confirming a diagnosis of corneal ulceration.

Courtesy of Fernando Malalana.

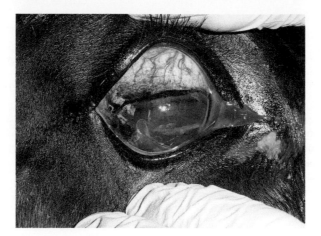

Figure 6.8   Evidence of keratomalacia ('melting ulcer') demonstrating the typical gelatinous appearance and blue/white discoloration of the cornea.

Courtesy of Derek Knottenbelt.

- there are no foreign bodies/other structures in contact with the cornea
- eyelid function and integrity
- corneal sensitivity
- ± take a swab for C&S from the periphery of the ulcer.
▶ The following information will assist follow-up/communication with a specialist:
  - ulcer position
  - depth (superficial or deep)
  - degree/extent of corneal vascularisation and oedema (mild/moderate/severe)

- evidence of keratomalacia ('melting') – gelatinous appearance, corneal swelling and appears blue/white colour (if melting is present – take corneal scrapes for cytology/ Gram staining)
- anterior chamber – any evidence of concurrent uveitis
- pupil size – normal/dilated (mydriasis)/contracted (miosis).

Initial treatment

▶ Surgical management may be required in certain cases – refer or seek specialist advice if there is evidence of:
  - a descemetocele
  - an ulcer that is moderate/severe in depth
  - a corneal stromal abscess
  - continued, progressive keratomalacia.
▶ Medical therapy is indicated in less severe cases:
  - treat the ulcer itself and any concurrent uveitis.
  - the 4 As:
    » antimicrobials
    » anti-inflammatories
    » ± atropine
    » anti-collagenases.
▶ Topical antimicrobials:
  - corneal ulcers are usually infected – fungal infections are unusual in the UK but do occur. In uncomplicated (non-melting) ulcers consider use of chloramphenicol or gentamicin
  - if a melting ulcer is present, initiate therapy with one of the following: gentamicin/ polymyxin B/amikacin/tobramycin/ciprofloxacin/ofloxacin/ticarcillin-clavulanate
  - base ongoing therapy on Gram stain and C&S results.
▶ ± Systemic antimicrobial therapy is indicated in severe corneal ulceration.
▶ Administer NSAIDs – flunixin meglumine 1.1 mg/kg IV initially.
▶ Administer topical atropine (1%) – maintain pupil dilation if evidence of miosis (see Anterior uveitis below).
▶ Initiate anti-protease therapy – essential in all but very superficial corneal ulcers:
  - serum, EDTA or acetylcysteine
  - 5 mL sterile water added to a commercial EDTA blood collection tube provides the easiest and most effective anti-collagenase medication; this is administered q. 2 h.

When to worry

▶ Rapid worsening of clinical signs.
▶ Development of a melting ulcer (keratomalacia) or stromal involvement.
▶ The ulcer does not show signs of healing – it should ideally reduce in size by 0.6 mm/d and should have healed in <7 d.

Anterior uveitis

This may develop as a consequence of trauma or corneal ulceration (ulcerative keratitis) or it may be an acute relapse of equine recurrent uveitis (ERU). In severe cases, inflammation can extend to involve the posterior parts of the eye. Uveitis also occurs in systemic diseases such as neonatal septicaemia (see Ch. 12) or *Strep. equi* var *equi* infection (strangles).

Clinical signs

▸ Lacrimation.
▸ Epiphora.
▸ Blepharospasm.
▸ Conjunctival hyperaemia ± involvement of deeper episcleral vessels.
▸ Corneal oedema.
▸ Aqueous flare.
▸ Miosis (constriction of the pupil).

Initial assessment

▸ Obtain a full history. Specific questions include:
  ▪ whether the horse has had previous ophthalmic problems (including episodes of uveitis) – the Appaloosa breed has an increased risk of ERU
  ▪ how long the clinical signs have been evident (or when the eye was LSN)
  ▪ if a known/suspected traumatic event occurred
  ▪ type, duration and frequency of administration of any ongoing medication (perhaps the eye has been seen by a colleague previously and you may be seeing it for the first time).
▸ Perform a full clinical examination. Specific assessment should include:
  ▪ any evidence of trauma and assessment of any traumatic injuries
  ▪ evidence of concurrent systemic illness, including pyrexia.
▸ Perform a complete ophthalmic examination:
  ▪ check fluorescein staining of the cornea even if an obvious ulcer is not visible – steroids must not be administered if there is any evidence of corneal ulceration
  ▪ if a known traumatic incident has taken place, check for concurrent ocular or periorbital injuries
  ▪ check for evidence of a previous episode of uveitis (iris hypopigmentation, synechiae [iris adhesions], granula iridica degeneration/rupture, cataract formation, retinal detachment, lens luxation).

Initial treatment

▸ Administer systemic analgesia/NSAIDs:
  ▪ flunixin meglumine 1.1 mg/kg IV initially
  ▪ If this is a recurrence of uveitis, place on a 4-week decreasing dose of oral NSAIDs and reassess periodically.
▸ Administer topical mydriatics such as atropine to provide analgesia and to reduce the risk of adhesions:
  ▪ Administer at intervals sufficient to maintain maximal pupillary dilation
  ▪ If the pupil does not dilate after administration of 2 atropine doses, it is unlikely to do so with atropine alone
  ▪ ± use of topical phenylephrine in this case (check no history of CV disease)
  ▪ monitor for GI signs with atropine – colic, reduced defecation
  ▪ check the contralateral eye – stop therapy if mydriasis develops in this eye (indicates systemic absorption).

- Administer topical corticosteroids:
  - only administer if there is no evidence of corneal ulceration
  - prednisolone/dexamethasone.
- Nursing care:
  - keep in a darkened stable out of direct sunlight
  - Protect the eye from further trauma; fly masks are fine if protective masks are not immediately available.
- Reassess q. 24 h initially.

When to worry

- Seek specialist advice/refer if there is:
  - no/poor response to treatment within 24 h
  - development of endophthalmitis.

Acute blindness

This is relatively uncommon in horses and may be caused by non-ocular pathology (see Table 6.2)

Approach

- Obtain a full history; specific questions that should be asked include:
  - recent general health of that horse and any horses on the yard
  - any previous ocular problems, e.g. uveitis
  - any trauma observed/suspected, e.g. rearing over backwards, blood noted around the head or disturbance of bedding in the stable.

Table 6.2 Potential causes of acute blindness

Infectious	Viral (togaviruses, rabies, WNV, JEV, EHV) Bacterial (e.g. bacterial meningitis) Protozoal (EPM)
Traumatic	Intracranial haemorrhage Optic neuropathy
Neoplastic	Intracranial mass
Toxic/metabolic	Hyperammonaemia Pyrrolizidine alkaloid- and thiaminase-containing plants
Vascular	Air embolism Ischaemia Perinatal asphyxia (neonates) Intracarotid injection Post-anaesthetic cerebral necrosis

▶ Observe the horse and assess its mentation, vision and whether it is neurologically normal or not.
▶ Perform a full clinical and neurological examination (see p. 128) to eliminate other causes of blindness.
▶ Perform a full ocular examination to identify ocular disease:
  ▪ check menace, dazzle and PLR reflexes
  ▪ check for obvious ocular pathology
  ▪ determine whether there is evidence of previous disease in that eye, e.g. ERU, glaucoma.
▶ Where there has been a known or suspected traumatic event in a previously normal, sighted horse and there is no previous history of ocular disease or evidence of other neurological causes for blindness, blunt trauma causing an optic neuropathy should be suspected. Typical findings on ocular examination include:
  ▪ globe usually intact
  ▪ pupils may be widely dilated
  ▪ visual defects, ranging from marked visual impairment to blindness.

Treatment

▶ Depends on underlying cause (see relevant sections).

Where blunt trauma causing optic neuropathy is suspected:

▶ Administer NSAIDs – flunixin 1.1 mg/kg IV q. 12 h initially.
▶ Administer systemic corticosteroids.
▶ Re-evaluate every few days initially – determine response to initial treatment with repeat neurological and ophthalmic assessment.
▶ Monitor for the development of optic nerve atrophy:
  ▪ changes may take 4–6 weeks to become evident.
▶ Euthanasia should be considered if the horse remains completely blind with no evidence of improvement in vision after 2 weeks (may consider sooner if acute deterioration with development of other neurological signs).

KEY TIP

Persistent mydriasis (dilation of the pupil) without prior administration of a mydriatic carries a poor prognosis for vision.

KEY TIP

An acutely blind horse is often distressed and can be very dangerous to deal with; handle carefully and with sympathy.

Acute exophthalmos

Anterior displacement of the globe within the orbit is a relatively uncommon but significant sign. Acute cases are usually traumatic or inflammatory in origin. In traumatic cases the degree of force may be severe enough to cause immediate exophthalmos (suspect significant damage to orbital and periorbital structures) or may be delayed by a few days due to progressive swelling of periorbital tissues or the development of cellulitis. Neoplasia and other space-occupying masses usually present with an insidious onset.

Clinical signs

▸ Usually unilateral (easier to assess using the normal side for comparison).
▸ Relative prominence of the globe – differentiate from enlarged globe (buphthalmos) or proptosis.
▸ Conjunctival hyperaemia and chemosis.
▸ Epiphora.
▸ Distorted eyelid contour.
▸ Distension of the supraorbital fossa.
▸ ± Pain on pressure around the eye (orbital cellulitis cases are often painful and dull).
▸ Mydriasis if damage to the optic nerve has occurred.

Initial assessment

▸ Obtain a full history. Specific information that should be obtained includes:
  ▪ duration of clinical signs
  ▪ history of known trauma or recent illness.
▸ Perform a full clinical examination. Specific evaluation should include:
  ▪ check T° – pyrexia
  ▪ check for other traumatic wounds/injuries.
▸ Perform a full ophthalmic examination and check specifically for:
  ▪ exposure keratitis – fluorescein/Rose Bengal staining
  ▪ position and movement of the globe (if abnormal, check for orbital fractures)
  ▪ other traumatic sequelae
  ▪ swollen eyelids or opacity in the anterior part of the eye may prevent full assessment – US evaluation indicated
▸ Perform US evaluation of both eyes (may consider hospitalisation/referral):
  ▪ check for disruption to the contour of the orbit/areas of increased hypoechogenicity between the globe and orbit
  ▪ discrete areas of hypoechogenicity – suspect local abscess.
▸ ± Radiography:
  ▪ perform if severe trauma known/further assessment of orbital rim fractures.
▸ ± CT evaluation:
  ▪ ideally performed standing rather than under GA (if available).
▸ ± Biopsy/FNA of abnormal tissue between the globe and orbit.

Treatment

▸ Depends on the underlying cause (see relevant sections):
  ▪ treatment of orbital fractures
  ▪ removal of foreign body(ies)
  ▪ treatment of orbital cellulitis/abscess formation
  ▪ treatment of corneal ulcers.

▶ Protect the exposed cornea – apply ocular lubricants q. 4h.
▶ Perform a temporary tarsorrhaphy to reduce exposure of the cornea whilst the inflammation is resolving:
 ▪ sedation and local anaesthetic nerve blocks (see p. 365)
 ▪ ± place SPL system if corneal medication is required
 ▪ place 2–3 horizontal mattress sutures of 2-0 or 3-0 monofilament nylon horizontal mattress sutures through the eyelids exiting at meibomian gland orifices (evident as a grey line across the eyelid)
 ▪ sutures must not penetrate the full thickness of the eyelid
 ▪ use stents made of cut pieces of rubber tube/buttons (more comfortable than cut pieces of drip tubing) to prevent suture pull-through
 ▪ just appose the eyelids – do not evert or invert
 ▪ tie in a bow so that sutures can be undone periodically to check the cornea.

Acute orbital cellulitis

This is quite common and can develop subsequent to a penetrating foreign body, direct trauma to the eye or as a result of systemic disease through septic emboli.

Clinical signs

▶ Blepharoedema and chemosis (Fig. 6.9).
▶ Swelling of the supraorbital fossa.
▶ Nictitans protrusion.
▶ Corneal oedema.
▶ ± Pyrexia, dullness.

Initial assessment

▶ Obtain a full history and perform a full clinical examination to rule out other causes of systemic disease.
▶ Examine the periorbital region carefully – where this has occurred following trauma, it may be possible to identify a small wound adjacent to the orbital rim.
▶ Check for evidence of a foreign body.
▶ ± Perform US assessment using the normal eye for comparison – it may be difficult to perform ophthalmic examination due to the degree of soft tissue swelling (Fig. 6.9).
▶ ± CT evaluation in severe cases.
▶ ± Aspiration of discrete abscess and submit for C&S.

Treatment

▶ If a discrete abscess has formed, perform drainage (ideally under GA) – hospitalise/refer:
 ▪ avoid iatrogenic damage
 ▪ it is more difficult to establish drainage compared to other species.
▶ If there is evidence of diffuse cellulitis, treat medically:
 ▪ BS antimicrobials – 5-d course initially
 ▪ administer NSAIDs.
▶ Monitor carefully for evidence of extension of infection into the globe (panophthalmitis).

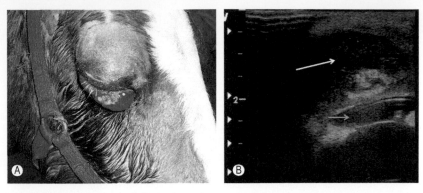

Figure 6.9 (A) Acute orbital cellulitis in a horse that sustained a puncture wound to the upper eyelid a few days earlier. (B) US evaluation of the eye and periorbital structures confirmed that an abscess had formed at the site (white arrow) which was subsequently drained (red and blue arrows – anterior chamber and lens).

Glaucoma

This is rare and the clinical signs are more subtle compared to other species which may result in acute cases being missed. It is usually chronic in nature, and secondary to ERU, but can develop following trauma.

Clinical signs of acute glaucoma

▸ Pain (photophobia, blepharospasm, lacrimation) – may be subtle unless concurrent uveitis is present.
▸ Diffuse corneal oedema.
▸ ± Mydriasis.
▸ Reduced menace response.

Treatment

▸ Seek specialist advice/refer.
▸ Confirm the diagnosis by measurement of IOP (>30 mmHg).
▸ Therapy:
  ▪ timolol maleate 0.5% or dorzolamide 2%, or combination of both, q. 8–12 h
  ▪ treatment of concurrent uveitis.
▸ Surgery if no response/deterioration (see specialist texts).

Chemical injuries

These are uncommon in horses and it is important to determine the chemical involved and whether it is alkali/acid in nature.

Immediate first aid

▸ Get the owner/carer to flush the eye with saline – human saline preparations used by contact lens wearers or warm water (if nothing else is available) can be used until you arrive.

▸ Do not put anything else in the eye.

Initial treatment

▸ Continue irritation with lukewarm sterile saline solution to ensure that the eye has been irrigated fully (e.g. 1 L attached to an IV fluid giving set).

▸ Perform a full ophthalmic examination and check for evidence of chemical burns elsewhere.

▸ Initiate treatment as for a complicated corneal melting ulcer (see p. 116).

▸ Wound management for burns if required (see p. 32).

▸ Alkali burns carry a much poorer prognosis compared to acid injuries.

References and further reading

• **Brooks, D.E., 2008.** Ophthalmology for the Equine Practitioner (second ed.). Teton New Media,

• **Brooks, D.E., 2010.** Equine conjunctival diseases: a commentary. Equine Vet. Educ. 22, 382–386.

• **Dallap Schaer, B., 2007.** Ophthalmic emergencies in horses. Vet. Clin. North Am. Equine Pract. 23, 49–65.

• **Dwyer, A.E., 2011.** Diseases and surgery of the globe and orbit. In: Gilger, B.C. (Ed.), Equine Ophthalmology (second ed.). Elsevier, St. Louis, Missouri, pp. 52–92.

• **Gilger, B.C., 2009.** Equine recurrent uveitis. In: Robinson, N.E., Sprayberry, K.A. (Eds.), Current Therapy in Equine Medicine (sixth ed.). Elsevier, St. Louis, Missouri, pp. 635–638.

• **Gilger, B.C., 2011.** Diseases and surgery of the globe and orbit. In: Gilger, B.C. (Ed.), Equine Ophthalmology (second ed.). Elsevier, St. Louis, Missouri, pp. 93–132.

• **Irby, N.L.,** Ophthalmologic emergencies. In: Orsini, J.A., Divers, T.J. (Eds.), Equine Emergencies Treatment and Procedures (third ed.). Elsevier, St. Louis, Missouri, pp. 379–409.

• **Matthews, A.G., 2009.** Ophthalmic antibicrobial therapy in the horse. Equine Vet. Educ. 21, 271–280.

• **Plummer, C.E., 2007.** Exophthalmos in the horse. Equine Vet. Educ. 19, 584–589.

• **Utter, M.E., Brooks, D.E., 2009.** Medical and surgical therapies for ulcerative keratitis. In: Robinson, N.E., Sprayberry, K.A. (Eds.), Current Therapy in Equine Medicine (sixth ed.). Elsevier, St. Louis, Missouri, pp. 648–651.

• **Wilkie, D.A., 2010.** Equine glaucoma: state of the art. Equine Vet. J. (Suppl. 37), 62–68.

Neurological emergencies

Approach to neurological emergencies

Equine neurological emergencies present with changes in mentation, posture or gait (including recumbency). Due to their size and temperament, some imaging modalities and parts of the neurological examination utilised in small animals may not be available or practical in horses with neurological diseases (apart from neonatal foals), which can make diagnosis challenging. Where neurological disease has resulted in recumbency, seizures, severe ataxia or changes in mentation causing horses to become fractious, management of these cases can be difficult and human safety must be taken into consideration (including the risk of potential zoonoses).

General approach

▶ If the horse is comatose/seizuring/collapsed, perform a rapid clinical examination, stabilise the patient (see relevant section) and obtain a brief history regarding the circumstances leading up the incident.
▶ Obtain a general history. Specific information that should be obtained includes:
  ▪ if there has been a change in the horse's mentation/behaviour
  ▪ if the signs seen are intermittent/continuous
  ▪ management changes that may have occurred around the time behaviour changed.
▶ Perform a full clinical examination. Specific clinical information that should be obtained includes:
  ▪ whether weakness/recumbency/dullness is secondary to another disease, e.g. endotoxaemia/SIRS
  ▪ evidence of any concurrent injuries
  ▪ pyrexia (infectious causes).

▸ Perform a neurological examination: (see below)
  ▪ determine if the horse has a neurological abnormality
  ▪ determine the likely location of a lesion.
▸ Create a list of possible diagnoses.
▸ Make a diagnostic and therapeutic plan.
▸ Assess response to therapy over time (including repeated neurological assessment).
▸ Revise diagnosis and treatment based on results of additional tests and response to therapy.

KEY TIP

Before administering any sedation in a seizing or severely ataxic horse, try to perform as much of a neurological examination as possible. This will help to narrow the list of possible diagnoses.

Neurological examination

▸ Be logical and consistent.
▸ Develop a routine and do it the same way each time – an examination checklist is useful.
▸ It may not be safe to perform a dynamic examination in a severely ataxic horse/not possible in the recumbent horse.
▸ Be aware of zoonotic risk in certain cases, e.g. rabies, viral encephalitides.
▸ Record the findings – this is essential for determining whether there has been an improvement/deterioration over time.
▸ Repeat neurological assessments – helps determine the likely diagnosis and prognosis.

OBSERVE GENERAL BEHAVIOUR, MENTATION AND POSTURE

- Best done before entering stable
☐ Assess general behaviour and look for abnormal behaviours, e.g. yawning, circling
☐ Determine the level of mentation
  ▪ *alert and responsive – varies between horses*
  ▪ *depressed – will react to environment*
  ▪ *encephalopathic – compulsive circling, head pressing, apparent blindness, seizures, depressed/lethargic*
  ▪ *hyperaesthetic – overly responsive to stimuli, jerk/tremors seen when stimulated*
  ▪ *stupor – appears asleep but will respond to sound, light and noxious stimuli (e.g. skin pinch)*
  ▪ *semicoma – partial responsiveness to stimuli*
  ▪ *coma – complete non-response to stimuli*
☐ Assess head and body posture – normal/abnormal
  ▪ *position and movement of head*
  ▪ *position and movement of limbs and trunk – evidence of defects in proprioception*

ASSESSMENT OF THE HEAD AND CRANIAL NERVES

☐ Assess horse's response as you enter the stable.

☐ Assess cranial nerve function (Table 7.1) starting by examination of the eyes for:

- size and symmetry of palpebral fissure
- eye position
- pupil size
- normal physiological nystagmus – nose elevated, head moved to each side
- prominence of the 3rd eyelid
- PLR – direct/consensual (swinging light response)
- palpebral reflex
- menace response
- evidence of vision.

Table 7.1 Function and assessment of the cranial nerves

Cranial nerve	Function	Assessment	Clinical signs seen in disease
I Olfactory	Smell	Difficult – very hard to remove visual/auditory stimuli	
II Optic	Vision	Menace response and pupillary light reflex	Blindness and loss of PLR Unilateral vs bilateral – direct and consensual
III Oculomotor	Extraocular muscles (dorsal, ventral, medial rectii; ventral oblique; levator palpebrae) Pupillary constriction	Pupillary light reflex Pupil size Medial movement of globe Eye position Palpebral fissure size	Dilated pupil Loss of PLR direct and consensual in affected eye Visual (normal menace) Lateral and ventral strabismus Ptosis Mydriasis
IV Trochlear	Extraocular muscle (dorsal oblique)	Eye position	Dorsomedial strabismus

(Continued)

Table 7.1 Function and assessment of the cranial nerves (Continued)

Cranial nerve	Function	Assessment	Clinical signs seen in disease
V Trigeminal	Motor – masticatory muscles Sensory head	Palpebral blink, nociception when head touched Chewing, jaw tone, masticatory muscle size	Loss of sensation and palpebral and corneal reflexes Atrophy and dropped jaw
VI Abducent	Extraocular muscles (retractor bulbi, lateral rectus)	Globe retraction and lateral movement of globe	Medial strabismus Loss of corneal reflex
VII Facial	Motor – muscles of facial expression Parasympathetics – salivary and lacrimal glands	Facial symmetry Palpebral blink Ear, muzzle and lip movement	Muzzle deviation Ptosis Ear droop Loss of palpebral reflex and blink, Dry eye
VIII Vestibulocochlear	Posture and balance Hearing	Head and eye position Hearing Balance Response to blindfolding on a soft surface	Head tilt/ Ventrolateral strabismus Nystagmus (in early stages, may not be present later in disease), Loss of balance (ataxia, exacerbated by blindfold), Circling/ falling to the side Deafness
XI Glossopharyngeal	Sensory and motor – pharynx and larynx	Ability to swallow (observation and endoscopy)	Dysphagia DDSP
X Vagus	Sensory and motor – pharynx and larynx	Ability to swallow Laryngeal function	Dysphagia Laryngeal paralysis DDSP
XI Spinal accessory	Motor – cervical muscles, larynx and oesophagus	Muscle atrophy	Muscle atrophy
XII Hypoglossal	Motor – tongue	Tongue strength and symmetry	Tongue atrophy and paralysis

☐ Assess the rest of the head for:
- evidence of a head tilt
- facial symmetry
- facial expression
- movement of ears, muzzle, lips and evidence of muscle fasciculations
- facial sensation
- Evidence of Horner's syndrome (pupillary constriction, ptosis of upper eyelid, protrusion of 3rd eyelid, sweating around base of ear and around eye).

☐ Open the horse's mouth:
- assess jaw tone and palpate masseter muscles for pain/stiffness
- assess tongue for tone, strength, symmetry and look for drooling of saliva.

☐ Observe the horse eating, drinking and swallowing.

☐ ± Endoscopic assessment of the pharynx and larynx to assess CN 9 and 10.

ASSESSMENT OF SPINAL REFLEXES AND MUSCLES

☐ Cervicofacial/auricular reflex (around C2) and local cervical reflex (C3–C6).

☐ Lateral flexion of neck in both directions – normal/reduced.

☐ Sway test – push at withers and horse should right itself quickly.

☐ Cutaneous trunci reflex.
- Assess for loss of skin sensation (hypalgesia or analgesia)/increased sensitivity (hyperaesthesia).

☐ Note any abnormal regions of sweating.

☐ Note any evidence of muscle atrophy.

☐ Tail carriage and tone.

☐ Perineal reflex.

☐ Anal tone.

DYNAMIC ASSESSMENT (IF SAFE TO PERFORM/NOT RECUMBENT)

☐ Assess for evidence of:
- ataxia
- paresis – deficiency of voluntary movement due to reduced muscular power (weakness)
- dysmetria – limb movements hypermetric (exaggerated range of movement/ excessive joint movement), spastic (increased muscle tone) or hypometric (limb stiffness, reduced joint flexion)

☐ Grade any gait abnormalities 0–5 (Table 7.2):
- walk in a straight line and serpentine
- walk with head elevated
- walk while pulling tail in each direction
- spin in tight circles
- walk backwards
- walk over uneven ground and up and down an incline
- trot in a straight line
- ± foot placement and hopping tests of FL (perform on soft surface)
- ± assessment following placement of blindfold (perform on soft surface).

Table 7.2 Grading of gait abnormalities

Grade	
0	No deficits
1	Abnormality just detectable at normal gait – worse when backed/turned/ pressure on HQ/neck extension
2	Easily detected at normal gait – worse as above
3	Very prominent at walk, buckles/falls when backed/turned/pressure on HQ/ neck extension
4	Stumbling, tripping, falling spontaneously
5	Horse recumbent

Adapted from Furr and Reed (2008a).

Neurological examination of the recumbent horse

▸ Used to rule in/out a possible neurological cause in the case of the recumbent/collapsed horse (see Table 7.5 and p. 313).
▸ These cases can be difficult to assess:
  ▪ fear/anxiety/exhaustion/dehydration/metabolic derangements may affect responses
  ▪ recumbency may cause peripheral neuropathies that are not part of primary disease.
▸ Assess withdrawal reflexes for each limb (spinal reflexes) and conscious pain perception (ascending spinal pathways).
▸ ± Assess biceps, triceps and patellar reflexes – can be difficult to interpret.

Assessment and plan

▸ Determine if the horse is neurologically normal/abnormal.
▸ If neurologically abnormal, determine the likely location of the lesion based on neurological examination (Tables 7.3–7.5):
  ▪ combinations of clinical signs that cannot be explained by one site of disease may be due to diffuse/multifocal disease.
▸ Decide what further diagnostic tests are required (Table 7.6).
▸ Make a provisional therapeutic plan based on the initial diagnosis.
▸ Revise the plan according to the results of diagnostic tests and repeat clinical and neurological assessment.

Traumatic injury to the CNS

Traumatic injuries to the head or vertebral column may occur during handling, exercise or competition where the type and location of impact are known or may be suspected in horses found recumbent (see p. 313). Prompt and appropriate first aid is essential to

Table 7.3 Clinical signs that assist localisation of a CNS lesion

Potential location of lesion	Clinical signs that may be observed
Cerebrum	Abnormal posture – mild weakness Seizures Altered mentation – depression, aimless wandering, head pressing, yawning Blindness (normal PLR)
Cerebellum	Hypermetria Intention tremor – worse when trying to eat Muscle hypertonicity Abnormal menace response
Brainstem	Ataxia/weakness/dysmetria/Narrow circling Spasticity Tetraparesis Depression/semicoma Cranial nerve deficits ± Dysphagia, anisocoria, dilated pupils
Vestibular system	Ataxia – worsened by blindfolding Head tilt Pronounced postural abnormalities Abnormal nystagmus/lack of physiological nystagmus Ventral strabismus when head elevated
Spinal cord/UMN	Mild/moderate paresis/ataxia/dysmetria ↑ Tone – spasticity prominent ↑ Reflex response Minimal muscle atrophy Muscle fasciculations absent
Peripheral nerves/LMN	Mild postural deficits/ataxia ↓ Tone – weakness predominates ↓ Spinal reflex response Profound muscle atrophy Muscle fasciculations present

Table 7.4 Clinical abnormalities that are associated with lesions affecting different spinal cord segments

Spinal cord segment	Clinical signs
C1–C5	Spastic gait, worse in HL Proprioceptive deficits Weakness ± Horner's syndrome

(Continued)

Table 7.4 Clinical abnormalities that are associated with lesions affecting different spinal cord segments (Continued)

Spinal cord segment	Clinical signs
C6–T2	Proprioceptive deficits, worse in FL Weakness, especially in FL Muscle atrophy FL Loss of FL spinal reflexes Loss of cutaneous trunci reflex ± Horner's syndrome
T3–L3	FL gait normal HL proprioceptive deficits/weakness/spasticity
L4–S2	Proprioceptive deficits/weakness in HL Loss of HL spinal reflexes
S3–S5	Normal FL and HL Urinary incontinence Faecal retention Hypalgesia tail and perianal region
Coccygeal	Normal FL and HL ↓ Tail tone Hypalgesia caudal to lesion

Modified from Furr and Reed (2008a).

Table 7.5 Clinical signs that may be used to determine the likely location of a neurological lesion in the recumbent horse

Clinical signs	Lesion localisation
Normal mentation	Suggests lesion caudal to C1
Can dog sit Good strength and co-ordination of FL	Likely caudal to T2
Loss of FL strength Can lift head and cranial neck	Likely lesion around C6–T2
↑ FL tone Flaccid paralysis HL (Schiff–Sherrington phenomenon)	Likely lesion around T2–L4
Abnormal spinal reflexes (FL, flexor, triceps and biceps reflexes; HL, patellar reflex)	Normal spinal reflex requires intact sensory nerve, spinal cord segment(s), peripheral motor nerve and muscle – reduced/absent if abnormal Exaggerated response – UMN disease cranial to site of spinal cord segments

Table 7.6 Diagnostic tests that may be useful in assessment of neurological emergencies

Test	Indications
Serum biochemistry and haematology	Suspected inflammation/infection Assessment of hepatic function ($\pm$ ammonia levels if they can be measured) in cases of altered mentation $\pm$ Serial evaluation of enzymes if recumbent
Serology for viral antibodies Nasopharyngeal swab for virus isolation (EHV)	Suspected infectious disease
Radiography	Assessment of bony trauma Myelography where spinal compression suspected
Endoscopy	Cranial nerve deficits or epistaxis Suspected temporohyoid arthropathy (THO)
CSF analysis	Suspected infectious disease or meningitis
CT/MRI	Assessment following traumatic injury to the head Standing CT where available (risk associated with GA)
Scintigraphy	Traumatic injury to head and vertebral column
US	Assessment of skull and cervical vertebral fractures

prevent further haemorrhage, ischaemia or infection that may limit restoration of neurological function and worsen the prognosis.

General approach to management

▶ Do not jump to immediate conclusions – concussed horses will have a dramatic onset of clinical signs but will recover quickly.
▶ Where traumatic injuries to the CNS occur during competition, do not be pressurised by riders/owners, officials or bystanders to make hasty decisions until you have assessed the horse fully.
▶ Determine whether the horse is neurologically normal/abnormal or whether collapse recumbency has occurred due to other causes, e.g. cardiovascular/musculoskeletal.
▶ Ongoing therapy is merited where there is continued clinical improvement.
▶ Consider euthanasia where there is evidence of clinical deterioration or if there is no improvement after 24h in a recumbent horse – prolonged recumbency of unexplained cause in adult horses usually has a grave prognosis.

Clinical signs

These depend on the location and severity of damage, and knowledge of how the injury occurred is useful. Injury to the vertebral column most commonly occurs in the cervical and thoracolumbar regions subsequent to rearing and falling over backwards, colliding with solid objects or other horses, kicks and slipping. Fractures of the sacrum and coccygeal verte-brae may occur following a horse falling violently backwards on the ground or against a solid object.

Head trauma

▸ Ataxia.
▸ Abnormal mentation.
▸ ± Cranial nerve deficits (see Table 7.1), epistaxis, blood/CSF from ear.
▸ Recumbency.
▸ Seizures.
▸ Altered consciousness, stupor – coma.

Spinal cord trauma (see Table 7.4)

▸ Ataxia.
▸ Recumbency.
▸ Cauda equina signs.
▸ Loss of conscious pain perception.

Initial assessment and treatment

Perform an initial rapid assessment and administer first aid treatment.

▸ Be aware of personal safety and secure the horse, e.g. place headcollar.
▸ Check airway, breathing and circulation – initiate CPR if required (see p. 185).
▸ Control seizures if present – diazepam 0.1–0.2 mg/kg IV.
▸ ± Administer sedation if the horse is attempting to stand but is not fully aware of surroundings/lacks co-ordination – xylazine 1 mg/kg IV. (avoid use of acepromazine – reduces seizure threshold)
▸ Assess the pattern of respiration.
▸ Control any haemorrhage or perform tracheotomy (p. 353) if suspected URT obstruction.
▸ ± Intubation if required.
▸ ± Supplementary oxygen 10–15 L/min.

Obtain a history. Specific questions that should be asked include:

▸ Evidence of any neurological abnormalities prior to traumatic incident.
▸ Description of traumatic incident if observed – when, how and where trauma was sustained.
▸ Description of any change in clinical signs since the episode occurred.

Perform a full clinical examination. Specific assessment includes:

▸ Check for concurrent traumatic injuries, including damage to peripheral nerves and injuries to the limbs/thorax/abdomen.
▸ Assess for epistaxis/evidence of CSF drainage from ear/obstruction of nasal passages where head trauma has been sustained.

Perform a neurological examination (see p. 128):

▸ Perform without sedation if possible.
▸ Important to perform a full evaluation including assessment of cranial nerves as a baseline measurement (can then judge if improving/deteriorating).
▸ Determine if neurologically normal or not.
▸ Localise the likely region of injury (see Tables 7.3–7.5).

▶ Depends on the clinical signs at the time of examination – if relatively stable, may wait until further diagnostic tests have been performed before administering further medication.
▶ Treat the direct effects of injury, secondary damage to nervous tissue and other concurrent traumatic injuries.
▶ Aggressive initial treatment is required if the horse is recumbent or exhibits altered levels of mentation.
▶ Use of corticosteroids, antioxidants and magnesium sulphate is controversial due to lack of evidence regarding effect on outcome.

Control pain and inflammation

▶ Administer NSAIDs (e.g. flunixin meglumine 1.1 mg/kg IV) – analgesia, anti-inflammatory and anti-pyretic properties.
▶ ± Administer corticosteroids (controversial):
  ▪ dexamethasone 0.1–0.2 mg/kg IV q. 6–8 h for first 24 h
  ▪ methylprednisolone 30 mg/kg IV if injury <4 h old.

Control cerebral oedema

▶ If deteriorating neurological status, (look for papilloedema) administer:
  ▪ 20% mannitol 0.25–2 g/kg slow IV (monitor blood glucose)
  ▪ DMSO 1 g/kg IV as 10% solution
  ▪ ± hypertonic saline IV (see p. 376) – use is controversial.

Maintain systemic blood pressure

▶ Administer isotonic, hypertonic or colloid solutions (see p. 374).
▶ Administer whole blood if significant haemorrhage has occurred (see p. 376).

Maintain blood oxygen levels

▶ Ensure adequate pulmonary ventilation.
▶ ± Intubate and ventilate/provide oxygen supplementation (10–15 L/min).

Other treatment

▶ Treat any concurrent wounds/injuries.
▶ Move to a quiet, safe (ideally well-padded) area that is a suitable temperature (warm, not too hot or cold).
▶ Monitor rectal temperature – can develop hyperthermia following head trauma (see p. 215).
▶ Surgical decompression is controversial – craniotomy can be performed as a last resort if there is ongoing deterioration following head trauma despite medical therapy.

▶ Decide whether further diagnostic investigation and treatment are required:
  ▪ depends on the clinical signs, location of CNS injury and facilities available.
▶ Determine if euthanasia is warranted or whether the horse should be hospitalised for further diagnostic tests and ongoing treatment/monitoring (seek specialist advice).
▶ Repeated clinical and neurological assessment is essential.

▶ The prognosis depends on the severity of injury and response to treatment – these vary from mild cases that recover quickly to horses that remain recumbent where the prognosis is poor – grave.
▶ Euthanasia should be considered where there is evidence of:
  ▪ dilated unresponsive pupils
  ▪ deteriorating vital signs – HR, BP
  ▪ abnormal respiratory pattern
  ▪ progressive loss of cranial nerve function
  ▪ opisthotonus
  ▪ seizures increasing in frequency/severity
  ▪ prolonged recumbency (>6h)
  ▪ loss of withdrawal reflex or conscious pain perception.

Peripheral nerve syndromes

These may be acute in nature, secondary to trauma, inflammation or occasionally following toxicosis. Following traumatic injury, return of nerve function is usually rapid (hours/days) where neurapraxia has occurred (concussion of nerve fibres with no morphologic change). Where there has been damage to the axon (axontmesis) or both axon and myelin sheath (neurotmesis) following severe blunt trauma/penetrating injury, there will be prolonged/permanent loss of function (see texts/seek specialist advice).

Cranial nerves

▶ The more distal a lesion on a cranial nerve (CN), the fewer clinical signs that are seen.
▶ Where >1 cranial nerve is involved, a more central lesion should be suspected – if altered mentation and limb paresis, likely to be a brainstem lesion.
▶ Vestibular disease – see Ataxia, next section.
▶ Guttural pouch disease (see Ch. 5) – multiple cranial nerves may be involved causing:
  ▪ dysphagia (CN IX, X)
  ▪ soft palate paresis and dorsal displacement (CN IX, X)
  ▪ laryngeal paralysis (CN X)
  ▪ Horner's syndrome (sympathetic trunk cranial cervical ganglion)
  ▪ tongue paralysis (CN XII)
  ▪ occasionally facial nerve paralysis (CN VII) and masseter muscle atrophy (CN V).
▶ Facial nerve and other peripheral nerves (see Table 7.7).

General approach to treatment of acute-onset peripheral nerve syndromes

▶ Administer NSAIDs – flunixin 1.1 mg/kg IV or phenylbutazone 4.4 mg/kg IV initially.
▶ Administer dexamethasone 0.05–0.1 mg/kg if recent (hours since injury), and no contraindication for their use.
▶ Surgical decompression if mass/haematoma is evident.
▶ ± Bandaging of limbs.
▶ ± Hydrotherapy.

Table 7.7 Peripheral nerve syndromes that may be seen in the horse

Peripheral nerve syndrome	Clinical signs	Causes	Specific treatment/ prognosis
Facial nerve paralysis	↓ Spontaneous and reflex movement of ears, eyelids, lips, external nares Unilateral: ear and lips on the side of lesion droop, muzzle pulled to opposite side	Pressure on side of face Laceration GP disease, including temporohyoid arthropathy Skull fracture EPM	Depends on cause Treatment for corneal ulceration/ corneal exposure (topical application of ophthalmic lubricant)
Suprascapular nerve paralysis (Sweeney)	Laxity of shoulder joint – subluxation during limb protraction	Usually subsequent to trauma to the shoulder ± May involve brachial plexus	Box rest Surgical decompression if no improvement in 3 months
Radial nerve paralysis	Poor extension of FL, normal protraction Depends on location of lesion Stand with dropped elbow, extended shoulder Inability to extend distal limb joints, scuffing toe Difficulty getting up and down	Trauma – fractured humerus, kicks/falls on lateral humerus Prolonged lateral recumbency Overstretching of nerve – fractured 1st rib/hyperextension FL Compression from enlarged axillary LN/ abscess in cranial thorax	Box rest Bandaging lower limb Treatment of concurrent myopathy Post anaesthetic – recovery in 24–48 h Other causes – guarded/poor prognosis Depends on location and extent of injury Poor – humeral fracture and radial nerve damage
Sciatic nerve paresis	HL hangs behind body, stifle dropped and extended Can bear some weight on the leg ± Cutaneous hypalgesia below stifle	Misplaced IM injections especially foals Local abscess formation at injection site Scandinavian knuckling syndrome (see texts)	Treat any abscesses Bandaging of lower limb Prognosis based on nature and severity of injury/response to treatment

(Continued)

Table 7.7 Peripheral nerve syndromes that may be seen in the horse (Continued)

Peripheral nerve syndrome	Clinical signs	Causes	Specific treatment/ prognosis
Femoral nerve paralysis	Bilateral – crouched HL position, difficulty rising from recumbency. Unilateral – inability to support weight on affected limb/ extends stifle, rests limb with all joints in flexion	Mares post foaling Post GA Occasionally after penetrating wound to flank	Prognosis guarded in unilateral cases, grave in bilateral cases (euthanasia indicated) ± Sling support
Stringhalt (equine reflex hypertonia)	Exaggerated flexion of limb during protraction Excessive hock flexion	Spinal cord/ peripheral nerve disease Lesions around lateral digital extensor tendon/hock Toxic – multiple causes, including plants (see Ch. 16)	Further assessment – removal from plants or radiography/US ± Surgery (see texts/seek specialist advice)

Ataxia

This is defined as a lack of co-ordination of motor movements, resulting in inconsistent (or irregular) movement of the head, neck, trunk and/or limbs (Fig. 7.1). This is a description of clinical signs rather than a specific diagnosis and there are many possible causes. Ataxia may be classified as cerebellar, vestibular or sensory (spinal) – see Table 7.8. The sensory form is most common in adult horses.

Initial stabilisation and assessment

Perform immediate stabilisation if the horse is severely ataxic/panicked and a danger to itself:

▶ Human safety is important – wear protective headgear.
▶ Avoid accessing ataxic horses on concrete/tarmac surfaces – perform in a stable with rubber matting and shavings bedding, a padded recovery box if in hospital facilities or in an open space with soft underfooting (e.g. grass).
▶ Perform initial neurological assessment prior to administration of sedatives – this helps to determine the likely location of a neurological lesion and assists diagnosis.
▶ Avoid administering sedation in an already ataxic horse unless required, e.g. evidence of panic/distress. If required:
   ▪ Administer xylazine 1 mg/kg IV if clinical signs of cerebral involvement are evident.

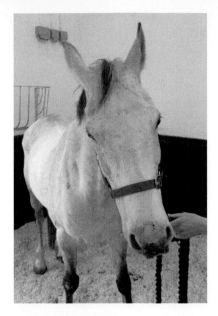

Figure 7.1 Head tilt in a horse with vestibular ataxia.

Courtesy of Fernando Malalana.

Table 7.8 Clinical signs used to differentiate between cerebellar, vestibular and sensory forms of ataxia

Cerebellar	Vestibular	Sensory (spinal)
Jerky, hypermetric gait Swinging head movements Head tremor ± Defective menace response No limb weakness	Usually head tilt and asymmetric ataxia Head tilt, ventro-lateral strabismus (usually towards side of lesion) Wide-based stance Short steps, unsteady gait ± Nystagmus (often transient/short-lived in horses), circling/falling Exacerbated when blindfolded Can be difficult to differentiate central vs peripheral vestibular signs Central – cranial nerve signs, depression, limb weakness, strabismus	Unpredictable gait, affecting one or more limbs Upper motor weakness Normal mentation, no cranial nerve deficits Most noticeable at changes of speed and direction Worsened when walked on a slope/with the head elevated

- Administer acepromazine 0.02 mg/kg IV for anxiolytic effects if there is no evidence of cerebral involvement.
▶ In cases of severe ataxia, consider sedation/anaesthesia prior to transport in a horse ambulance to hospital facilities for further evaluation and stabilisation if appropriate/ available (discuss with referral centre first/seek specialist advice).

Obtain a detailed history. Specific questions that should be asked include:
▶ Recent medications administered.
▶ Recent illness/trauma.
▶ Type of feed/forage.
▶ Recent import/travel (consider EPM in horses in USA/imported from USA).
▶ Illness in any in-contacts, including pyrexia, respiratory disease, abortion.
▶ When clinical signs first seen and circumstances, e.g. known trauma.
▶ Speed of onset (acute/more gradual).
▶ Subtle signs of ataxia before traumatic incident.
▶ Recent signs of difficulty eating.

Perform a general clinical examination. Assessment should include:
▶ Rule out conditions that may be confused with CNS disease, e.g. myopathy/laminitis.
▶ Evidence of systemic illness.
▶ Palpate the base of the ears and check inside the ears.
▶ Check for evidence of trauma, including haemorrhage/CSF leakage from external ear/nares.

Perform a full neurological examination:
▶ Make a list of possible causes of ataxia based on the clinical signs and neuroanatomical diagnosis (Table 7.9).

Further assessment and treatment

▶ Consider the likelihood of infectious disease as a cause of signs seen (see Ch. 15):
- obtain blood samples (heparinised blood, clotted blood/serum) and nasal/ nasopharyngeal swabs for virus isolation, PCR and serology
- sample in-contacts
- implement necessary biosecurity measures (see p. 387).
▶ Decide if further diagnostic tests need to be performed, including referral if warranted/ available:
- radiography ± myelography
- endoscopy
- ± MRI/CT
- CSF analysis
- ± scintigraphy.
▶ Initiate treatment as appropriate:
- NSAIDs
- BS antimicrobials
- ± corticosteroids (controversial)
- ± antioxidants, including DMSO, vitamin E.
▶ Provide nursing and other supportive care – determine if hospitalisation/referral for ongoing care is needed:
- care as for recumbent horse (see p. 314)

Table 7.9 Possible causes of ataxia in adult horses

Cerebellar	Head trauma
	Toxic – tremorgenic mycotoxins
	Cerebellar abiotrophy – foals <6 months, Arabian bloodlines
Vestibular	*Central CNS disease*
	Infectious/abscess
	Neoplasia
	Peripheral disease
	Otitis media/interna
	Temporohyoid osteoarthropathy
	Skull fractures
	EPM
	Polyneuritis equi
	Idiopathic (rare)
Spinal (sensory)	CVM
	Equine herpes virus myeloencephalopathy
	Fractured vertebrae
	Spinal cord trauma
	Verminous encephalomyelitis
	Spinal cord neoplasia
	Soft tissue lesions
	Dorsal articular process arthritis
	EPM/protozoal myeloencephalitis
	Viral meningoencephalitis (WNV, EEE, VEE, WEE, rabies – other encephalitis viruses)
	Bacterial meningitis
	Synovial cysts
	Toxins (e.g. stinging nettles, fluphenazine, moxidectin)
	Vertebral osteomyelitis
	Equine degenerative myeloencephalopathy
	Discospondylitis
	Cauda equine neuritis/polyneuritis equi
	Fibrocartilagenous embolism
	Air embolism
	Intracarotid injection
	Post-anaesthetic haemorrhagic myelophathy

- vestibular ataxia – keep outside (they rely heavily on vision)
- confine if mild ataxia – covered arena/small paddock with good footing.
▸ Revise treatment plan and prognosis based on the results of additional diagnostic tests and response to treatment.

Prognosis

▸ Depends on underlying cause and initial response to treatment.

Equine herpes myeloencephalitis

EHV-1 is a pathogen that has widespread distribution and usually results in subclinical infection and respiratory disease and less commonly abortion and neonatal death (see p. 284). Equine herpes myeloencephalitis (EHM) can develop in some individuals and usually occurs in horses aged >3–5 years of age.

History, clinical signs and diagnosis

▶ Often history of recent pyrexa/pyrexia in in-contacts.
▶ HL ataxia and weakness (although all 4 limbs can be involved).
▶ Urinary incontinence/faecal retention, lack of anal and tail tone.
▶ Can progress to paresis and recumbency.
▶ Diagnosis – virus isolation/PCR/ paired serology (see p. 284).

Treatment and prognosis

▶ BS antimicrobials (secondary bacterial infection) – e.g. trimethoprim sulphonamides.
▶ ↓ Inflammatory response:
   - flunixin 1.1 mg/kg q. 12 h IV 3–5 d
   - dexamethasone 0.1–0.2 mg/kg IV q. 24 h for 3 d (use is controversial)
   - DMSO 0.5–1.0 g/kg IV or PO 3 d
   - ± aspirin 10 mg/kg PO q. 48 h
   - ± valacyclovir (valaciclovir) 30–40 mg/kg q. 8–12 h PO for 7 d (better bioavailability than acyclovir (aciclovir)).
▶ Nursing care if recumbent (see p. 314).
▶ Biosecurity procedures must be implemented, including isolation of affected horses, segregation and monitoring of in-contacts (see p. 387 and HBLB codes of practice (http://codes.hblb.org.uk) – useful to give these to the clients too).
▶ Morbidity 10–90%, depending on outbreak – between 5 and 30% show neurological signs.
▶ Recumbency for >24 h is associated with a poor prognosis – consider euthanasia on welfare grounds. Gait deficits are often lifelong.

Seizures

Adult horses have a relatively high seizure threshold (unlike neonates – see p. 241), requiring considerable insult to the forebrain to induce convulsions. These most commonly occur secondary to trauma, hepatoencephalopathy or toxicosis (Table 7.10). Where seizure activity is not present at the time of examination, it is important to obtain a good history, including a description of the clinical signs seen to rule out potential confusion with collapse/syncope or struggling.

Clinical signs

▶ Variable – from mild alterations in consciousness and focal muscle fasciculations, such as facial twitching, to recumbency (petitmal to grand mal seizures).
▶ Prodromal phase – restless/distracted/change in mentation.

Table 7.10 Possible causes of seizures in adult horses

Trauma	Causes
Metabolic	Hepatoencephalopathy Hyperammonemia Hypocalcaemia Hyponatraemia Hypoglycaemia Hyperthermia Pregnancy

Toxic	Plants/mycotoxins (see Ch. 16):
	  Nardoo fern
	  Swainsona
	  Locoweed
	  Datura
	  Buckeye
	  Solanum spp.
	  Mouldy grain
	  Metaldehyde

Infectious	Viral encephalitis Verminous encephalitis EPM Bacterial meningitis/abscess
Iatrogenic	Intracarotid injection Adverse drug reactions (moxidectin, enrofloxacin, fluphenazine) Post myelography Post-anaesthetic cerebral necrosis Air embolism
Neoplasia	Adenocarcinoma etc.
Idiopathic	Idiopathic epilepsy in young Arabians

▸ Tonic–clonic movements for ≥30 s – stiff hypertonic limbs, repetitive and rhythmic muscle movements.

▸ Non-arousable during seizure – unconscious for seconds.

▸ Depressed and quiet ± blind following seizure.

▸ Head trauma very common, especially around eyes due to prominent positioning. Owner may have assumed the horse has been cast previously if not observed during seizure.

Advice to owner/carer over the telephone

▸ Do not try to enter stable to control the horse – keep the horse quiet, minimise noise in the immediate vicinity, remove any objects the horse may injure itself on in the environment and await vet's arrival.

Control seizures if the horse is actively convulsing:

▶ Administer diazepam 0.1–0.2 mg/kg IV, phenobarbitone 8–32 mg/kg IV or can use standard doses of α2 agonists.

▶ Alternatives include phenobarbital 12 mg/kg IV, then 6.6 mg/kg IV q. 12 h or pentobarbital 2–20 mg/kg IV or q. 4 h as required (do not use euthanasia solutions/those with other active ingredients)

▶ If convulsions cannot be controlled with these, consider general anaesthesia – euthanasia should also be considered in these cases.

▶ Do not use acepromazine (reduces seizure threshold).

Obtain a thorough history. Specific questions that should be asked include:

▶ Age and breed.

▶ Recent/current medications.

▶ Recent illness.

▶ Vaccination history.

▶ Recent travel/import.

▶ Description of clinical signs observed and circumstances surrounding the episode (if not ongoing):

　▪ differentiate from acute collapse/syncope – fatigue, loss of unconsciousness for seconds, no tonic/clonic movements, recovery almost immediate.

Perform a full clinical examination. Specific information that should be obtained includes:

▶ Rule out other underlying problem.

▶ Pyrexia (possible infectious diseases/exhaustion syndrome, see p. 212).

▶ Evidence of trauma (e.g. blood from nares/ears).

Perform a neurological examination (see p. 128).

Take samples for further tests:

▶ Haematology.

▶ Serum biochemistry, including glucose (especially pregnant/obese/potentially hyperlipaemic animals), ± ammonia (if available).

▶ Electrolytes (including Ca^{2+} and Mg^{2+}).

▶ ± Serology if suspected infectious disease (see Ch. 15).

▶ ± Blood gas analysis (if available).

▶ Determine on the basis of clinical examination and result of initial tests if extracranial/intracranial disease is present and narrow the list of potential causes.

▶ Decide on further tests that need to be performed – a diagnosis should be pursued if ≥1 episode of seizures of unknown cause occurs (consider referral/seek specialist advice):

　▪ investigation of hepatic disease, e.g. liver biopsy

　▪ endoscopy of GP

　▪ radiographs of head – DV, lateral

　▪ CSF analysis (TP/cell counts, culture, serology)

　▪ ± EEG

　▪ ± CT/MRI.

▸ Treat/correct underlying disease (if determined).

▸ Ongoing anticonvulsant medication is recommended if status epilepticus has occurred (>30 min continuous seizure) or ≥2 sequential seizures without full recovery of consciousness (see texts).

Encephalitis

Consider in any horse with acute-onset behavioural change (ranging from depression to diffuse CNS signs) with concurrent pyrexia. Viral encephalitis, including alphaviruses (EEE, WEE, VEE), WNV, louping ill virus, Hendra virus and rabies (see Ch. 15), should be considered in endemic regions (Fig. 7.2).

> **KEY TIP**
>
> Consider the risks to your safety and that of any handlers and be aware of potential zoonotic conditions such as rabies, VEE and Hendra virus.

Management

▸ General supportive care until the diagnosis is confirmed – euthanasia may be undertaken if disease such as rabies (Fig. 7.2) is considered highly likely based on clinical signs and region (cannot confirm antemortem).

▸ Dexamethasone 0.1–0.2 mg/kg IV q. 12–24 h over 24–48 h if progressive deterioration in neurological signs evident.

▸ NSAIDs.

▸ Control of seizures (see previous section).

▸ IV fluids.

▸ Nutrition – enteral feeding if tolerated.

▸ Protection from trauma.

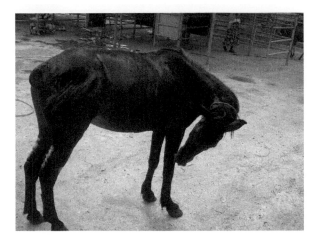

Figure 7.2 Self-mutilation in a horse with the spinal form of rabies.

Courtesy of Derek Knottenbelt.

▸ Report to relevant vet/human health agencies where appropriate (see Ch. 15).
▸ Take appropriate precautions when handling cases/performing PM examination.

Meningitis

Meningitis is uncommon in the mature horse and occurs more commonly in the neonate. It can be secondary to viral encephalitis/bacterial infection that has extended into the CNS from an adjacent structure or via the haematogenous route. Early recognition and treatment is essential and cases can be associated with high mortality.

Clinical signs

▸ Pyrexia.
▸ Depression.
▸ Anorexia.
▸ Neck stiffness, hyperaesthesia.
▸ ± Sudden limb extension, hypertonicity on passive flexion of the head/neck.
▸ ± Seizures.

Diagnosis and treatment

▸ Evidence of viral/bacterial infection and clinical signs consistent with possible meningitis.
▸ Check the guttural pouches for temporohyoid osteoarthropathy.
▸ Obtain CSF sample – WBC, TP, bacterial growth on culture (gold standard for diagnosis).
▸ General supportive treatment and systemic antimicrobials – ideally based on C&S results from CSF (see texts/seek specialist advice).

Tetanus

Clostridium tetani spores are commonly found in the environment and may gain entry into the body via wounds, the umbilicus (foals) or the urogenital tract (immediately after foaling). Toxins that are produced prevent neurotransmitter release (tetanospasmin), resulting in ↑ muscle tone and spasm, and cause further tissue necrosis (tetanolysin) and growth of the bacteria. Horses are particularly sensitive to its effects and it is a major cause of mortality in areas of the world where vaccination is not routinely performed. Tetanus vaccination status should always be determined in at-risk horses.

Clinical signs and progression

▸ Variable time between entry of bacteria and the development of clinical signs – around 7–10 d.
▸ Rigidity/spasm of the head muscles causing difficulty/inability to eat or drink.
▸ ± Unable to open mouth ('lockjaw').
▸ Facial muscle spasm – grimace.
▸ Prolapse of the 3rd eyelid (Fig. 7.3).
▸ Flared nostrils and erect ear carriage.

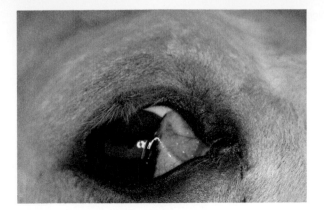

Figure 7.3 Prolapse of the third eyelid in a horse with tetanus.

Courtesy of Derek Knottenbelt.

▸ Rigid extension of the neck, back, legs and an elevated tailhead ('sawhorse stance').
▸ Stiff gait.
▸ May progress to recumbency.
▸ Hyperthermia.
▸ Tetanic spasms are initiated by stimuli including light, noise, and touch – these can cause panic, recumbency and secondary musculoskeletal trauma.
▸ Death – respiratory muscle involvement or secondary to other complications, e.g. aspiration pneumonia, prolonged recumbency, GIT dysfunction.

Diagnosis

▸ Obtain a full history. Specific questions that should be asked include:
  ▪ if the horse has been fully vaccinated against tetanus and when the last vaccination was given (see p. 25)
  ▪ whether the horse has recently sustained a wound/been lame due to a foot abscess.
▸ Clinical signs in an unvaccinated horse/vaccinations out of date – difficult to confirm by laboratory methods.

Treatment

Eliminate the source of toxin

▸ Lavage the wound thoroughly (if it can be located).
▸ Remove necrotic tissue.
▸ Administer systemic antimicrobials IV initially:
  ▪ penicillin or metronidazole (penicillin use considered controversial by some specialists).

Neutralise unbound toxin and stimulate an immune reaction

▸ Administer tetanus antitoxin locally and IM, SC or IV (will not have any effect on already bound toxin).
▸ Administer tetanus toxoid vaccine at a separate site (minimise risks of serum hepatitis).
▸ ± Intrathecal administration of tetanus antitoxin (see texts).

Provide analgesia and control muscle spasms

▶ Flunixin meglumine 1.1 mg/kg q. 12 h IV.
▶ Acepromazine 0.02–0.1 mg/kg IV q. 6–12 h.
▶ Where severe tetanic spasms are evident:
  ▪ diazepam 0.1–0.2 mg/kg IV (as required) ± xylazine 0.25–0.6 mg/kg IV or IM (only use short term as prolonged use will result in CNS and respiratory depression)
  ▪ ± phenobarbital 12 mg/kg IV over 20 min followed by 6.0–9.0 mg/kg IV q. 8–12 h or 11 mg/kg PO q. 24 h.

Supportive and nursing care

▶ Place in large, well-bedded stable with good footing ± padded walls.
▶ Keep the area quiet and dimly lit ± place cotton wool earplugs (provided these do not cause distress).
▶ Keep feed and water easily accessible ± IV fluids and nutritional support (e.g. gruel fed via stomach tube).
▶ Appropriate nursing if recumbent (see p. 314).

Prognosis

▶ Mortality rates of around 60%.
▶ Long, costly treatment in more severely affected cases and full recovery can take weeks or months (due to irreversible binding of toxin, new nerve terminals have to grow).
▶ Indicators of likely poor prognosis:
  ▪ severe clinical signs at presentation
  ▪ rapid progression of clinical signs (<2 d between development of clinical signs and tetanic spasms)
  ▪ lack of any previous tetanus vaccination
  ▪ umbilical and uterine infections.

Botulism

Clostridium botulinum spores are found worldwide in soil and produce neurotoxins (usually types B and C). These neurotoxins bind to presynaptic membranes at the neuromuscular junctions, irreversibly blocking acetylcholine release and causing flaccid paralysis. Botulism in adult horses is usually due to ingestion in forage, e.g. spoiled hay or silage with pH >4.5. Toxico-infectious disease can occur in foals (Shaker foal syndrome, see p. 242).

Clinical signs

▶ Dysphagia.
▶ Excessive salivation.
▶ Weak tongue (Fig. 7.4), eyelid and tail tone.
▶ Exercise intolerance and muscular weakness.
▶ Progression to muscle tremors, carpal buckling and ataxia.
▶ Increased respiratory rate but shallow respiration – due to paralysis of intercostal muscles and diaphragm.
▶ Progression to recumbency.
▶ Death – respiratory muscle paralysis and cardiac failure.

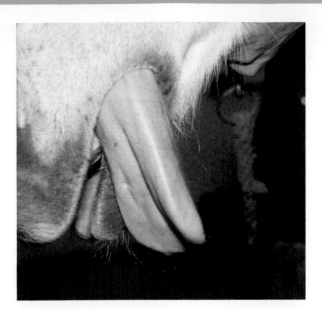

Figure 7.4 Tongue weakness in a horse with botulism.

Courtesy of Derek Knottenbelt.

Initial approach and diagnosis

▶ Obtain a full history. Specific questions that should be asked include:
  ▪ duration of clinical signs and progression
  ▪ clinical signs in other horses/animals on the premises.
▶ Perform a full clinical and neurological examination (see p. 128):
  ▪ toxins will affect the cranial nerves but not the CNS – ↑ suspicion in horse with symmetrical cranial nerve deficits but normal mentation.
▶ Diagnosis based on history and clinical signs:
  ▪ laboratory confirmation of diagnosis is difficult
  ▪ progression of neurological signs whilst the horse remains bright.

Treatment and prognosis

▶ Administer polyvalent antitoxin if available:
  ▪ may have little effect in severely affected animals.
▶ BS antimicrobials (vs aspiration pneumonia):
  ▪ avoid ones that may cause neuromuscular blockade, e.g. aminoglycosides.
▶ Nursing care as for recumbent horse (see p. 314).
▶ Prognosis depends on the amount of toxin absorbed and clinical signs evident:
  ▪ recumbency – poor prognosis
  ▪ mild clinical signs – can recover fully.

References and further reading

- De Pennington, N., Colles, C., Dauncey, E., 2011. Australian stringhalt in the UK. Vet. Rec. 169, 476.

- Furr, M., Reed, S., 2008a. Neurologic examination. In: Furr, M., Reed, S. (Eds.), Equine Neurology. Wiley Blackwell, Chichester, W Sussex, pp. 65–75.

- Furr, M., Reed, S., 2008b. Differential diagnosis of equine spinal ataxia. In: Furr, M., Reed, S. (Eds.), Equine Neurology. Wiley Blackwell, Chichester, W Sussex, pp. 95–99.

- Hahn, C., 2006. The wobbly horse: differential diagnoses. In Pract. 28, 8–13.

- Hahn, C., 2008. Common peripheral nerve disorders in the horse. In Pract. 30, 322–329.

- Hillyer, M., 2009 Head injuries and recumbency. In: Proceedings of the 48th British Equine Veterinary Association Congress, Birmingham, UK, 10–12 September, pp. 188–189 (also available via <http://www.ivis.org>).

- Johnson, A.L., 2010 How to perform a complete neurologic examination in the field and identify abnormalities. AAEP Proceedings, Baltimore, Maryland, vol. 56 pp. 331–337 (also available via IVIS at <http://www.ivis.org>).

- Kay, G., Knottenbelt, D.C., 2007. Tetanus in equids: a report of 56 cases. Equine Vet. Educ. 19, 107–112.

- Lacombe, V., Furr, M., 2008. Differential diagnosis and management of horses with seizures or alterations in consciousness. In: Furr, M., Reed, S. (Eds.), Equine Neurology. Wiley Blackwell, Chichester, W Sussex, pp. 77–93.

- MacKay, R.J., 2004. Brain injury after head trauma: pathophysiology, diagnosis and treatment. Vet. Clin. North Am. Equine Pract. 20, 199–216.

- Mitchell, E., Furr, M.O., McKenzie, H.C., 2006. Bacterial meningitis in five mature horses. Equine Vet. Educ. 18, 249–255.

- Mitchell, E., Furr, M.O., McKenzie, H.C., 2007. Antimicrobial therapy for bacterial meningitis. Equine Vet. Educ. 19, 316–323.

- Morresey, P.R., 2006. Management of the acutely neurologic patient. Clin. Tech. Equine Pract. 5, 104–111.

- Newton, S.A., 1998. Suspected bacterial meningoencephalitis in two adult horses. Vet. Rec. 142, 665–669.

- Nout, Y.S., Reed, S.M., 2005. Management and treatment of the recumbent horse. Equine Vet. Educ. 19, 324–336.

- Reed, S.M., 2007. Head trauma: a neurological emergency. Equine Vet. Educ. 19, 365–367.

- Schwarz, B., Piercy, R.J., 2006. Cerebrospinal fluid collection and its analysis in equine neurological disease. Equine Vet. Educ. 18, 243–248.

- Stewart, A.J., 2009. Ataxia. In: Robinson, N.E., Sprayberry, K.A. (Eds.), Current Therapy in Equine Medicine (sixth ed.). Elsevier, St. Louis, Missouri, pp. 609–614.

- Tennent-Brown, B.S., 2007. Trauma with neurologic sequelae. Vet. Clin. North Am. Equine Pract. 23, 81–101.

- Weese, J.S., 2009. Clostridial diseases. In: Robinson, N.E., Sprayberry, K.A. (Eds.), Current Therapy in Equine Medicine (sixth ed.). Elsevier, St. Louis, Missouri, USA, pp. 158–166.

Reproductive emergencies

These are common in the horse and are most frequently encountered in the mare, either immediately before, during or after parturition. Reproductive emergencies occur less frequently in male horses but are most common in colts and stallions. Many of these conditions have potential consequences for future fertility which may be of critical importance in high-value broodmares and breeding stallions. Complications that occur following castration and which require emergency management are covered in Ch. 14.

Approach to emergencies in the pregnant/postpartum mare

A variety of emergency situations may arise in the mare during pregnancy, parturition and the postpartum period. These are often related to the urogenital tract but can involve

Table 8.1 Common causes of complications during pregnancy, parturition and immediately postpartum

Complications during pregnancy/ parturition	Complications immediately postpartum
Haemorrhage	Retained foetal membranes
Colic	Colic
Uterine torsion	Perineal bruising and haematomas
Placentitis	Perineal lacerations
Prepubic tendon rupture	Rectovaginal fistula
Hydrops	Haemorrhage
Abortion	Vaginal lacerations
Dystocia	Partial uterine inversion
	Uterine prolapse
	Bladder prolapse/eversion
	Bladder rupture
	Rectal prolapse
	Postpartum eclampsia (lactation tetany)
	Mastitis

other organ systems, most commonly the GIT (Table 8.1). Certain clues may also indicate impending problems during pregnancy and parturition (Table 8.2).

Dystocia 🔊

This is relatively uncommon (1 and 10% of foalings) but is a true emergency where time is critical in delivering the foal before foetal hypoxia and subsequent death occurs. Most cases are a result of foetal malposture/skeletal deformities and, unlike in other species, foetal oversize is uncommon. The long neck and limbs of the foal, relatively limited space for manoeuvre and power of maternal contractions also present extra challenges. In addition to risking the life of both the foal and potentially the mare, trauma to the reproductive tract during correction of dystocia must be minimised if the mare's future fertility is to be preserved.

Advice to client

▶ If a velvety red bag (chorioallantois) is evident at the vulva (Fig. 8.1) this should be ruptured immediately with a clean pair of kitchen scissors and the foal delivered (stay on the telephone to guide them through this if they are inexperienced).
▶ If the foal is obviously malpresented (e.g. only a head or a head and one leg is visible) keep the mare walking until you arrive (to avoid further straining and the foal becoming more impacted into the pelvic canal).
▶ Get them to start organising transport if the mare might need to be taken quickly to clinic/ referral facilities.

Get there ASAP!

▶ Take a foaling kit with equipment/medications for dealing with dystocia and performing CPR on the foal (see p. 223).

Table 8.2 Normal pregnancy and parturition and indications for veterinary assessment

	Normal	Indications for veterinary assessment
Normal gestation	Variable depending on breed/ individual mare Usual range 332–342 d (average 335 d)	Vaginal discharge Premature lactation Sudden onset abdominal distension/change in abdominal wall contour Signs of colic
Parturition		
1st stage	Relaxation of the cervix and uterine contractions start Highly variable in duration Ends with rupture of the chorioallantois and expulsion of urine-like allantoic fluid	Very prolonged Signs of uterine contractions start then diminish/disappear
2nd stage	Forceful contractions and delivery of foal in 20–30 min	Appearance of allantochorion (red bag delivery) Obvious evidence of malpresentation, e.g. head and no limbs Foal not delivered in 20–30 min
3rd stage	Expulsion of foetal membranes Up to 3 h (average 1 h)	Foetal membranes not passed after 3 h

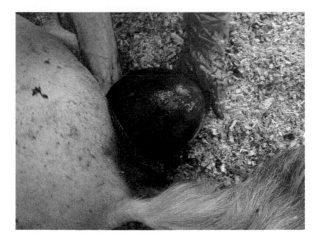

Figure 8.1 Premature separation of the chorioallantois ('red bag delivery').

▶ This must be rapid but thorough and should take no longer than 15 min – make a note of the time that you start examination or get someone to time it.
▶ Obtain a succinct history, including:
  ▪ when the mare was due to foal
  ▪ if she has foaled previously and if problems were encountered
  ▪ description of signs of labour seen and when they started
  ▪ duration of 2nd-stage labour
  ▪ any interventions already performed (e.g. by stud personnel).
▶ Perform a quick assessment of the mare's CV status:
  ▪ MM colour, HR, hydration.
▶ ± Sedate the mare if trying to get up and down/trying to kick (e.g. xylazine).
▶ Bandage the tail and clean the perineum with diluted antibacterial scrub solution.
▶ Put on rectal gloves or use ungloved hands provided they have been adequately cleaned (be as hygienic as possible).
▶ Check that the mare is appropriately restrained.
▶ Perform a brief vaginal examination to determine:
  ▪ any dryness/oedema of the vaginal wall (gives an idea of how long parturition has been progressing for)
  ▪ whether the mare's pelvic conformation is normal/abnormal.
▶ Determine whether the foal is still alive:
  ▪ obvious foetal movements, response to a stimulus or apex heart beat palpated over the thorax.
▶ Palpate the foal to determine the cause of dystocia:
  ▪ presentation (anterior/posterior/transverse)
  ▪ posture and position (normal/abnormal, what the problem is)
  ▪ twins/gross foetal deformities (Fig. 8.2).
▶ Attempt to deliver the foal if this can be performed quickly (e.g. simple repositioning of a limb).
▶ ± If the foal's nose is visible or palpable and the foal is still alive 'EXIT' (ex utero intrapartum treatment) can be attempted:
  ▪ 7–10-mm internal diameter cuffed endotracheal tube passed via the foal's nares into the trachea and ventilation initiated
  ▪ however it can be very difficult to perform unless experienced in using the technique (particularly ensuring that the tube is correctly positioned in the trachea) and may result in further delays in delivering the foal.
▶ Discuss possible options for correction as assessment is being performed – further decisions will be based on a number of factors, including: economics, hospital/referral facilities available and distance away, owner wishes, whether the foal is alive or dead and the health of the mare.

▶ There is no 'right way' for all dystocias to be corrected but sensible, quick decisions must be made.
▶ Even if the foal is already dead, the sooner it is delivered with least trauma, the better the prognosis for future fertility and for saving the mare's life.

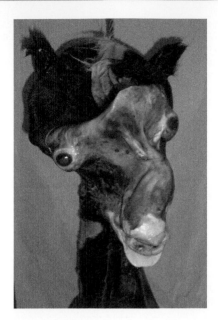

Figure 8.2 Gross foetal malformation requiring a Caesarean section to be performed in a mare that presented with dystocia.

Assisted vaginal delivery (AVD)

▶ Try this first if vaginal delivery is considered possible.

▶ If severe malformations/transverse presentation are evident, skip to Caesarean section/ embryotomy options.

▶ ± Administer sedation if required (NB will have effects on the foal's cardiovascular system if it is still alive).

▶ ± Administer clenbuterol 200 μg (for 500-kg horse) by slow IV or IM injection to ↓ uterine spasm.

▶ ± Perform epidural anaesthesia – this will take a little bit of time and does not completely eliminate straining (might be best to proceed to CVD/referral if straining precludes repositioning and delivery of a foal that is still alive).

▶ ± Pump additional lubrication into the uterus using a sterile stomach tube, stirrup pump and obstetric lubricant if the foal/inside of the uterus feels very dry.

▶ Place a head rope and apply ropes to both forelimbs just above the fetlocks (can also apply to both hind limbs in case of posterior presentations).

▶ If referral for Caesarean section is an option and the clinic is nearby, do not spend more than 10–20 min attempting this prior to getting the mare to the clinic.

Controlled vaginal delivery (CVD)

▶ This is where vaginal delivery is performed with the mare anaesthetised (reduces straining and aids repositioning of the foal) and ideally with the mare's hindquarters elevated (this is important but can be difficult to achieve outside clinic facilities).

▶ This may be an option where vaginal delivery is considered possible but AVD has failed.

▶ Decide if this should be performed at referral facilities (if nearby):

  ▪ CVD will be attempted there whilst the mare is being prepared for a Caesarean section.

- If referral is not an option or the foal is still alive but the referral facilities are a distance away (and the foal may have died anyway by the time the mare has arrived at the clinic), this can be performed on site.
- Once the mare is anaesthetised (see p. 361 for GA protocols) and the hindquarters elevated, proceed as for AVD.
- If still unsuccessful and the foal is alive, decide whether Caesarean section is an option (regardless of whether the foal is still alive by the time the mare arrives at the clinic).
- If the foal is dead, consider Caesarean section/embryotomy.

Caesarean section

- Consider immediately if it is obvious that vaginal delivery is impossible/likely to be very difficult.
- Even if the foal is dead, this may the best course of action where AVD has not been successful (unless experienced in performing embryotomy and this is considered likely to be quick and easy to perform).

Embryotomy

- Perform only if the foal is dead, you have suitable experience and equipment and where Caesarean section would not be a better alternative (if this is an option).
- Should require no more than 1–3 cuts – if not, severe trauma may be sustained to the mare's reproductive tract.
- If unsuccessful, consider Caesarean section/euthanasia.

If all else fails

- Can consider performing a terminal Caesarean section, e.g. if the foal is valuable/mare has existing health problems – need to consider the issues related to rearing an orphan foal (see p. 245):
  - anaesthetise the mare, deliver the foal via a midline incision and euthanase the mare immediately (unless willing to perform heroic surgery to save the mare's life in the field – likely to be unsuccessful unless you have suitable surgical expertise/the mare is small).
- Alternatively, perform euthanasia of the mare (and consequent euthanasia of the foal *in utero*).

Aftercare

- Assess the foal immediately following delivery and perform resuscitation if required (see p. 224).
- Repeat vaginal and uterine examination:
  - check for a second foal (highly unlikely but just in case….).
- Check for uterine or vaginal tears/invagination of the tip of the uterus (uterine tears can be very difficult to palpate).
- ± Assist delivery of the foetal membranes by administering low-dose oxytocin (5 IU IM) – ideally wait 1–2 h before administering, as the mare may show signs of colic if given before this.
- Can also perform chorioallantoic distension for removal of the membranes:
  - using a clean nasogastric tube, hold the exposed membranes tightly around the tube, infuse 12–15 L of warm water or sterile saline and tie off the opening with umbilical tape
  - the membranes are usually passed 5–30 min later.
- Treat as for RFM if the foetal membranes are not passed within 3 h (see p. 160).

Abortion/stillbirth

These may present as emergencies related to dystocia (see p. 154) or retained foetal membranes (see p. 160). Urgent investigation of the cause may be required, particularly if an infectious aetiology (e.g. EHV-1) is suspected/unproven to limit potential spread of disease and prevent further foetal losses in other pregnant mares (Table 8.3).

▶ Stillbirth (the loss of a full-term foetus/delivery of non-viable offspring after 310–320 d of gestation) is often related to complications that occur during parturition.

▶ Abortion (earlier foetal losses, most commonly occurring <day 40 or during the last few months of gestation) is usually associated with foetal infections or conditions affecting the foetal membranes.

Action following abortion/stillbirth of unknown cause

▶ Prevent further potential abortions:
  ▪ isolate the mare in the stable/paddock where she aborted
  ▪ move other mares to a clean paddock and keep in an isolated group until the cause is known.
▶ Obtain a general history. Specific information that should be obtained includes:
  ▪ any recent abortion/stillbirth in other mares on the premises
  ▪ any recent respiratory/neurological illness in other horses on the premises
  ▪ stage of gestation that abortion occurred
  ▪ any previous pregnancy losses
  ▪ illness during pregnancy
  ▪ general health in the few days prior to abortion/stillbirth.
▶ Perform a full clinical examination of the mare. Specific evaluation should include:
  ▪ reproductive examination – retention of twin foetus, RFM.

Table 8.3 Possible causes of abortion/stillbirth

Maternal	Infectious	Non-infectious
Age	*Viral*	Umbilical cord torsion
Endotoxaemia	EHV-1, rarely EHV-4	Excessively short umbilical cord
Uterine torsion	EVA	Twinning
Uterine artery rupture	*Bacterial/fungal*	Placental infarction
Body wall hernias	Ascending placentitis	Premature placental separation
	Haematogenous	Dystocia/delayed delivery/
	Atypical (nocardioform)	perinatal asphyxia
		Body pregnancy
		Fescue toxicosis
		Mare reproductive loss
		syndrome
		Congenital abnormalities
		Idiopathic

▶ Perform treatment if required – e.g. septic metritis (see p. 161).
▶ Investigate the cause:
  ▪ obtain a blood sample from the mare (serology)
  ▪ send the foetus and placental membranes to a suitable laboratory or perform assessment on site (see p. 388).
▶ Further action will depend on the results – rule in/out infectious cause and take appropriate action.

Retained foetal membranes (RFM)

This is a common postpartum complication, particularly subsequent to dystocia, abortion/stillbirth or Caesarean section. Failure to pass all the placenta within 3 h postpartum requires prompt treatment to prevent the development of metritis and subsequent laminitis.

Initial assessment

▶ Determine the duration of time since delivery of the foal and how much (if any) placenta has been removed or whether any of the placenta is missing (Fig. 8.3).
▶ Check tetanus status.
▶ Assess HR, evidence of digital pulses/warm hooves, check T°.
▶ If partial retention is suspected, disinfect the perineum, put on rectal gloves and perform examination of the uterus (remnants are usually retained at the non-gravid horn) – if

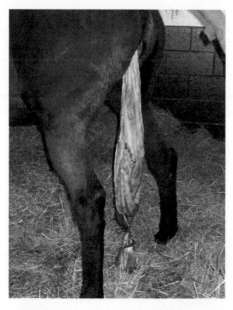

Figure 8.3 Retained foetal membranes in a mare following parturition.

Courtesy of Barbara Schmidt.

unsure, treat as for RFM, until the uterus involutes sufficiently to be able to palpate the tip of the uterine horns.

▸ Determine if there is evidence of concurrent metritis.

Treatment

▸ Do not forcibly extract the membranes:
  ▪ they usually tear and retained portions remain firmly attached
  ▪ this can also result in inversion of the tip of the uterine horn.
▸ Tie the placental remnants in a loose knot above the mare's hocks.
▸ If small pieces are retained at the tip of a uterine horn, can try to gently remove them.
▸ Administer oxytocin 10–20 IU IV or IM or as IV infusion (30–60 IU in 1L saline/LRS over 30–60 min).
▸ Administer tetanus toxoid/antitoxin if required (see p. 23).
▸ If the foetal membranes are still not passed in a further 2 h, re-administer oxytocin:
  ▪ can increase the dose by 10–20 IU every 2 h
  ▪ most will be passed after 1–2 doses.
▸ If retained beyond around 6 h:
  ▪ administer BS antimicrobials and NSAIDs
  ▪ treat as for metritis (next section).
▸ If still not passed within 12 h, try gentle traction and twisting to remove them.

Metritis

This is a common sequel following RFM that requires prompt, aggressive medical treatment to prevent the development of septicaemia, endotoxaemia and laminitis. Even if the metritis and septicaemia can be subsequently resolved, severe laminitis can have irreversible, life-threatening consequences.

Clinical signs

▸ Foul-smelling red/brown vaginal discharge.
▸ Pyrexia.
▸ Anorexia/depression.
▸ Congested (hyperaemic) MM.
▸ ± Bounding digital pulses, laminitic gait.

Initial assessment and treatment

▸ Assess the mare's MM, HR, T°, hydration.
▸ Check for evidence of ↑ digital pulses/laminitic gait and stance.
▸ Determine the severity of laminitis if evident (Obel grade – see p. 46).
▸ Administer BS antimicrobials – penicillin, gentamicin IV ± metronidazole.
▸ Administer flunixin 1.1 mg/kg IV.
▸ Administer tetanus toxoid/antitoxin if required (see p. 23).
▸ Start IV fluid therapy if required – consider hospitalisation/referral in severe cases.
▸ Lavage the uterus with warm, clean water or sterile saline/LRS:

- use a sterile nasogastric tube (ideally with several fenestrations at the side to prevent the end becoming blocked)
- clean the perineum first with diluted antimicrobial scrub and put on rectal gloves
- use a cupped hand to pass the end of the stomach tube into the uterus to prevent perforation of the uterus (the uterine wall may be inflamed and friable)
- Perform in 3–6 L flushes, siphon off the fluid and repeat until the retrieved fluids are clear

▶ ± Administer oxytocin to assist uterine involution.
▶ Initiate treatment for laminitis:
   - ice therapy of the feet (see p. 67)
   - foot support (see p. 46).
▶ Reassess and lavage the uterus q. 12 h until clinical signs have resolved.

> **KEY TIP**
> Check whether the foal is hungry and requires supplemental feeding (a mare's milk production may ↓ as a consequence of systemic illness).

Periparturient haemorrhage

This is more common in older, multiparous mares immediately after foaling, but can occur during late pregnancy. Haemorrhage usually originates from the uterine artery (less frequently from the ovarian or iliac arteries) and, if contained, e.g. within the broad ligament, may be self-limiting. However, if the haematoma ruptures or if there is free, uncontrolled haemorrhage into the abdominal cavity, the mare will collapse and die quickly. Intrauterine haemorrhage may also be seen. Surgical intervention is not usually practical or possible.

Clinical signs

▶ Mild/moderate signs of colic.
▶ Pale MM.
▶ Trembling.
▶ ± Sweating – feels cold.
▶ ± Distress, collapse, death.

Initial approach

▶ Minimise any stress to the mare – keep the foal nearby (unless the mare is close to collapse) and do not move her.
▶ Evaluate CV signs (MM, HR, pulse quality, warmth of extremities).
▶ ± Perform rectal examination:
   - if the mare is obviously tachycardic and has pale MM, the risk may outweigh any benefits
   - perform if unsure of the diagnosis, e.g. to rule out gastrointestinal causes of abdominal pain such as LCT
   - asymmetric swelling of broad ligament is palpable if haemorrhage is contained within it.
▶ ± Perform abdominocentesis if free haemorrhage into the abdomen is suspected (confirm blood within abdomen with a PCV that is the same as the systemic PCV).

▸ ± Transabdominal/transrectal US.
▸ Check the vulvar region for swelling and haemorrhage in case there is a dissecting haematoma along the vaginal wall (see p. 167) or uterine haemorrhage:
  ▪ uterine haemorrhage – usually self-limiting provided there is no uterine tear.

Stabilisation

▸ Can be difficult – each situation is different, based on presenting clinical signs, economics, facilities and expertise available.
▸ Have to balance the risks of expanding blood volume, ↑ BP and disturbing clot formation if fluid therapy is performed vs not doing anything if active haemorrhage is ongoing.
▸ If the mare is stable and has mild signs of haemorrhagic shock:
  ▪ conservative approach (extreme hypotension) may offer the best chance of survival
  ▪ keep in a quiet, darkened stable and with minimal disturbance
  ▪ ± minimal fluid therapy (see p. 186)
  ▪ ± administer oxytocin (postpartum mare) to ↓ the weight of the uterus 10–20 IU IV or IM
  ▪ administration of analgesia ± low-dose sedation if required.
▸ If haemorrhagic shock is evident or the mare is deteriorating rapidly, treat as for severe, ongoing haemorrhage (see p. 186).
▸ Monitor carefully, e.g. development of pyrexia that may indicate impending infection.

Uterine torsion

This is relatively uncommon but should be considered in a mare that is presented with signs of colic during the last trimester of pregnancy (8 months onwards). Occasionally uterine torsion may be associated with dystocia.

Clinical signs

▸ Depression.
▸ Occasional pawing, flank watching (moderate, intermittent colic).
▸ Only slight ↑ HR and ↑ RR.
▸ Normal GIT sounds.
▸ Dystocia (if occurs at time of foaling – uncommon).

Diagnosis

▸ Rectal examination:
  ▪ uterine ligament on the side of the rotation is pulled down and under the uterine body – the other one runs over the uterine body towards the side of rotation then downward
  ▪ rule out GIT cause of abdominal pain, e.g. large colon distension.
▸ Vaginal examination:
  ▪ check cervical tone and evidence of dilation/abnormal discharge
  ▪ uterine torsion usually occurs cranial to the cervix.
▸ ± Transabdominal US:
  ▪ assess foetal viability.

▸ This will be dictated by economics, availability of hospital/referral facilities, stage of pregnancy and foetal viability.

▸ If uterine torsion occurs at term and the cervix is dilated, manual correction via the cervix can be attempted.

▸ Consider referral for correction by ventral midline laparotomy (treatment of choice).

▸ Alternatively, a standing flank laparotomy can be performed (see texts).

▸ If surgery is not an option – can consider correction by rolling the mare under GA as a last resort (not recommended).

Uterine prolapse

Risk of this occurring is greatest following dystocia, RFM and abortion but it can occur after an apparently normal foaling. Uterine prolapse can also occur secondary to straining, tenesmus and colic and is more common in multiparous mares.

Clinical signs

▸ Oedematous uterus evident, extending from the vulva (sometimes to the ground; see Fig. 8.4).

▸ Mare may be recumbant/standing.

▸ ± Distress, shock.

▸ ± Rupture of uterine blood vessels, haemorrhage and death.

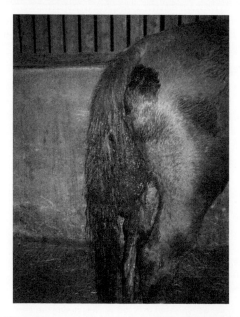

Figure 8.4 Uterine prolapse that occurred in a mare immediately following parturition.

Courtesy of Fiona Jones.

Advice to owner/carer over the telephone

▶ Keep the mare quiet and standing (if possible).
▶ Place the uterus in a clean, large plastic bag and elevate the uterus to the level of the vulva (can also use a board to keep the uterus elevated).

Initial assessment and treatment

▶ Quickly check the mare's HR, MM and pulse quality for evidence of haemorrhagic shock.
▶ Sedate the mare if required (depending on CV status, temperament and degree of pain).
▶ Administer NSAIDs – flunixin 1.1 mg/kg IV.
▶ ± Administer epidural anaesthetic (they can still strain).
▶ If the mare is fractious, strains excessively or becomes violently uncomfortable, consider GA.
▶ Bandage the tail and lavage the surface of the endometrium with warm water/saline.
▶ Confirm the diagnosis – DDx rectal prolapse, evisceration of intestine via a vaginal laceration, bladder prolapse or eversion.
▶ Remove any placental remnants not adhered to the uterine wall.
▶ Check for evidence of full-thickness tears – these should be repaired using absorbable suture material (3.5–4 metric).
▶ Check there is no involvement of bladder/GIT within the everted uterus – US can be helpful:
  ▪ if bladder, can drain with large needle and syringe
  ▪ intestinal involvement – exploratory laparotomy may need to be considered.
▶ It is best to replace the uterus within the abdomen on the premises rather than transporting to a clinic (risks additional tearing/uterine compromise).

Replacement of the uterus within the abdomen

▶ If possible, stand the mare on an incline with HQ slightly higher than the rest of the body.
▶ Apply obstetric lubricant over the uterus.
▶ Identify the everted tip of a uterine horn and, using a closed fist or the flat of the hand, kneed the uterus back through the vagina and through the cervical ring.
▶ Once the uterus has been replaced, distend the uterus with sterile saline (or clean warm water if economics dictate) and walk the mare (down a slope is ideal).
▶ Alternatively, fill a rectal sleeve with water, tie the end off and use it as a probe to push the uterine tip into its normal position.
▶ Check positioning of the uterus per rectum.
▶ Siphon fluid off and administer oxytocin 10–20 IU IV or IM.
▶ ± Place vulvar retention sutures (except ventrally) – 5 metric suture/umbilical tape, remove in 24 h.
▶ If unsuccessful, GA the mare, ideally hoist the HL and replace the uterus.
▶ If the prolapsed uterus cannot be replaced or there is evidence of severe systemic compromise in the mare, euthanasia is warranted (see p. 329).

> **KEY TIP**
> Take care to avoid damage to the uterine blood vessels during uterine repositioning as this may result in severe, potentially fatal haemorrhage.

▸ ± Fluid therapy if evidence of haemorrhagic/hypovolaemic shock (see p. 374).
▸ ± Check Ca^{2+} levels – if low/hypocalcaemia is considered likely, administer 40% calcium borogluconate by IV infusion (see p. 215).
▸ Continue NSAIDs.
▸ Administer BS antimicrobials.
▸ Check tetanus status.
▸ Monitor carefully for evidence of:
  ▪ discomfort, straining – risk of re-prolapse
  ▪ endotoxic shock/SIRS – uterine necrosis (obtain peritoneal fluid – see p. 341).
▸ Remove retention sutures 24 h later.
▸ Perform uterine lavage (± treat as for metritis see p. 161).
▸ Prognosis if the uterus can be replaced:
  ▪ good if no tears in the uterus and the uterine arteries have not been damaged
  ▪ very good for future fertility.

Uterine tears

These are usually sustained during parturition and may be detected during uterine palpation following correction of dystocia or affected mares may subsequently develop clinical signs consistent with peritonitis. Rarely uterine tears may occur in mares during late pregnancy following blunt trauma to the abdomen.

Initial diagnosis and treatment

▸ Assess as for peritonitis (see p. 75).
▸ If peritonitis is confirmed, and there is no cytological evidence of gastrointestinal rupture, a uterine tear is the most likely diagnosis.
▸ ± Perform hysteroscopy to evaluate the location and size of the tear (see texts).
▸ Small tears – medical management may be successful:
  ▪ NSAIDs, BS antimicrobials
  ▪ oxytocin 10–20 IU IV or IM q. 2 h – promote uterine involution
  ▪ ± fluid therapy.
▸ Large tears/no response to medical therapy in smaller tears – surgical exploration and repair indicated (consider referral/seek specialist advice).

Vaginal tears

These are more common in primiparous mares when sustained during normal parturition, or may occur following correction of dystocia or during mating. These should be considered where there is evidence of haemorrhage from the vagina or where signs consistent with peritonitis develop (see p. 75). If full-thickness tears are sustained in the peritoneal portion of the vagina, there is also risk of evisceration of intestine or prolapse of the bladder through the defect.

Initial assessment

▶ Perform a vaginal examination (± vaginoscopy):
- assess degree of haemorrhage ± ligate any obvious source of haemorrhage
- assess depth (full/partial thickness) and location (most are retroperitoneal) of tear
- if tear is ventral, pass a urinary catheter to check urethral integrity.

▶ Perform abdominocentesis (see p. 341).

Treatment

▶ If only partial thickness/extraperitoneal tears where there is no damage to the urethra, conservative management is indicated.

▶ If intestinal herniation occurs, assess intestine, clean and replace within the abdomen:
- if intestinal viability is in doubt – exploratory laparotomy/serial abdominocentesis is warranted (consider referral/seek specialist advice)
- repair the tear under sedation and epidural anaesthesia (see p. 362)
- 3.5/4 metric absorbable suture
- perform Caslick's procedure following repair.

▶ Alternatively can keep the mare cross-tied until the tear has healed.

▶ Administer NSAIDs, BS antimicrobials and check tetanus status.

▶ ± Perform serial abdominocentesis (intraperitoneal tears).

Perineal injuries

These are common, especially in primiparous mares or following delivery of a large foal, and range from perineal bruising to extensive tears.

▶ Differentiate a vaginal haematoma from more severe haemorrhage following rupture of larger uterine or vaginal arteries which can dissect along the vagina and exit at the vulva.

▶ Assess degree of laceration/evidence of rectovaginal fistula:
- first degree – involve mucosa of vestibule and skin of vulva
- second degree – involve vestibular mucosa, submucosa and extend into the muscularis of the perineal body
- third degree – complete disruption of the rectovestibular shelf (communication between vestibule and rectum) and anal sphincter
- rectovaginal fistula – as for third degree but there is no disruption of the anal sphincter.

▶ Check tetanus status.

▶ Initial conservative management is indicated (surgical repair immediately following injury usually results in dehiscence of the site):
- BS antimicrobials
- NSAIDs
- laxative diet ± oral administration of fluids/mineral oil.

▶ Surgical repair in around 6 weeks' time (except first-degree lacerations, which usually heal without surgical intervention).

▶ ± Drainage of a haematoma in 7–10 d if there is no significant reduction in size.

Mastitis

This is very uncommon and usually occurs after weaning or during lactation if the foal does not suckle normally. Mastitis is usually bacterial in origin (occasionally fungal infections can occur) but can be caused by trauma, frostbite or avocado poisoning.

Clinical signs

▸ Swollen, hot mammary gland that is painful on palpation.
▸ ± HL lameness, ventral oedema.
▸ DDx – abscess, oedema, trauma, neoplasia (US can be helpful).

Treatment

▸ Check the foal:
  ▪ rule out illness in the foal (if it has stopped sucking, mastitis may have been 2° to this)
  ▪ if the foal is healthy and is hungry and there is insufficient milk, supplemental feeding may be required (see p. 245).
▸ Sedate the mare.
▸ Clean the mammary gland.
▸ Try to obtain a sample of milk – submit for C&S and cytology.
▸ Administer NSAIDs.
▸ Administer BS antimicrobials for 5–7 d.
▸ ± Hotpacking, stripping (may be too painful).
▸ ± Infuse a lactating cow intramammary preparation into the gland at the end of the antimicrobial course.

Failure of milk letdown

▸ Agalactia – domperidone 1.1 mg/kg PO q. 12–24 h most commonly used agent.
▸ If adequate mammary development and milk supply – can give oxytocin 5–10 IU IV or IM and try to manually express milk to promote milk letdown.
  ▪ Acepromazine promotes milk let-down and anecdotally feeding the mare cocoa powder does too (see texts).
  ▪ Ensure the mare has free access to water.
▸ Check hydration status of foal and administer supplemental milk/fluid therapy if required.

Postpartum eclampsia (lactation tetany)

This is very rare and mares at greatest risk include those who are lactating heavily (especially Draft breeds but can occur in other breeds) and who have undergone recent stress, e.g. change in surroundings.

Clinical signs

▸ Restless,↑ RR, twitching, muscle tremors.
▸ Clonic spasms progressing to tonic spasms.
▸ Recumbency.
▸ DDx tetanus – 3rd eyelid is not prolapsed as in tetanus cases.

▶ Clinical signs.
▶ Confirm by Ca^{2+} measurement – hypocalcaemia.
▶ Treat as for hypocalcaemia (see p. 214).

Prepubic tendon rupture and body wall hernias

These result in an abrupt change in the contour of the abdominal body wall outline (Fig. 8.5) and in severe cases shock, haemorrhage and death may occur.

Clinical signs

▶ Abdominal discomfort – can be severe.
▶ ↑ HR, ↑ RR.
▶ Reluctance to move.
▶ Ventral oedema.
▶ Flattened mammary glands.
▶ Softening/pain on palpation of the body wall.
▶ Severe – colic, haemorrhage, shock and death.

Diagnosis and treatment

▶ Based on history and clinical signs.
▶ Differentiate from colic of gastrointestinal origin or hydrops conditions.
▶ ± Transabdominal US.
▶ Administer flunixin 1.1 mg/kg IV.
▶ If the degree of pain can be controlled, conservative management is indicated:
  ▪ box rest – keep in area with good footing
  ▪ ± large abdominal support bandage
  ▪ ongoing analgesia and foetal monitoring (see texts)
  ▪ ± IV fluid therapy.
▶ Euthanasia should be considered in severe cases where the degree of pain cannot be controlled.
▶ Warn the owner that tears/ruptures can suddenly and catastrophically deteriorate.
▶ Ensure the mare is closely monitored at parturition – assisted vaginal delivery will be required.
▶ Induction of parturition may be indicated if the mare's condition is deteriorating.
▶ If a live foal is successfully delivered, may need to provide nutrition for the foal – oedema around the mammary gland may prevent foal from suckling.
▶ Rebreeding is not recommended (can be used as embryo transfer donor mare).

Hydrops conditions

These are relatively uncommon but require emergency, prompt action to save the mare. Hydrops conditions usually occur during the last trimester of pregnancy and are most commonly related to excessive allantoic fluid accumulation (hydrops allantois). These conditions are usually progressive and few mares reach term and deliver a live foal. Rebreeding can be undertaken in these mares.

Clinical signs

▶ Sudden-onset abdominal distension.
▶ Progressive lethargy and inappetance.
▶ ± Dyspnoea, cyanotic MM.

Diagnosis and management

▶ Clinical examination to differentiate from body wall rupture/prepubic tendon rupture (see previous section) – sometimes these can occur as a result of hydrops or develop subsequently.
▶ Rectal examination:
  ▪ large fluid-filled uterus
  ▪ the foetus cannot be palpated due to the amount of fluid present.
▶ ± Transrectal/transabdominal US – confirm diagnosis.
▶ Induction of parturition is indicated where there is severe CV compromise of the mare/the mare's condition is deteriorating:
  ▪ place an IV catheter and set up IV fluids (sudden-onset hypovolaemia can develop once large quantities of fluid are released from the uterus)
  ▪ administer oxytocin 10 IU IV or IM initially q. 30 min (as little as 2.5 IU may be sufficient near term) – increase the dose if no response

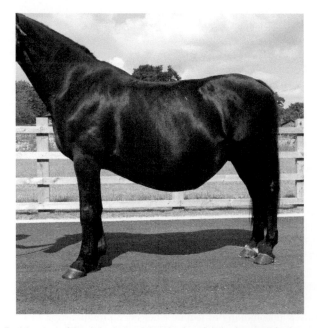

Figure 8.5 Partial rupture of the abdominal wall that developed during late gestation in a pregnant mare.

- remove foetal fluids using a sterile stomach tube once the foetal membranes have ruptured (may be a rapid expulsion of vast quantities of fluid – try to avoid)
- increase IV fluid rate to maintain the mare's systemic BP
- assist delivery of the foetus if required (as for dystocia)
- monitor CV system carefully
- treat any postpartum complications, e.g. RFM.

Trauma to the penis and prepuce

This is more common in colts/stallions and is usually a result of them trying to mount mares over fences, attempting to jump over stable doors to get to mares or being kicked during breeding when the penis is erect. Marked swelling develops quickly and haematomas and cellulitis can result. Any lacerations sustained are usually relatively superficial but occasionally can result in transection of the urethra.

Clinical signs

▶ Acute-onset preputial swelling.
▶ Paraphimosis in severe cases.
▶ ± Penile haematoma.
▶ ± Wounds to prepuce/penis.

Assessment and treatment

▶ Assess the degree of swelling/paraphimosis (Fig. 8.6).
▶ Assess any lacerations – depth and structures involved:
  - check that the urethra is intact (endoscopy of the urethra is indicated if this is unclear on clinical examination).
▶ Superficial lacerations – can be sutured if indicated (fresh/extensive) or left to heal by secondary intention.
▶ Deep lacerations/urethral laceration – surgical management under GA indicated.
▶ Monitor to ensure normal urination occurs.
▶ Treatment as for paraphimosis (see next section).

Penile prolapse, priapism and paraphimosis

Early treatment of these cases is required to prevent permanent penile paralysis. This is especially important in breeding stallions so that they can maintain their breeding function. Persistent penile prolapse from the effects of sedative drugs is more common than priapism (persistent penile erection). Both can progress to paraphimosis (inability to retract the protruded penis into the prepuce) if the penis is not replaced quickly within the prepuce. Paraphimosis can also develop following preputial trauma and other conditions causing dependent oedema.

Priapism

▶ Aim to replace and maintain the penis within the prepuce or, if not, keep it slung firmly against the body wall (see Fig. 8.7).

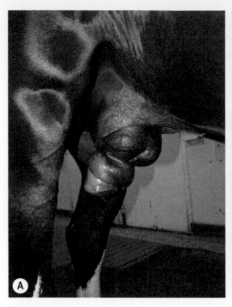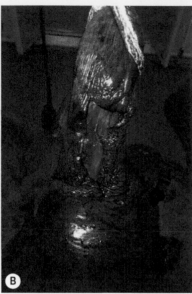

Figure 8.6   (A) Paraphimosis in a gelding. This can be secondary to trauma such as (B) a colt that sustained a penile laceration.

▸ Can GA the horse and try and apply a bandage tightly around the penis, starting at the glans and working towards the base of the penis to evacuate as much blood as possible prior to removing the bandage, pushing the penis back into the prepuce and suturing the prepuce closed temporarily.

▸ Flushing the corpus cavernosum penis with heparinised saline and creation of surgical shunts have been described – consider referral/see specialist texts.

Penile prolapse following sedation

▸ If the penis has not returned back into the sheath 30 min after the horse has recovered normal levels of alertness, push the penis back into prepuce.

▸ The penis can be kept inside the prepuce with a small soft towel/clean sock with a tennis ball inside it/soft paper towelling and the horse monitored closely – remove this every 30 min to check retractor penis muscle function and remove the packing temporarily if the horse postures to urinate.

▸ If this is not possible, sling the penis against the body wall, as for paraphimosis (Fig. 8.7).

Paraphimosis

Following swelling of the penis and internal lamina, the preputial ring becomes a constricting cuff, resulting in a vicious cycle of worsening oedema, exudation of fluid from exposed tissues, excoriation of the exposed epithelium, infection and cellulitis. Treatment involves controlling oedema and preventing further trauma:

▸ Retain the penis within the external preputial lamina using sutures/towel clamps.

▸ If this is not possible, sling the penis against the body wall – a pair of tights is a cheap, easy-to-fashion sling that allows the horse to urinate and can be changed daily (Fig. 8.7).

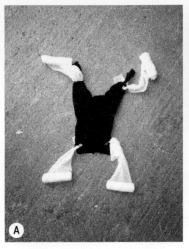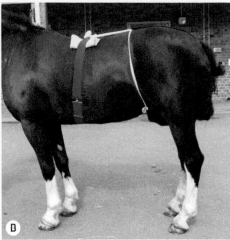

Figure 8.7 (A,B) Cut the ends off a large pair of tights, knot these ends; then thread knitted bandage through each corner and tie. This is a simple way to sling the penis/preputial tissues against the body wall, reducing development of further dependent oedema.

▸ Apply emollient cream (e.g. udder cream) to the exposed tissues.
▸ ± Massage and hydrotherapy.
▸ It can take 2–3 weeks for severe priapism to resolve fully.
▸ The prognosis is generally good if the penis is not permanently damaged/paralysed.

Inguinal herniation

This should always be ruled out in any stallion that develops acute, severe signs of colic. Inguinal herniation (also referred to as scrotal herniation) may occur following breeding/exercise and is reported to be more common in certain breeds, e.g. Standardbreds, draft breeds. Herniation usually involves small intestine and, unlike inguinal hernias in neonates, usually results in intestinal strangulation requiring prompt surgical treatment (Fig. 8.8).

Clinical signs

▸ Acute-onset moderate/severe abdominal pain.
▸ Scrotal enlargement.

Diagnosis

▸ Assess as for acute colic (see p. 59).
▸ Palpable scrotal enlargement.
▸ Palpation of small intestine entering the inguinal canal on rectal examination.
▸ US of scrotum – can see intestine sitting adjacent to spermatic cord and vaginal tunic.

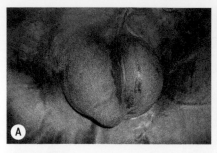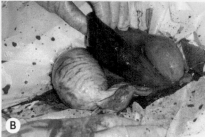

Figure 8.8 (A,B) Unilateral scrotal swelling in a stallion that presented with signs of colic. A loop of ischaemic small intestine can be seen adjacent to the testicle.

Treatment

▸ Referral for surgical management indicated.

Torsion of the spermatic cord

This is extremely uncommon but can cause colic and acute scrotal enlargement in stallions. Rotation of >360° results in congestion of the testicle and spermatic cord progressing to infarction. It is important to note that it is normal for the testicle to rotate 180°.

Diagnosis

▸ Enlargement of the affected testicle and spermatic cord and pain on palpation.
▸ Rule out inguinal herniation (more common cause of colic and scrotal swelling):
  ▪ rectal examination
  ▪ US of the scrotum.

Treatment

▸ Surgical management – unilateral castration and orchiopexy of contralateral testicle.

References and further reading

- **Arnold, C.E., Payne, M., Thompson, J.A.,** et al. 2008. Periparturient hemorrhage in mares: 73 cases (1998–2005). J. Am. Vet. Med. Assoc. 232, 1345–1351.

- **Boller, M., Fürst, A., Ringer, S.,** et al. 2005. Complete recovery from long-standing priapism in a stallion after propionylpromazine/xylazine sedation. Equine Vet. Educ. 17, 305–311.

- **Frazer, G.S.,** 2009. Postpartum complications in the mare. In: Robinson, N.E., Sprayberry, K.A. (Eds.), Current Therapy in Equine Medicine (sixth ed.). Elsevier, St. Louis, Missouri, pp. 789–797.

- **Frazer, G.S., Perkins, N.R., Embertson, R.M.,** 1999. Correction of equine dystocia. Equine Vet. Educ. 11, 48–53.

- **Lu, K.G., Barr, B.S., Embertson, R.,** et al. 2006. Dystocia – a true emergency. Clin. Tech. Equine Pract. 5, 145–153.

- **McDonnell, S.M.,** 2005. Managing the paralysed penis, priapism or paraphimosis in the horse. Equine Vet. Educ. 17, 310–311.

- **McGladdery, A.,** 2001. Dystocia and postpartum complications in the mare. In Pract. 23, 74–80.

- **MacPherson, M.L.,** 2003. Induction of parturition. In: Robinson, N.E. (Ed.), Current Therapy in Equine Medicine (fifth ed.). Elsevier, St. Louis, Missouri, pp. 315–317.

- **Palmer, J.E.,** 2009. Rescuing foals during dystocia. In: Robinson, N.E., Sprayberry, K.A. (Eds.), Current Therapy in Equine Medicine (sixth ed.). Elsevier, St. Louis, Missouri, pp. 848–850.

- **Parker, N.A., Howard, R.D., May, K.A.,** 2001. Severe scrotal pain associated with herniation of the testis and epididymis in an Arabian stallion. Equine Vet. Educ. 13, 172–174.

- **Riggs, E.,** 1996. Diagnosis and treatment of penile conditions in horses. In Pract. 18, 488–495.

- **Schumacher, J.,** 2012. Penis and prepuce. In: Auer, J.A., Stick, J.A. (Eds.), Equine Surgery (fourth ed.). Elsevier, St. Louis, Missouri, pp. p840–866.

- **Spirito, M.A., Sprayberry, K.A.,** 2011. Uterine prolapse. In: McKinnon, A.O., Squires, E.L., Vaala, W.E., Varner, D.D. (Eds.), Equine Reproduction (second ed.), vol. 2. Wiley Blackwell, Chichester, W Sussex, pp. 2431–2434.

- **Taylor, A.H., Bolt, D.M.,** 2011. Persistent penile erection (priapism) after acepromazine pre-medication in a gelding. Vet. Anaesth. Analg. 38, 523–525.

- **Vasey, J.R., Russell, T.,** 2011. Uterine torsion. In: McKinnon, A.O., Squires, E.L., Vaala, W.E., Varner, D.D. (Eds.), Equine Reproduction (second ed.), vol. 2. Wiley Blackwell, Chichester, W Sussex, pp. 2435–2439.

- **Wilkins, P.A.,** 2009. Complications in the peripartum mare. In: Robinson, N.E., Sprayberry, K.A. (Eds.), Current Therapy in Equine Medicine (sixth ed.). Elsevier, St. Louis, Missouri, pp. 785–788.

Urinary tract emergencies

These emergencies are relatively uncommon in the horse. Urinary tract involvement might not be immediately obvious as these cases may present with relatively non-specific clinical signs or where clinical signs are related to the urinary tract (e.g. abnormal urine colour), the primary disease process may be related to other organ systems.

Acute urine discoloration

A variety of conditions may cause acute change in the colour of urine to a red/black or brown colour. This may be an indication of other systemic disease and where haemoglobin or myoglobin is present, acute renal failure can develop unless prompt treatment is performed.

Possible causes of urine discoloration

▶ RBC.
▶ Haemoglobin.
▶ Myoglobin.
▶ Oxidising agents.
▶ Plant-derived pigments.
▶ Drug induced (rifampicin, phenothiazines, doxycycline).

> **HANDY TIP**
> Always ask if the urine was seen to be discoloured as the horse urinated – sometimes normal pigments within normal-looking urine can cause urine to turn red on exposure to snow/bedding materials (get a free catch urine sample to be sure).

Table 9.1 Ways in which haematuria, haemoglobinuria and myoglobinuria may be differentiated

Test	Haematuria	Haemoglobinuria	Myoglobinuria
Initial visual assessment	May see blood clots	Red/brown colour	Red/brown colour
Visual assessment after centrifugation of urine	Layer of RBC covered by clear urine	Urine remains discoloured	Urine remains discoloured
Microscopic examination of urine	Abundance of RBC/RBC 'ghosts'*	Absence of RBC	Absence of RBC
Visual assessment of serum	Normal	Evidence of pink tinge to plasma (haemoglobinaemia)	Normal
Serum biochemistry	Normal/abnormal (depends on underlying disorder)	Normal/abnormal Often increased bilirubin	Usually elevated CK (several thousand U/L)

*If there is a delay of more than 1–2 h assessing sample, RBC may haemolyse in urine – may see RBC 'ghosts' on microscopic examination.

Initial approach

▶ Obtain a full history. Specific questions that should be asked include:
  - when urine was first noticed to be abnormal/when LSN
  - frequency/amount of urination, straining during urination, ↑ water intake
  - any other abnormal clinical signs noted/recent illness
  - any current drug administration
  - any recent exposure to known urinary tract toxins (see p. 300).
▶ Perform a full clinical examination. Specific assessment should include:
  - assessment for evidence of another primary disease, e.g. severe myopathy (Fig. 9.1) or acute anaemia.
▶ Obtain a urine sample (ideally free catch/by catheterisation – if α2 agonists administered, urine must be obtained immediately due to subsequent dilution and glucosuria):
  - assess urine colour (normal/abnormal) – normal urine is pale–dark yellow and may be relatively viscous
  - look for obvious blood clots in the sample (haematuria).
▶ Obtain a blood sample and place in plain, EDTA, lithium heparin ± sodium citrate tubes.

Further investigation and treatment

▶ Perform further urinalysis within 30 min of sample collection – if not, keep in fridge (Tables 9.1, 9.2).
▶ Measure specific gravity – assess renal function (SG <1.020).

177

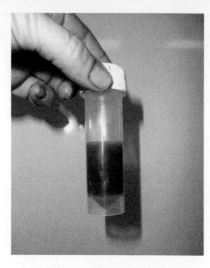

Figure 9.1 Myoglobinuria in a urine sample obtained from a horse with atypical myopathy.

Table 9.2 Potential causes for haematuria, haemoglobinuria and myoglobinuria

Haematuria	Haemoglobinuria	Myoglobinuria
Urolithiasis	Infectious disease (EIA, piroplasmosis, equine ehrlichiosis)	Exertional rhabdomyolysis
Neoplasia		PSSM
Urethral rents (gelding – haemospermia in stallions)	Toxic, e.g. red maple leaf, onions	Toxic drugs, e.g. monensin or plants (coffee senna/white snake root)
Urethritis (*Draschia/Habronema*)	Immune mediated (see p. 197)	
Bacterial cystitis		Atypical myopathy (see p. 56)
Pyelonephritis	Adverse drug reactions (see p. 267)	
Idiopathic haematuria (Arabs)		Immune-mediated myopathy
Verminous nephritis		
Blister beetle (cantharidin) toxicosis		
Chronic administration NSAIDs		
Vascular anomalies		
Secondary to purpura haemorrhagica/systemic bacterial toxins		
Bladder haematoma (neonatal foals)		

▶ Urine dipstick assessment for blood:
  ▪ negative – plant-derived pigments are most likely cause
  ▪ positive – due to presence of RBC/haemoglobin or myoglobin.

▸ Centrifuge urine sample:
- ▪ assess for layer of RBC (haematuria) or if discoloration remains after centrifugation (haemoglobinuria/myoglobinuria).
▸ Examine urine sample under microscope:
- ▪ check for presence of any casts, RBC or WBC
- ▪ large numbers of calcium carbonate crystals are common.
▸ Perform full haematology and serum biochemistry:
- ▪ check for evidence of myopathy (see p. 55) and rule in/out other systemic disease
- ▪ assess renal function (urea and creatinine).
▸ Assess serum for discoloration (Table 9.1).

Further assessment and treatment

If haemoglobinuria/myoglobinuria is diagnosed:

▸ Identify and treat underlying disease – see Table 9.2 for a list of possible causes.
▸ Start treatment as for ARF (see next section).

If haematuria is diagnosed:

▸ Determine if blood is seen at certain points during urination or if it is associated with exercise:
- ▪ start of urination – more likely to be distal urethra in origin
- ▪ end of urination – more likely to be proximal urethra/bladder neck in origin
- ▪ if only seen after exercise – most likely to be due to bladder calculus.
▸ Assess for any evidence of tenesmus/grunting at the end of urination.
▸ Perform rectal palpation ± US per rectum (5MHz linear transducer):
- ▪ assess size, thickness of bladder, urethra over pelvic brim and palpable masses
- ▪ determine whether there is evidence of a bladder calculus (usually small, intrapelvic bladder – hand only needs to be passed to wrist level)
- ▪ thickened material palpable in bladder may be indicative of sabulous cystitis (confirm by cystoscopy).
▸ Examine the vestibule and vagina in mares.
▸ Perform endoscopic assessment of the urethra and bladder and assessment of urine from each ureter (can catheterise separately) – see texts.
▸ US ± renal biopsy if haematuria evident in sample obtained from ureters (advanced procedure).
▸ Perform further urinalysis and urine culture:
- ▪ check for evidence of WBC in urine sample (normal is <5 WBC and RBC per high-powered field catheterised; <8 if free-flow)
- ▪ if UTI suspected, obtain urine sample by catheterisation and send for quantitative urine culture (UTI if >10 000 CFU/mL urine).
▸ Submit urine sample for cantharidin analysis if toxicosis suspected (geographic region).
▸ Assess PCV, TP and renal function (BUN, creatinine, electrolytes) and provide supportive therapy as required (see Acute blood loss, p. 186 and Acute renal failure, next section).
▸ Submit blood in EDTA and sodium citrate tubes for coagulation tests if nothing abnormal found on other tests to rule out clotting disorders (uncommon).

Acute renal failure (ARF)

Renal disease is less common in horses compared to other veterinary species. The presenting signs of renal failure may be relatively vague and non-specific and it may only be identified when serum biochemistry is performed. Where subtle signs of chronic renal failure have been present for a while and missed by owners, affected horses can present as an acute emergency when the kidney can no longer compensate (>70% nephrons compromised).

Pathogenesis

▸ ARF is usually due to decreased perfusion of the kidneys (pre-renal failure) or direct damage to the kidney itself (intrinsic renal failure), e.g. by toxins, or progressive renal damage as a result of pre-renal failure.

▸ Post-renal failure due to disruption of the lower urinary tract or urinary obstruction is relatively uncommon except for ruptured bladder in the neonate (see p. 243).

▸ Horses at high risk for acute renal failure (ARF) include:
  ▪ acute, severe illness causing hypovolaemia or endotoxaemia, e.g. colic, exhaustion, haemorrhage
  ▪ development of haemoglobinuria/myoglobinuria
  ▪ history of treatment with nephrotoxic drugs (aminoglycosides, NSAIDs).

Clinical signs

These are usually referable to the primary problem (e.g. acute rhabdomyolysis) and ARF may only be diagnosed after serum biochemistry has been performed.

▸ Depression and anorexia (rarely encephalopathy) due to uraemia.

▸ Oliguria/anuria/polyuria – variable in ARF.

▸ Dehydration.

▸ Tachycardia.

▸ Injected/hyperaemic MM.

▸ ± Mild colic.

▸ ± Evidence of chronic renal failure – oral ulcers, excess dental tartar, weight loss.

Initial assessment and diagnosis

▸ Take a full history. Specific questions that should be asked include:
  ▪ any recent administration of potentially nephrotoxic drugs (e.g. aminoglycosides, NSAIDs) or exposure to known nephrotoxins (see p. 300)
  ▪ recent illness
  ▪ evidence of altered water intake/urination.

▸ Perform a thorough clinical examination to rule in/out other systemic disorders.

▸ Take blood samples for haematology and serum biochemistry.

▸ Obtain a urine sample (free-flow or by catheterisation).

▸ Diagnosis of ARF confirmed by biochemistry and urinalysis:
  ▪ renal azotaemia (↑ BUN,↑creatinine)
  ▪ failure to concentrate urine (SG <1.020) in the face of azotaemia
  ▪ fractional urinary excretion of Na^+ (>1%)
  ▪ evidence of proteinuria, pigment and casts.

▸ Massive proteinuria and severe hypoalbuminaemia indicates a likely primary glomerular problem.

▸ For optimal care, hospitalisation/referral is required (see texts/seek specialist advice)

▸ IV or frequent oral fluid therapy is critical and can be performed where there are limited facilities if this is not an option (see p. 339, 374).

▶ If anuric/oliguric administer full rate bolus of Hartmann's solution/LRS (at least 10 L) and/or 2 ml/kg hypertonic saline then at least 2 x maintenance rates until creatinine decreases significantly (can take 2–3 d to reduce fully).

  ■ ± administer furosemide (1– 2 ml/kg IV) – only with concurrent fluid therapy
  ■ withhold nephrotoxic drugs
  ■ regularly monitor for signs of fluid volume overload and monitor PCV, TP, serum creatinine, electrolytes and urine volume and concentration.

▶ The prognosis depends on the underlying cause but is likely to be significantly worse if initial treatment is delayed.

Urinary tract obstruction

This is usually due to obstruction of the urethra by a urolith (calculus) and is more common in male horses. This may be mistakenly diagnosed as colic of gastrointestinal origin if careful clinical assessment is not performed; evidence of persistent penile protrusion and willingness to eat in a horse showing signs of colic should increase suspicion of a potential urinary tract obstruction.

Clinical signs

▶ Abdominal discomfort (colic).
▶ Frequent posturing to urinate but failure to pass urine.
▶ Persistent penile protrusion (Fig. 9.2).
▶ Constant dripping of urine.

Initial approach

Obtain a general history. Specific questions that should be asked include:

▶ Duration of signs or when LSN.
▶ Evidence of any prior haematuria.

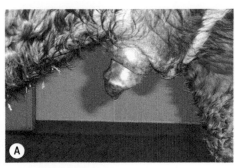
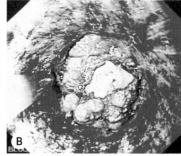

Figure 9.2 Urethral calculus in a horse. (A) The horse presented with signs of colic, which was suspected to be gastrointestinal in nature – evidence of persistent penile protrusion, constant dripping of urine and a distended bladder on rectal examination indicated that a urinary tract obstruction was more likely; this diagnosis was confirmed by failure to pass a urinary catheter and (B) endoscopic examination of the urethra.

Perform a general clinical examination. Specific assessment should include:

▶ Elevate the tail and look for distension of urethra below anus – often there is moderate/severe distension if the obstruction is distal to this.

▶ ± May be able to palpate obstructing mass percutaneously.

Carefully check the sheath and urethral fossa for smegma accumulations/maggot infestation – these can cause altered urination/discomfort. 🔲

Perform a rectal examination:

▶ Rule out any distension of gastrointestinal viscera as a cause of colic.

▶ The bladder will be turgid and full.

Pass a urinary catheter:

▶ Suspect an obstruction if a catheter cannot be passed into the bladder and urine obtained (measure catheter at the point where it cannot be passed further to get a rough idea of the level at which the obstruction has occurred).

Further evaluation and treatment

▶ Confirmation of diagnosis by endoscopy – direct visualisation of site of obstruction.

▶ Surgical removal – depends on location of obstruction (hospitalisation/referral indicated).

▶ Laser/electrohydraulic lithotripsy may be indicated if suitable equipment is available.

▶ Can progress to bladder rupture.

Bladder eversion

This is uncommon but can occur in mares following excessive straining, e.g. dystocia, retained foetal membranes (Fig. 9.3).

Clinical signs

▶ Bladder is everted via urethra (DDx bladder prolapse, 'red bag' delivery see p. 154).

▶ Visualisation of exposed bladder mucosa and ureteral openings.

▶ Urine can be seen dripping from the surface.

Treatment

▶ Replacement of the bladder (see texts/seek specialist advice).

▶ Consider hospitalisation/referral – can perform in the field if this is not an option.

▶ Sedation and administration of epidural anaesthetic (see p. 362).

▶ Cleanse surface with sterile saline/LRS and repair any tears.

▶ Check that no herniated intestinal contents are present within the bladder (US useful).

▶ Resect part of the bladder wall if localised necrosis is evident.

▶ Manually replace the bladder into its correct anatomic position:

  ▪ ± incise urethral sphincter to replace and suture afterwards

▶ Place a Foley catheter, lavage the bladder and confirm successful replacement (rectal examination).

Aftercare

▶ BS antimicrobials.

▶ NSAIDs.

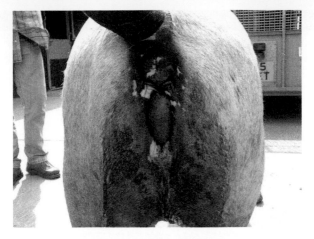

Figure 9.3 Bladder eversion in a mare.

Courtesy of Fernando Malalana.

▶ Check tetanus status.

▶ Treat underlying cause of straining.

Bladder displacement/prolapse

This is rare and usually causes urinary obstruction. In mares the bladder can be forced up through a vaginal laceration and is usually secondary to repeated straining. It is very rare in males but scrotal herniation of the bladder has been reported.

Clinical signs

▶ Serosal surface of the bladder can be seen (if via tear).

▶ DDx – bladder eversion.

▶ Bladder rapidly becomes distended with urine.

Diagnosis and treatment

▶ Surgical intervention depends on location of the bladder and adjacent structures involved – seek specialist advice/referral.

▶ If the bladder is prolapsed through a vaginal tear, correction can be performed under standing sedation and epidural anaesthesia.

▶ May need to drain urine from the bladder via a needle first prior to replacing bladder in its correct position.

▶ Treatment of vaginal laceration by suturing if possible (see p. 166).

▶ Assess and treat the underlying cause of any straining, e.g. colic, retained foetal membranes.

▶ Aftercare:

  ▪ BS antimicrobials

  ▪ NSAIDs

  ▪ check tetanus status.

Ruptured bladder

▶ Uncommon in adults – more frequent in foals (see p. 242).

▶ Can occur after foaling, subsequent to urinary tract obstruction (e.g. urolithiasis, penile haematoma) or following blunt abdominal trauma.

▶ Diagnosis similar to bladder rupture in the neonatal foal:
  ▪ vague initial presenting signs – anorexia, lethargy, pollakiuria/anuria
  ▪ azotaemia – ↑ BUN, ↑ creatinine
  ▪ altered serum electrolytes ↓ Na^+, ↓ Cl^-, ↑ K^+.

▶ Confirmation by:
  ▪ abdominal US – ↑quantities of hypoechoic fluid identified
  ▪ abdominocentesis – peritoneal:serum creatinine ratio >2:1
  ▪ endoscopic examination of the bladder – identification of defect.

▶ Treatment – surgical repair (seek referral/specialist advice).

Acute-onset urinary incontinence

▶ Urine is seen to be passed without the horse posturing to urinate.

▶ A large bladder is usually palpable on rectal examination and urine is made to overflow easily when pressure is placed on the bladder.

▶ Acute-onset incontinence may be associated with:
  ▪ dystocia/recent foaling – damage to urethral sphincter
  ▪ neurological illness (see Ch. 7)
  ▪ musculoskeletal problems (see Ch. 3)
  ▪ sabulous cystitis.

▶ Treatment depends on underlying cause (see relevant sections/texts).

References and further reading

• **Almy, F.S., LeRoy, B.E., Barton, M.H.,** 2009. Clinical pathology of renal disease. In: Robinson, N.E., Sprayberry, K.A. (Eds.), Current Therapy in Equine Medicine (sixth ed.). Elsevier, St. Louis, Missouri, pp. 748–752.

• **Edwards, G.B.E., Archer, D.C.,** 2011. Urolithiasis. In Pract. 33, 2–10.

• Geor R.J. Acute renal failure in horses. Vet. Clin. North Am. Equine Pract. 23, 577–591.

• **Schmitz, D.G.,** 2007. Toxins affecting the urinary system. Vet. Clin. North Am. Equine Pract. 23, 677–690.

• **Schott II, H.C., Woodie, J.B.,** 2012. Bladder. In: Auer, J.A., Stick, J.A. (Eds.), Equine Surgery (fourth ed.). Elsevier, St. Louis, Missouri, pp. 927–939.

• **Schumacher J.** Hematuria and pigmenturia of horses. Vet. Clin. North Am. Equine Pract. 23, 655–675.

Cardiovascular emergencies

Cardiovascular emergencies are generally less common in horses compared to other species. Presenting signs include severe haemorrhage, dyspnoea, collapse and occasionally sudden death or less specific signs such as lethargy and weakness.

Cardiac arrest

This may occur following destabilisation of a cardiac dysrhythmia or following drug administration, e.g. during anaesthesia or following accidental intracarotid injections (see p. 270). In reality, outside clinic facilities, treatment options are relatively limited and where cardiac arrest has occurred due to a primary cardiac problem, resuscitation is often unsuccessful. Resuscitation is more likely to be effective in drug-induced cardiac arrests and in the foal immediately following parturition (see p. 223). For details of resuscitation of anaesthetised horses in clinic facilities, see specialist texts.

CPR of adult horses/ponies

1. Check if a pulse is present and auscultate the heart – if there is no heartbeat (asystole), start CPR immediately.

2. Make a note of the time.

3. Start the ABCD of resuscitation:

Airway

• Insert a nasotracheal tube (if available).

• Perform a tracheotomy if a URT obstruction is suspected.

Breathing

- If oxygen with demand valve/anaesthetic machine is available, start ventilation (4–6 breaths/min).
- If only oxygen and tubing are available, start intranasal oxygen at 10–15 L/min and occlude the other nostril and mouth.

Circulation

- Start chest compressions – stand on the sternal side of the chest (be careful as this is a dangerous place to be if a horse starts to kick vigorously).
- Use your knees (hands only if small pony) to deliver 60–80 chest compressions/min – this is very tiring and requires a team of people doing this for 1–2 min each.

Drugs

- Administer adrenaline 0.01–0.02 mg/kg IV (up to 0.2 mg/kg) *followed by at least 50–100 mL of sterile saline/LRS in order for it to reach the myocardium* (this is very important) and continue CPR attempts.
- Volume of 1:1000 adrenaline = 1 mg/mL to administer.

300 kg	400 kg	500 kg	600 kg
3 mL	4 mL	5 mL	6 mL

4. Place an IV catheter while resuscitation is continuing and start fluid therapy.

5. Other drugs should not be administered unless an ECG is available (if so treat any dysrhythmias as appropriate).

6. Re-evaluate whether there is a heart beat/evidence of PLR every 1–2 min.

7. Adrenaline can be administered every 3 min.

8. If there is no response after 15 min, stop CPR efforts – the horse is unlikely to survive even if subsequently resuscitated.

Severe haemorrhage

The origin and severity of haemorrhage may be obvious where external blood loss has occurred (Table 10.1). However, where internal haemorrhage occurs, diagnosis and control of haemorrhage may be more challenging. A 500-kg horse has a circulating blood volume of around 45 L (around 80–90 mL/kg or 8–9% of their body weight). Healthy horses can cope with acute loss of 15–25% of their blood volume and in the short term can even survive losses of up to 40% of total blood volume (but need urgent fluid therapy). The aim is to identify and control haemorrhage where possible and provide cardiovascular support where required.

Clinical signs

▶ ± External haemorrhage.

▶ ↑ HR, ↓ pulse quality, ↓ CRT.

▶ Altered MM colour – pale.

▶ Cool extremities.

▶ ± Epistaxis (respiratory tract haemorrhage).

▶ ± Abdominal pain (intra-abdominal haemorrhage).

▶ ± ↑ RR/dyspnoea (intrathoracic haemorrhage).

Table 10.1 Possible causes of severe haemorrhage

Trauma	Laceration/rupture of vein or artery
	Laceration/rupture of spleen/liver/heart/lung/pregnant uterus
	Muscle rupture
	Fractures
Pregnancy/parturition	Rupture uterine/vaginal arteries
	Umbilical cord haemorrhage and rib fractures in foals (see p. 239)
Spontaneous/idiopathic	Guttural pouch mycosis (see p. 99)
	Aortic/pulmonary artery rupture/aortocardiac fistula
	Mesenteric vessel rupture
	Rupture of neoplastic mass
	Severe EIPH/pulmonary haemorrhage (see p. 103)
	Severe clotting disorders (secondary to DIC/other underlying coagulopathy)
Iatrogenic	Trauma to ethmoturbinates (see p. 264)
	Haemorrhage post-castration (see p. 265)
	Haemorrhage at surgery site, e.g. enterotomy/ovariectomy/hysterotomy

▶ ± Swelling around large muscle masses (e.g. long bone fracture that has lacerated an adjacent large blood vessel).

▶ ± Trembling and sweating.

▶ ± Bradycardia, collapse and death – ongoing, untreated severe haemorrhage.

Advice to the owner/carer

▶ Apply external pressure directly to the site if possible/safe to do so.

▶ Keep the horse quiet and do not move it unless it is in imminent danger.

▶ Warn the owner that the horse may collapse and can behave violently if severe haemorrhage is ongoing – ensure human safety and, if possible, confine to a safe area.

Initial first aid

▶ Immediately clamp/ligate an obvious source of haemorrhage or pack the site with one or more sterile gauze bandages.

▶ Assess the surroundings to get a rough idea of how much blood has been lost (where external haemorrhage has occurred).

▶ Determine whether the horse is showing signs of cardiovascular shock (HR >60 beats/min, ↑ RR, poor arterial pulse quality, ± pale MM).

▸ Obtain an EDTA blood sample for assessment of PCV/TP – this will act as a baseline measurement (note: PCV/TP values will not change immediately in acute haemorrhage).
▸ Obtain a succinct history about the events leading up to development of clinical signs, the signalment of the horse and any recent illness:
  ▪ traumatic incident – what happened, if the impact was seen, where on the body this occurred
  ▪ older stallions – consider aortocardiac fistula
  ▪ late pregnancy/immediately postpartum in multiparous mare – consider uterine/vaginal artery rupture (see p. 162)
  ▪ previous episodes of epixtaxis in the preceding days/weeks – consider GPM (for Assessment of epistaxis, see p. 97)
  ▪ recent castration (see p. 265).
▸ Perform a thorough clinical examination to determine the origin of haemorrhage if this has not been identified so far.

If the source of haemorrhage has been identified and haemorrhage controlled:
▸ Determine whether fluid therapy is required and the type of fluids that should be administered:
  ▪ 10–15% blood loss (around 4–6 L in a 500-kg horse) – crystalloids (e.g. LRS)
  ▪ 15–25% blood loss (6–11 L in a 500-kg horse) – colloids
  ▪ >25% blood loss (>11 L in a 500-kg horse) – whole blood (see p. 376).
▸ Administer intranasal oxygen if the horse is in severe CV shock (10–15L/min) and place an IV catheter prior to starting fluid therapy (see p. 374).
▸ Where a blood transfusion is required, colloid therapy can be initiated until blood has been obtained.

If the source of haemorrhage has not been identified and controlled:
▸ If the horse is very anxious but is not showing evidence of cardiovascular shock (HR <60 beats/min, good pulse quality), administer acepromazine 0.02 mg/kg IV to ↓ BP and reduce anxiety:
  ▪ do not administer if the horse is in CV shock, as the reduction in BP will precipitate collapse.
▸ Do not move the horse or induce stress (avoid ↑ BP).
▸ Administer intranasal oxygen (if available) 10–15L/min.
▸ Administer analgesia to control signs of pain if evident (not α2 agonist).
▸ ± Administer tranexamic acid 5–25 mg/kg slow IV/IM/SC or aminocaproic acid 20–40mg/kg IV diluted 1:9 in saline and given over 30–60min (see texts/website).
▸ If a traumatic episode preceded haemorrhage, check for other injuries, including neurological signs associated with trauma to the head, possible limb fractures/synovial structure involvement in lacerations to the legs and penetrating injuries to the abdominal/thoracic cavities (see relevant sections).
▸ Further diagnostic tests will be based on the likely source of haemorrhage (history, findings on further diagnostic tests).
▸ Abdominal haemorrhage suspected:
  ▪ rectal examination
  ▪ abdominocentesis (see p. 341)
  ▪ abdominal US (see Fig. 10.1/website).
▸ Thoracic haemorrhage suspected:
  ▪ auscultation and percussion
  ▪ ± pleurocentesis (see texts/website)

- ± thoracic US
- ± radiography.

▶ Upper limb haemorrhage suspected:
  - visual assessment for muscle/pelvic asymmetry
  - rectal palpation (pelvis)
  - US
  - ± radiography.

Further assessment and treatment

▶ Reassess the horse's cardiovascular signs and determine whether there is evidence of continued haemorrhage or if the horse's condition remains relatively stable:
  - PCV/TP will not change for 4–6h following the start of haemorrhage and will not stabilise until 24h after haemorrhage has stopped
  - PCV/TP will then start to increase after 4–6d
  - systemic lactate measurement is a good way of assessing peripheral perfusion.

▶ Where there is evidence of ongoing haemorrhage that cannot be controlled and there is a traumatic aetiology, referral for potential surgical investigation should be considered (contact referral facility asap to discuss).

▶ If there is no history of trauma, surgical intervention is less likely to be required (except in certain conditions e.g. GPM) – stress should be avoided if the source of haemorrhage has not been identified and controlled in these cases (e.g. transport).

▶ In cases of ongoing haemorrhage the risks associated with conservative management on site has to be weighed against the benefits of hospitalisation for more regular monitoring and treatment – seek specialist advice if necessary.

▶ The risks of performing aggressive fluid therapy (which may result in ↑ BP and may restart haemorrhage if it has abated) have to be weighed against the detrimental effects of hypovolaemia and subsequent sequelae (e.g. compromised renal function).

▶ Do not drain blood from body cavities unless essential (e.g. marked respiratory distress).

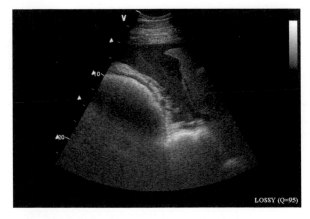

Figure 10.1 Transcutaneous US evaluation of the abdomen of a horse that had sustained blunt trauma to the region. Large quantities of fluid material of mixed echogenicity that had a 'swirling' appearance were identified, consistent with blood (haemoperitoneum).

Courtesy of Fernando Malalana.

189

▶ Ideally, aim to keep BP 60 mmHg (mean arterial pressure (MAP)), systolic <90 mmHg – this is impractical to measure in most situations, so can administer IV fluid (crystalloids) at 2–3 mL/kg/h until haemorrhage stops.

▶ ± Administer blood/plasma (can perform autotransfusion too – see texts).

> **HANDY TIP**
>
> Simple assessment of haemostasis (clotting function) can be performed by obtaining a sample of venous blood, placing it into a plain blood tube and keeping it at body temperature. Normal blood should clot within ~5–7 min (investigate further if >10 min).

Cardiac dysrhythmias

Cardiac dysrhythmias (arrhythmias) are frequent in the horse and may be clinically significant (pathological) or not (physiological). In general many bradydysrhythmias are physiological and occur in normal horses (due to high resting vagal tone) and will disappear after exercise or when excited. Dysrhythmias can also be transient, e.g. horses with colic. In general, most tachydysrhythmias are pathological and may cause collapse at rest or exercise or result in sudden death (see p. 326) (Table 10.2).

Initial assessment

▶ Take a general history. Specific questions that should be asked include:
- whether a heart murmur or abnormal rhythm has previously been identified
- any recent illness or current medication
- recent signs of collapse or exercise intolerance
- potential ingestion of ionophores (e.g. monensin).

▶ Assess the horse's general demeanour and perform a full general clinical examination:
- determine whether there is a potential non-cardiac problem (Table 10.3) or whether this can be ruled out
- consider whether systemic disorders that may cause myocardial failure are present (Table 10.4).

▶ Measure the HR:
- normal, ↓ or ↑.

Table 10.2 Dysrhythmias that may occur in the horse

Bradydysrhythmias	Tachydysrhythmias
2° AV block (physiological)	Supraventricular premature polarisations and tachycardia
Advanced 2° AV block	
Complete 3° AV block	Atrial fibrillation
Sinus bradycardia, sinus arrhythmia, SA block/SA arrest (physiological)	Ventricular pre-excitation
	Ventricular premature depolarisation
Sick sinus syndrome	Ventricular tachycardia

Table 10.3 Cardiac and non-cardiac causes of dysrhythmias

Cardiac	Non-cardiac
Valvular disease	Electrolyte and fluid imbalances, e.g. colic, exhaustion
Congenital defects	
Pericardial disease	Hypoxia
Myocardial pathology:	SIRS, septicaemia, endotoxaemia
– myocarditis	Drug induced
– monensin toxicity	Altered catecholamines/autonomic tone
– myocardial ischaemia/fibrosis	
– cardiomyopathy	
– neoplasia	

Table 10.4 Potential causes of myocardial failure

Viral	EHV-1 (see p. 284)
	EI (see p. 283)
	AHS (see p. 280)
	Mobilivirus
Bacterial	Streptococcal infections
Parasitic	Piroplasmosis
Toxic	Ionophores
	Snake envenomation (e.g. rattlesnakes, see p. 304)
	Plants (see Ch. 16)
	Cantharidin (blister beetle)
	Rodenticides (sodium fluoroacetate)
	Atypical myopathy
Neoplasic	Haemangiosarcoma
	Lymphosarcoma
	Melanoma
	Mesothelioma
Nutritional	Vitamin E/selenium deficiency
	Copper deficiency
	Excess molybdenum/sulphites
Genetic	Glycogen branching enzyme deficiency
Idiopathic	Dilated cardiomyopathy, amyloidosis

Adapted from Marr (2010).

▶ Characterise the heart rhythm:
- regular
- regularly irregular
- irregularly irregular.

▶ Assess peripheral pulse quality and whether synchronous with the heart beats.

▶ Examine jugular and saphenous veins for distension ± pulsation.

▶ Auscultate the heart:
- ID heart sounds (S1, S2 ± S3, S4)
- determine whether any cardiac murmurs are present and characterise these (intensity/ timing/duration/PMI/radiation of sounds).

▶ Auscultate lungs ± with rebreathing bag (caution in cases with HF/tachypnoea).

Initial treatment

▶ If a concurrent non-cardiac cause is suspected, initiate treatment for this accordingly.

▶ If the horse is in HF, provide emergency stabilisation (see below).

▶ Do not administer any specific antidysrhythmic agents without first obtaining a diagnosis by performing an ECG.

▶ In an emergency magnesium sulphate (which has some antidysrhythmic properties even if systemic Mg^{2+} is normal) can be administered – 4 mg/kg IV give slowly q. 2 min, not to exceed 50 mg/kg total dose.

Further investigation and treatment

▶ Perform ECG to characterise dysrhythmia (see texts/website):
- this should be performed asap in horses with evidence of HF/distress/recent collapse
- +ve electrode (LA) over apex of heart
- −ve electrode (RA) on right jugular groove
- earth (LL) placed anywhere
- lead I, 25 mm/s, 10 mm/mV.

▶ ± Echocardiography.

▶ Measure electrolytes, serum biochemistry – including cardiac troponin I.

▶ Specific antidysrhythmic therapy may be required and is specific for each dysrhythmia.

▶ Identification and treatment of myocarditis.

Heart failure

This occurs when abnormal cardiac function results in failure of the heart to fill with or eject sufficient quantities of blood to meet the metabolic requirements of the body. Horses have a large cardiac reserve, so cardiac disease may have been present for some time (and owners may have missed subtle abnormalities) until overt signs of heart failure (HF) develop and the horse is presented as an emergency. In other instances a well-tolerated cardiac problem such as mitral valve insufficiency may acutely deteriorate due to rupture of a chorda tendinae, causing cardiac decompensation and rapid development of HF.

These largely depend on whether heart failure results in reduced cardiac output (usually left-sided heart failure) or circulatory congestion (usually right-sided heart failure) (see Tables 10.5, 10.6).

Table 10.5 Clinical signs of heart failure that arise due to reduced cardiac output or circulatory congestion

Reduced cardiac output	Circulatory congestion
↑ HR	*Congestion of the pulmonic circulation*
Weakness	↑ RR
Exercise intolerance	Dyspnoea
Pale MM	White/pink-tinged frothy nasal discharge (pulmonary oedema)
↓ Arterial pressure	
Ataxia	± Coughing (rare)
Syncope	*Congestion of the systemic circulation*
Weight loss	Generalised venous distension
Cold extremities	Jugular pulsation > lower ⅓ neck
	Peripheral oedema – ventrum, prepuce, muzzle, limbs

Table 10.6 Cardiac lesions that may result in the development of heart failure

Signs of left-sided heart failure/both sides predominate	Signs of right-sided heart failure predominate
Congenital cardiac disorders	Congenital cardiac disorders
Mitral valve insufficiency	Pericarditis/pericardial effusion
– ruptured CT	Tricuspid valve insufficiency
– endocarditis	– rupture of CT
– degenerative lesion	– endocarditis
– secondary to dilation of valve annulus	– degenerative lesions
Aortic valve insufficiency	Pulmonic valve insufficiency
– severe degenerative lesions	– rupture of valve leaflet
– endocarditis	– degenerative lesion
– ruptured valve leaflet	
Myocardial disease	
– myocarditis	
– myocardial fibrosis/ischaemia	
– dilated cardiomyopathy	

Approach

▸ Obtain a general history. Specific questions that should be asked include:
  ▪ any recent illness
  ▪ history of prior cardiac disease, e.g. murmur previously identified
  ▪ signalment – consider ventricular septal defect in a young TB/Welsh pony
  ▪ any evidence of recent exercise intolerance/lethargy
  ▪ any current medications/recent drug administration or ingestion of toxins.
▸ Perform a thorough clinical examination:
  ▪ consider differential diagnoses for non-cardiac causes of peripheral oedema (e.g. neoplasia, protein-losing enteropathy), lung disease (e.g. pneumonia) and ↓ cardiac output (e.g. acute haemorrhage).
▸ Perform detailed auscultation of the heart:
  ▪ characterise any murmurs evident.
▸ Emergency stabilisation:
  ▪ furosemide 1.0–2.0 mg/kg IV q. 8–12 h
  ▪ intranasal oxygen 10–15 L/min if available.
▸ Treat any identified underlying cause (see relevant sections/texts).
▸ Euthanasia may be warranted at this stage if further investigation and treatment cannot be undertaken or if the horse's condition is deteriorating rapidly (Fig. 10.2).

Further assessment and treatment

▸ Echocardiography.
▸ ± ECG if accompanying cardiac arrhythmias.
▸ ± Thoracic radiography.
▸ Thoracic/abdominal US – assess for evidence of pleural effusion, hepatic congestion, ascites.
▸ Evaluation of electrolytes/organ function:
  ▪ haematology, serum biochemistry (± troponin I), blood gas analysis, urinalysis, serology (where infectious aetiology).

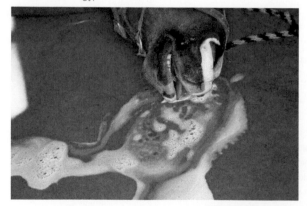

Figure 10.2 Collapse and death in a horse following rupture of a chorda tendinae. Large quantities of frothy, white fluid can be seen at the nares as a consequence of development of severe pulmonary oedema.

▶ Ongoing therapy to reduce congestion and improve cardiac output:
- furosemide
- ± digoxin
- ± vasodilators, e.g. hydralazine/ACE inhibitor.

Prognosis

▶ Usually grave unless the underlying cause is potentially reversible (e.g. pericarditis/endocarditis).
▶ Where non-reversible (e.g. structural abnormality) most horses die or are euthanased in <12 months if in HF.

Endocarditis

This is rare in horses but suspicions should be raised in a horse that is tachycardiac, pyrexic and has a new/changing cardiac murmur. This is also more commonly seen in young (<3 years old), male horses. Presenting signs are related to infection of the cardiac valves compromising cardiac function and dissemination of septic embolisation fragments to other organs causing sepsis at distant sites.

Clinical signs

▶ Dullness.
▶ Pyrexia (can be intermittent).
▶ ↑ HR.
▶ Cardiac murmur.
▶ ± Cardiac dysrhythmias/other signs of heart failure.
▶ ± Lameness/thrombophlebitis/diarrhoea/cough/seizures.

Initial approach

▶ Obtain a general history. Specific questions that should be asked include:
- identification of a heart murmur previously
- any recent illness (usually no predisposing factors identified).
▶ Perform a full clinical examination, including detailed auscultation of the heart:
- identify any systemic evidence of sepsis
- characterise the murmur present and the likely valve affected; the mitral valve is most commonly involved, followed in decreasing order by aortic > tricuspid > pulmonic
- occasionally a murmur might not be evident if the bacterial infection involves the myocardium/chordae tendinae.
▶ Take a blood sample for haematology and serum biochemistry:
- haematology – usually ↑ WBC, ↑ neutrophils, ↑ globulins, ↑ fibrinogen, ± ↓ RBC, ↓ PVC (anaemia of chronic disease)
- biochemistry – ± ↑ organ enzymes (depends if/where sepsis has developed); ↑ CKMB (most specific enzyme for myocardial disease).
▶ Stabilisation if evidence of acute HF (see p. 192).

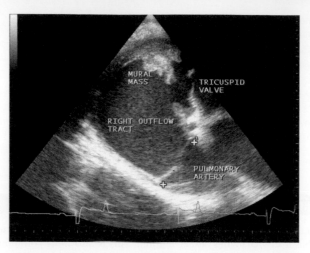

Figure 10.3 Echocardiographic image confirming a diagnosis of endocarditis in a horse.
Courtesy of Rachael Conwell.

Further assessment and treatment

▸ Echocardiography – gold standard for diagnosis (Fig. 10.3).
▸ ± ECG if arrhythmias present.
▸ Once a diagnosis is confirmed, aggressive long-term antimicrobial therapy is required:
  ▪ ideally obtain 3 × sterile blood samples over a 24-h period and only start after blood has been taken for culture
  ▪ IV antibiotics – bactericidal, prolonged and ideally based on culture and sensitivity. If nothing cultured, start on penicillin/gentamicin IV for 1–2 weeks followed by oral antimicrobials.
▸ ± Anti-thrombotics, e.g. aspirin 5–20 mg/kg PO q. 12–48 h.
▸ ± Treatment of HF if present/dysrhythmias of clinical significance.

Prognosis

▸ Generally poor where lesions are on the left side of the heart; guarded for those on right side.

Pericarditis/pericardial effusion

This is uncommon but should be ruled out in horses presenting with tachycardia and muffled heart sounds. These cases can present acutely with collapse or signs of acute HF or may be more gradual in onset depending on the quantity of fluid that accumulates in the pericardial sac and how quickly this occurs. Early recognition and appropriate treatment are important for the best chance of a successful outcome. Cardiac tamponade (where fluid accumulates rapidly in the pericardial sac, preventing expansion of the ventricles) can result in rapid death unless treated.

Clinical signs

▶ Depression, lethargy and ↓ appetite.
▶ ↑ HR.
▶ Muffled cardiac sounds.
▶ ± Pyrexia, jugular pulsation/distension, weak arterial pulse, pale/cyanotic MM, pericardial friction rubs, ↑ RR , dullness in the cranioventral thorax on auscultation, weight loss.

Initial approach

▶ Obtain a full history. Specific information that should be obtained includes:
  ▪ any recent history of trauma or transport
  ▪ any concurrent/recent illness
  ▪ illness in other in-contact horses including mare reproductive loss syndrome.
▶ Perform a full clinical examination and thorough cardiac auscultation.
▶ Take blood samples for haematology and serum biochemistry:
  ▪ haematology – ↑ WBC, ↑ fibrinogen
  ▪ biochemistry – dehydration (↑ PCV), variable changes in TP, altered electrolytes, evidence of organ damage (↑ enzymes).
▶ Emergency stabilisation if required:
  ▪ intranasal oxygen 10–15 L/min
  ▪ keep quiet and minimise stress
  ▪ DO NOT ADMINISTER FUROSEMIDE.

Further evaluation and treatment

▶ ECG to rule out other causes of tachycardia:
  ▪ low-amplitude QRS complexes visible ± electric alternans.
▶ Echocardiography – gold standard to confirm diagnosis (Fig. 10.4).
▶ ± Drainage of pericardial fluid under US guidance (advanced procedure).
▶ Prognosis if identified and treated appropriately:
  ▪ good in viral/immune-mediated/idiopathic cases
  ▪ fair if septic
  ▪ poor if traumatic/neoplastic/aorto-cardiac fistula.

Acute haemolytic anaemia

Acute anaemia is most likely to be related to severe blood loss or haemolysis. Where the cause is unknown, differentiation is based on the fact that acute blood loss usually results in ↓ of both PCV and TP, whereas haemolytic anaemia results in ↓ PCV but normal TP and evidence of jaundice or haemoglobinuria. The most common causes of haemolysis in the horse are immune-mediated disease, oxidant-induced damage to RBC and infectious diseases (depending on geographic location) – see Table 10.7.

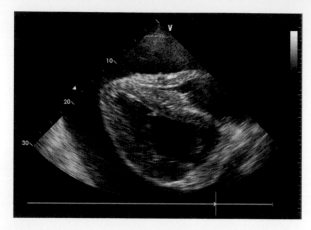

Figure 10.4   Echocardiographic image of a horse with pericardial effusion. A large quantity of hypoechoic fluid can be seen between the ventricles and the pericardium.

Courtesy of Fernando Malalana.

Table 10.7 Possible causes of haemolytic anaemia

Immune mediated	Autoimmune
	Bacterial infection
	Viral infections
	Neoplasia
	Drug reaction (e.g. tetracyclines, penicillin)
	NI (foals, see p. 242)
Infectious diseases	Piroplasmosis
	EIA (see p. 283)
Oxidative injury	Phenothiazines
	Onion toxicity
	Red maple leaf toxicity
Toxic	Bacterial toxins (e.g. *Clostridium*)
	Oak
	Burn injuries
	Snake bite
Miscellaneous	Hepatic disease (usually end-stage)
	DIC (usually secondary to severe underlying disease)

Clinical signs

▶ ↑ HR, ↑ RR.
▶ Weakness/lethargy.
▶ ± Systolic heart murmur (↓ blood viscosity, turbulence).
▶ ± Haemorrhagic shock if severe.
▶ ± Pyrexia.
▶ ± Jaundice.
▶ ± Petechial haemorrhages.
▶ ± Haemoglobinuria.
▶ ± Weight loss.

Initial assessment

▶ Obtain a complete history. Specific questions that should be asked include:
  ▪ recent illness/medication
  ▪ recent importation/travel abroad (see Ch. 15)
  ▪ known toxicosis/snake envenomation (see Ch. 16).
▶ Perform a full clinical examination. Specific assessment includes:
  ▪ rule in/out other systemic illnesses as the underlying cause.
▶ Take a blood sample and place into EDTA, plain, lithium heparin and sodium citrate tubes:
  ▪ look for evidence of haemoglobinaemia (pink plasma)
  ▪ haematology – PCV, Hb, MCHC
  ▪ serum biochemistry – evidence of organ damage/azotaemia
  ▪ new methylene blue stain – asses for Heinz bodies (oxidative RBC damage)
  ▪ stain for parasites/intracellular bacteria with Giemsa (*Babesia/Anaplasma* spp.)
  ▪ ± direct Coombs' test (or autoagglutination in EDTA tube)
  ▪ if EIA is possible, submit serum sample for Coggins' test (contact relevant laboratory).
▶ Obtain a urine sample:
  ▪ assess urine colour – if red/brown, determine if due to haematuria/haemoglobinuria/ myoglobinuria (see p. 176).

Further investigation and treatment

▶ Consider a blood transfusion if PCV ≤12% or <15% if PCV falling rapidly (see p. 376).
▶ Specific therapy depends on whether any underlying cause can be identified and appropriate specific/supportive treatment administered.
▶ Haemoglobinuria can cause acute renal failure (see p. 179).
▶ If nothing obvious can be found, consider performing a bone marrow biopsy to rule out causes of ↓ RBC production.

Vasculitis

This is an inflammatory process that originates primarily in the blood vessel wall, often as a sequel to an underlying infection.

Table 10.8 Possible causes of vasculitis

Viral	EHV-1
	EVA (see p. 285)
	EIA (see p. 283)
	AHS (see p. 280)
Bacterial	Salmonellosis
Parasitic	Ehrlichiosis – *Anaplasma phagocytophilum*
	Strongylus vulgaris
Immune-mediated	Purpura haemorrhagica secondary to *Strep.*
	equi var *equi* infection
	Adverse drug reactions
	Neoplasia (paraneoplastic vasculitis)
	Systemic lupus erythematosus-like syndrome
	Idiopathic
Physical	Trauma-induced vasculitis
	Photo-activated vasculitis
	Pastern and cannon leucoclastic vasculitis

Clinical signs

▶ Petechial and ecchymotic haemorrhage – MM, sclera.
▶ Subcutaneous oedema – head, ventral abdomen, limbs.
▶ ± Colic.
▶ ± Dyspnoea.
▶ ± Lameness/ataxia.

Possible causes

Vasculitis may be primary in origin (often directly associated with an infectious disease) or secondary to another underlying disorder – see Table 10.8/texts.

Diagnosis and treatment (Fig. 10.5)

▶ Diagnose and treat underlying cause based on history and further diagnostic tests.
▶ Definitive diagnosis : biopsy and histopathological examination of affected tissues.
▶ ± Corticosteroid administration, e.g. dexamethasone 0.1 mg/kg q. 24 h for 2–3 d.
▶ ± Blood/plasma transfusion if severe hypoproteinaemia/haemorrhage.
▶ Other supportive treatment as required, e.g. bandaging of distal limbs, walking in-hand.

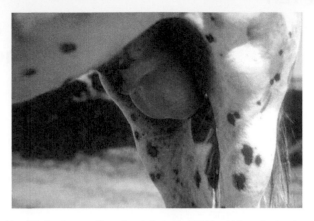

Figure 10.5 Vasculitis in a horse with equine viral arteritis (EVA) in which marked oedema of the scrotum is evident.

Courtesy of Peter Timoney via: http://www.ivis.org/special_books/Lekeux/timoney/IVIS.pdf

References and further reading

- **Bowen, M.,** 2007 Cardiac emergencies in the horse: In Proceedings of the 46th British Equine Veterinary Association Congress. Edinburgh, UK, 12–15 September 2007, Equine Veterinary Journal Ltd., Newmarket, UK, pp. 378–380.

- **Dugdale, A.,** 2010. Fluid therapy. In: Dugdale, A. (Ed.), Veterinary Anaesthesia: Principles to Practice. Blackwell Publishing Ltd, Chichester, UK

- **Fiege, K.,** 2009. Coagulopathies. In: Robinson, N.E., Sprayberry, K.A. (Eds.), Current Therapy in Equine Medicine (sixth ed.). Elsevier, St. Louis, Missouri, pp. 227–231.

- **Gardner, S.Y.,** 2009. Congestive heart failure. In: Robinson, N.E., Sprayberry, K.A. (Eds.), Current Therapy in Equine Medicine (sixth ed.). Elsevier, St. Louis, Missouri, pp. 204–206.

- **Jesty, S.A.,** 2009. Infective endocarditis. In: Robinson, N.E., Sprayberry, K.A. (Eds.), Current Therapy in Equine Medicine (sixth ed.). Elsevier, St. Louis, Missouri, pp. 212–215.

- **Knottenbelt, D.C.,** 2002. Vasculitis: just what does it mean? Equine Vet. Educ. 14, 247–251.

- **Marr, C.M.,** 2010. Heart failure. In: Marr, C.M., Bowen, M. (Eds.), Equine Cardiology (second ed.). Elsievier, St. Louis, Missouri, pp. 239–252.

- **Piercy, R.J., Marr, C.M.,** 2010. Collapse and syncope. In: Marr, C.M., Bowen, M. (Eds.), Equine Cardiology (second ed.). Elsevier, St. Louis, Missouri, pp. 227–237.

- **Reef, V.B., Marr, C.M.,** 2010. Dysrhythmias: assessment and medical management. In: Marr, C.M., Bowen, M. (Eds.), Equine Cardiology (second ed.). Elsevier, St. Louis, Missouri, pp. 159–178.

- **Sellon, D.C., Wise, L.N.,** 2010. Disorders of the hematopoietic system. In: Reed, S.M., Bayly, W.M., Sellon, D.C. (Eds.), Equine Internal Medicine (third ed.). Elsevier, St. Louis, Missouri, pp. 730–767.

- **Stainsby, D., MacLennan, S., Thomas, D.,** et al. 2006. Guidelines on the management of massive blood loss. Br. J. Haematol. 135, 634–641.

Hepatic, endocrine and metabolic emergencies

Acute hepatic disease

This can be difficult to diagnose and treat due to the fact that clinical signs may be diverse and highly variable, depending on the extent and duration of disease (Table 11.1), and are not usually seen until ≥70–80% of the liver is affected. Therefore by the time a diagnosis is reached, hepatic disease may be advanced and possibly irreversible. Hepatic encephalopathy (abnormal mental status that accompanies severe hepatic insufficiency) is potentially reversible, depending on the underlying cause of hepatic disease.

Clinical signs of hepatic disease

Table 11.1 Clinical signs seen in cases of hepatic disease

Common	Less common
Dullness	Dehydration
Anorexia	Photosensitisation
Colic	Respiratory distress (bilateral laryngeal paralysis)
Hepatic encephalopathy	Haemorrhage (↓ production clotting factors)
Weight loss	Diarrhoea
Jaundice	Peripheral oedema
	Dermatitis and pruritus
	Colic – gastric impaction/rupture
	Collapse (*C. novyi* hepatitis)

Clinical signs of hepatic encephalopathy

A variety of abnormal behaviours may be seen, including:

▸ Depression.
▸ Aggression/somnolence.
▸ Yawning.
▸ Pacing/aimless wandering.
▸ Blindness.
▸ Head pressing (Fig. 11.1).
▸ Ataxia.
▸ Recumbency and death.

Initial assessment

▸ Administer first aid if required:
  ▪ treat seizures if present (see p. 144)
  ▪ perform tracheotomy if evidence of respiratory distress (see p. 356).
▸ Obtain a full history. Specific information that should be obtained includes:
  ▪ what abnormal signs have been evident and speed of progression (sudden/gradual)
  ▪ any recent illness/medications
  ▪ potential ingestion of ragwort or other pyrrolizidine alkaloid plants or access to toxins (see Table 11.2).
▸ Perform a full clinical examination. Specific assessment should include:
  ▪ rule in/out disease in other body systems (e.g. hyperlipaemia)
  ▪ suspect cholangiohepatitis if pyrexia, colic and jaundice evident.
▸ Take blood samples for serum biochemistry and haematology (Table 11.3):
  ▪ key enzymes to measure: AP, AST, GLDH, γGT.

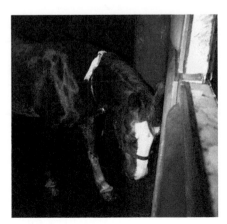

Figure 11.1 Hepatic encephalopathy in a pony that also presented with signs of respiratory distress due to bilateral laryngeal paralysis.

Table 11.2 Possible causes of hepatic disease

Toxins	Pyrrolizidine alkaloid toxicity (see p. 299 for a list of plants containing these alkaloids)
Severe metabolic disease	Hypoxia Hyperlipaemia
Infectious disease	Ascending infection from GIT causing cholangitis/cholangiohepatitis
Neoplastic	e.g. Adenocarcinoma
Immunological	Parenteral administration of products of equine origin
Obstructive	Cholelithiasis

Table 11.3 Results of serum biochemistry and haematology that can assist diagnosis of hepatic disease

Test	Liver specific
ALP (↑)	x
AP (↑)	x
AST (↑)	x
GLDH (↑)	✓
γGT (↑)	x - mostly, rarely pancreas
SDH (IDH) (↑)	✓
LDH (↑)	x
Bilirubin (↑)	x
Bile acids (↑)	✓
Albumin (↓)	x
Globulins (↑)	x
Glucose (↓ – rare)	x

▶ ± US of liver (see texts/consider referral):
  ▪ size, outline and echogenicity of the liver
  ▪ identification of focal areas of ↑/↓ echogenicity (site for biopsy).
▶ ± Liver biopsy (see texts/consider referral):
  ▪ gold standard for confirmation of the presence of significant hepatic disease
  ▪ assists determining prognosis, specific therapy and may help to identify the aetiology.
▶ ± Gastroscopy to investigate potential gastric impaction if signs of inappetance/mild colic.

Initial treatment for hepatic encephalopathy (if present)

▶ May be a result of irreversible hepatic disease (acute/chronic) but treatment is warranted whilst awaiting the results of diagnostic tests and assessing response to therapy.
▶ Administer sedation if required – xylazine 0.5 mg/kg IV, detomidine 0.01 mg/kg IV or acepromazine 0.02 mg/kg IV (do not administer acepromazine if seizures evident):
  ▪ use reduced dose – ↓ ability of liver to metabolise these agents
  ▪ avoid benzodiazepines.
▶ Treat cerebral oedema if evident:
  ▪ hypertonic saline 2–4 mL/kg IV (use is controversial)
  ▪ mannitol 0.25–1.0 g/kg – warm first, crystallises if cold.
▶ Reduce ammonia absorption from GIT:
  ▪ administer oral lactulose 0.3 mL/kg q. 6 h, reducing to q. 12 h, then q. 24 h, depending on response to therapy (this is usually seen within 24 h if it is going to be effective)
  ▪ ± administer metronidazole 15 mg/kg PO loading dose, then 7.5 mg/kg PO q. 6 h or neomycin 15 mg/kg q. 6 h.
▶ Other supportive treatment for hepatic disease (see below).

Initial supportive treatment

▶ Fluid therapy if the horse is dehydrated and unwilling to drink:
  ▪ oral fluids by stomach tube (oral rehydration solutions) – GI motility and no reflux
  ▪ IV fluid therapy – no GI motility in more severe cases.
▶ Nutritional support:
  ▪ allow free access to grass/grass hay (avoid alfalfa)
  ▪ offer a suitable concentrate feed (low protein levels) – split daily requirement into 4–6 feeds/d
  ▪ be careful with vitamin supplements – avoid supplements containing iron
  ▪ parenteral therapy if not willing to eat (see Hyperlipaemia, next section).
▶ ± Antimicrobial therapy:
  ▪ indicated if ↑ T°, haematology suggests systemic infection (↑ or ↓ WBC), neutrophils evident in biopsy sample
  ▪ start on trimethoprim sulphonamides or penicillin, gentamicin and metronidazole for 5 d initially, assess response to therapy.
▶ NSAIDs – if indicated (↑ T°, signs of colic) and once fluid deficits corrected.

Ongoing monitoring and treatment

▶ Depends on severity of clinical disease, response to therapy and results of US/biopsy of liver.

Prognosis

▶ Usually poor unless the disease process is acute and liver regeneration is already occurring.

▶ Liver enzymes can correlate poorly with outcome and it may be worth treating first and assessing clinical response to treatment (see texts for prognostic indicators).

Hyperlipaemia

Hyperlipaemia is most common in sick, anorexic ponies, miniature horses and donkeys (see p. 255) and disease can progress rapidly (usually 1–10 d between the onset of clinical signs and death). Even with treatment, this condition can be associated with high mortality. Therefore early diagnosis and appropriate, aggressive treatment is essential.

Pathogenesis

▶ Hepatic glycogen is a major source of plasma glucose.
▶ Where the body's energy supply is limited (anorexia) or metabolic demands are ↑ (pregnancy, lactation, maintaining body temperature in cold weather), depletion of glycogen stores results in release of fatty acids from adipose tissues.
▶ Release of fatty acids can overwhelm the liver's capacity for gluconeogenesis, resulting in release of triglycerides (TG) into the circulation.
▶ A variety of disorders of lipid metabolism (dyslipidaemias) can arise as a consequence of this, the most severe being hyperlipaemia.

> **HANDY TIP**
>
> A simple test that can be performed where TG cannot be measured easily or quickly is to allow a plain blood sample to stand and examine the serum or plasma for evidence of turbidity – this confirms the likely diagnosis (but hyperlipaemia cannot be excluded if the plasma/serum looks grossly normal) (Fig. 11.2).

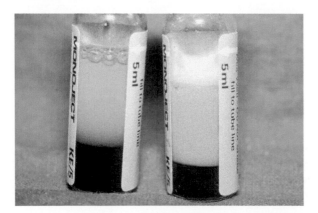

Figure 11.2   Blood sample from a normal (left) and hyperlipaemic pony (right). Gross turbidity of plasma is evident in the sample on the right due to high circulating levels of triglycerides.

Courtesy of Derek Knottenbelt.

Factors that increase the risk of hyperlipaemia

- Breed: ponies (particularly Shetlands), miniature horses and donkeys (see Ch. 13).
- Obesity.
- Pregnancy/lactation.
- Anorexia due to concurrent disease.
- Recent severe stress (illness/management change/feed restriction).
- PPID (Cushing's disease).

Clinical signs

▸ Anorexia.
▸ Depression and lethargy.
▸ ↓ GI motility and faecal output.
▸ Weakness.
▸ ± Diarrhoea.
▸ ± Ventral oedema.
▸ ± Proceeded by/complicated by other concurrent underlying disease:
  ▪ hepatic failure (see p. 202)
  ▪ renal failure – PU/PD, ↑ HR, congested MM, halitosis.
▸ Terminal – recumbency, abortion, altered mentation, convulsions and death.

Diagnosis

▸ Cloudy appearance to plasma (lipaemia – see Fig. 11.2).
▸ ↑ Plasma TG >5.6 mmol/L.

KEY TIP

Serum TG should always be measured in high-risk individuals that have become dull and anorexic even if the plasma looks grossly normal.

Initial assessment

▸ Obtain a full history. Specific information that should be obtained includes:
  ▪ any recent illness/unusual behaviour or major change to normal routine
  ▪ whether pregnant or lactating.
▸ Perform a full clinical examination to check for the underlying cause (1° hyperlipaemia is rare):
  ▪ rule out laminitis, severe dental disease, GI parasitism, PPID, colic
  ▪ check GIT sounds.
▸ Obtain a blood sample for serum biochemistry and haematology:
  ▪ confirm diagnosis

- assess hydration status (PCV/TP)
- assess hepatic and renal function: γGT, AP, AST, bile acids, creatinine, BUN, electrolytes (± ammonia, see p. 338)
- ± measure blood glucose levels.

▶ In severe cases, consider hospitalisation/referral (advanced care).
▶ Less severe cases can be managed on site (see below).

Management of mild/suspected cases of early hyperlipaemia

▶ Initiate treatment for any underlying disease.
▶ Bring inside if out in cold weather (↓ energy demands).
▶ Offer water and a selection of good-quality, palatable feeds (e.g. fresh cut grass, chopped forage, concentrate mix, sugar beet pulp) and check to see if they are willing to eat/drink:
  - feeding by hand and warming feed can be valuable in encouraging them to eat.
▶ If they will not eat but have evidence of GIT motility (i.e. no reflux on passage of a stomach tube, GIT sounds audible on auscultation) a variety of different types of feed can be administered via a stomach tube q. 8–12h:
  - Weetabix (20 biscuits for a 250-kg pony, 35 for a 450-kg horse q. 8h) – mix with 1–2 L lukewarm water (swells if too warm), blend (using a hand-blender) and administer immediately (have water ready to clear any blockages)
  - Ready brek (300 g for a 250-kg pony, 500 g for a 450-kg horse q. 8h) and administered as above
  - can supplement with glucose powder/syrups
  - alternatively can mix a complete pelleted feed into a gruel and administer by stomach tube q. 8–12h (can be difficult to get down a narrow stomach tube – hand-blender essential).
▶ Supportive treatment as for hepatic disease if present (see p. 205).
▶ Monitor carefully; reassess clinical signs and repeat serum TG measurement q. 12–24h initially.
▶ If there is no improvement/deterioration occurs, advanced care (or euthanasia) is required.

Advanced care of cases with severe clinical signs and no GIT motility

▶ Obtain a urine sample if possible prior to starting fluid therapy:
  - check for pre-renal azotaemia (SG >1.020 and ↓ after fluid therapy) or renal failure (SG 1.008–1.012).
▶ Start IV fluid therapy (see p. 374):
  - supplement IV fluids with 0.25 ml/kg/h of 50% dextrose solution.
▶ Administer 0.25 mg/kg flunixin IV q. 8h if endotoxic.
▶ Monitor clinical signs and blood glucose q. 4–8h.
▶ Start enteral nutrition once GIT motility returns.
▶ Monitor serum TG daily and continue treatment until they have returned to normal levels.

If no improvement (consider hospitalisation/referral):

▶ Total/partial parenteral nutrition using commercial solutions (see texts/seek specialist advice).
▶ Insulin therapy (see texts/seek specialist advice).

Severe starvation

Starvation may be acute or chronic in nature and may be encountered in horses following adverse climatic conditions/natural disasters or, more commonly, in cases of neglect (see Approach to assessment of the welfare case, p. 321). Severe cases may present as emergencies and it is essential that prompt assessment and treatment (if euthanasia is not warranted) is performed. Initial nutritional management of the chronically starved horse must be performed carefully to avoid a refeeding syndrome (observed in humans), which can lead to further metabolic derangements and death.

Clinical signs

▶ These are summarised in Table 11.4.
▶ Acutely starved horses (those deprived of all food) become inappetant before showing evidence of severe emaciation.
▶ Measurement of total bilirubin is a good indicator of starvation duration (>48 h if elevated).

Initial assessment and first aid treatment

▶ Before embarking on any examination and treatment, consider whether the case is likely to give rise to legal proceedings under Animal Welfare legislation (see p. 321).
▶ Obtain a full history. Specific details that should be obtained include (if known):
  ▪ duration of clinical signs
  ▪ feeding history
  ▪ general health, including previous/recent illness
  ▪ prophylaxis against intestinal parasites.
▶ Assess surroundings and evidence of feed available (look at feed type and quality too).

Table 11.4 Clinical signs of acute and chronic starvation

Acute starvation	Chronic starvation
Variable BCS	Low BCS (see www.newc.co.uk)
Severe depression	Lack of body fat;↓ Muscle mass
Inappetance	Poor hair coat
Signs of hepatic disease/ hyperlipaemia	Bone/joint deformities in growing horses
	Evidence of impaired wound healing and immune function
Jaundice	Ravenous appetite
Muscle fasciculations	Recumbency:
Weakness	<48h recumbency – will maintain appetite and attempt to eat food offered
Ventral oedema	
Ataxia	>48h recumbency – unwilling to eat, comatose
Seizures and death	Death within 72–96h of recumbency

▶ Perform a full clinical examination and assess for concurrent disease/injury:
  ▪ if recumbent, determine whether due to weakness or other another underlying condition (see p. 313).
▶ Determine whether treatment can be initiated; euthanasia should be considered in severe cases with a hopeless prognosis (see p. 328).
▶ Move to a thermoneutral environment (if outside in extreme cold/hot or humid conditions).
▶ Determine the degree of dehydration (see p. 375), body condition score (see p. 323) and estimate the horse's weight (if possible on a weigh scale or if not using a measuring tape).
▶ Offer 2–4 L of water every 30 min.
▶ If the horse is unwilling to drink and is dehydrated, pass a nasogastric tube, check for presence of reflux and, if no reflux is present, administer 5 L of oral electrolyte solution/water.
▶ If evidence of reflux, mild signs of colic or severe dehydration, start IV fluid therapy (see p. 374).
▶ Take blood samples for haematology, serum biochemistry and tapeworm ELISA.
▶ Take faecal samples for worm egg counts.
▶ Acute starvation:
  ▪ similar to treatment of hyperlipaemia in the acute stage (see previous section).
▶ Chronic starvation:
  ▪ initiation of nutritional support needs to be carefully undertaken to avoid refeeding syndrome – overfeeding is potentially more harmful than slight underfeeding.

Initial nutrition of the emaciated horse following chronic starvation

▶ Determine the horse's current body weight (usually >25% BW lost).
▶ Calculate resting energy requirements for current body weight (see website for an example diet plan):
  ▪ maintenance energy requirement – Mcal (DE)/d = 0.0333×body weight (kg)
  ▪ resting energy requirement = 0.7×maintenance energy requirement
  ▪ days 1–2: 25% of resting energy requirement
  ▪ days 3–4: 50% of resting energy requirement
  ▪ days 5–7: 75% of resting energy requirement
  ▪ days 7–14: 100% resting energy requirement. If tolerated:
  ▪ days 14–21: gradually increase to maintenance energy requirements for optimal body weight (at least 125% of initial body weight).
▶ Work out best feed to give; needs to be high in protein and fat but relatively low in non-structural carbohydrates:
  ▪ hay (soaked)
  ▪ vegetable oil (100–150 mL/feed – introduce gradually)
  ▪ high-fibre cubes
  ▪ chopped forage
  ▪ chopped fresh grass (preferably walk to graze if possible)
  ▪ avoid haylage/grain/concentrate feeds for at least 3 weeks, then introduce a low-protein coarse mix.
▶ Enteral nutrition best if the horse is willing to eat and has a functioning GIT:
  ▪ ensure access to fresh water at all times
  ▪ split feeds into 4–6 meals daily initially to prevent bolting of feed (then 2–3×daily).
▶ If able to walk, allow to graze for 30 min/d initially, increasing by 10 min each day after 7 d.

▶ If the horse had a functioning GIT but is unwilling to eat, slurried feed can be given via an indwelling/repeatedly placed stomach tube:
  ▪ equine commercial pelleted feed (high fibre) – work out calculated daily amounts as above and horse's fluid intake for the day (60 mL/kg/d)
  ▪ grind pellets before adding water/use kitchen blender after adding water, to make a slurry
  ▪ can use Weetabix or Ready brek mixes too (see Hyperlipaemia, p. 208)
  ▪ check that the slurry will run through a stomach tube (9–13 mm internal diameter, single-ended bore) and is no more than 3 L in volume for that feed (initially) to prevent overfilling of the stomach (can increase to 6 L in adult horse over several days)
  ▪ check for reflux (<2 L fluid retrieved from stomach fine)
  ▪ administer slurry – if becomes blocked, can flush with carbonated water
  ▪ flush stomach tube with 1 L water
  ▪ push a small amount of air through if tube indwelling to ensure tube is clear.
▶ If GIT non-functioning, will require IV fluids and parenteral nutrition (see p. 208).

Ongoing care and monitoring

▶ Nursing care as for the recumbent horse (see p. 315):
  ▪ put on deep bedding with lots of padding over the hips
  ▪ keep in sternal recumbency if possible
  ▪ place rugs and leg bandages if cold – less body fat to maintain heat
  ▪ wounds take longer to heal in these horses.
▶ Monitor clinical parameters daily for first 14 d, then weekly until fully recovered:
  ▪ vital signs (TPR)
  ▪ body weight and BCS
  ▪ faecal output and consistency
  ▪ digital pulses.
▶ Repeat biochemistry and haematology daily for first 10 d, then as required.
▶ Re-evaluate nutritional requirements and gradually increase to maintenance energy requirements for ideal body weight over at least 14 d.

Prognosis

▶ Poor if loss of >45–50% of body weight, recumbent for 72 h.
▶ 20% mortality in severely malnourished horses in first 19 d due to refeeding type syndrome.
▶ Recovery time is 2–3 months in cases of moderate starvation, 6–10 months in cases of severe starvation.

Exhaustion syndrome

This most commonly occurs in competition horses undergoing athletic activity for prolonged periods, particularly in conditions of extreme heat and humidity. However, this can occur in any horse pushed beyond its level of fitness in extremes of heat and humidity, including working equids (particularly if not acclimatised to these conditions). Mild lameness and other underlying conditions can also contribute to earlier onset of fatigue. It is important to recognise and treat this condition early and appropriately.

Clinical signs

Vary depending on severity, speed of onset and physiological reserve of the horse.

▶ Unable to continue to exercise.
▶ ↑ HR and ↑ RR.
▶ ↑ T° 40.0–42.0°C (104–107.6°F).
▶ Weak peripheral pulses and tacky MM.
▶ Dehydration.
▶ Depressed, lethargic, anorexic and unwilling to drink.
▶ Muscular soreness.
▶ ± Rhabdomyolysis and recumbency (severe cases).
▶ ± Synchronous diaphragmatic flutter – electrolyte alterations (see next section).
▶ ± Colic.
▶ ± Arrhythmias – atrial fibrillation most common.
▶ ± Neurological signs – ataxia, circling, seizures.

Diagnosis

▶ History and clinical signs.
▶ Differentiate from a tired horse whose HR and RR will return to normal more quickly (e.g. HR <60 beats/min, RR <40 breaths/min within 30 min) and will not have a persistently ↑ T°.

Initial treatment

▶ Must be aggressive and prompt – can result in multiple organ failure, shock, DIC and death if untreated.
▶ Stop exercise – may be sufficient in mild cases.
▶ Initiate cooling (see p. 215) and monitor T°.
▶ Offer 5 L oral fluids initially (selection of normal water and water with electrolytes) and 5–8 L every 30–60 min afterwards.
▶ If the horse will not drink, pass a nasogastric tube, check no reflux is present and administer 5 L isotonic fluids (oral rehydration fluids).
▶ Start IV fluids if there is no evidence of GIT sounds/the horse is showing signs of mild colic or if there is reflux.
▶ ± Administer butorphanol 0.01–0.04 mg/kg if the horse is showing signs of pain/distress (do not administer NSAIDs until the horse is rehydrated).
▶ Take blood samples for haematology and serum biochemistry.
▶ Re-evaluate the horse frequently (q. 20 min initially):
  ▪ assess mentation, HR, RR, T°, evidence of muscle soreness/exertional rhabdomyolysis syndrome (see p. 55) or synchronous diaphragmatic flutter.
▶ Administer NSAIDs if there is evidence of musculoskeletal pain once the horse is rehydrated/has urinated.

Treatment of more severe cases:

▶ If severe CNS signs:
  - administer intranasal oxygen 15 L/min (4 available)
  - if seizuring, administer diazepam 0.1–0.2 mg/kg IV or phenobarbital 2–10 mg/kg IV q. 8–12 h
  - ± administer prednisolone sodium succinate 1–10 mg/kg IV.
▶ Assess results of haematology/biochemistry, including electrolytes (if available):
  - ↑ PCV, ↑ RBC (endurance horses may have PCV as high as 50–67%)
  - ↑ TP, ↑ albumin (as high as 140 g/L and 45 g/L, respectively, in endurance horses)
  - ↑ plasma lactate
  - ↓ Cl^-, ↓ Ca^{2+}, ↓ Na^+
  - ↑ serum muscle enzymes – mild to marked elevations
  - azotaemia – pre-renal/toxic insult to kidneys
  - ± hypoglycaemia
  - + acid–base abnormalities.
▶ Start IV fluid therapy:
  - may need up to 30–60 L in severe cases
  - 12G catheter
  - administer extracellular fluid volume replacement solutions, e.g. 0.9% NaCl, LRS
  - do not use hypertonic saline
  - maximum fluid rate of 10–20 mL/kg/h (5–10 L/h for 500-kg horse)
  - add a total of 250 mL 40% calcium gluconate (see next section) and 100 mL of 50% dextrose to the fluids given in the first 2–3 h, then reassess (measurement of electrolytes and glucose useful; base further therapy on the results of these).
▶ Monitor urination and comfort:
  - administer NSAIDs once the horse has urinated.
▶ Monitor for signs of:
  - leucopenia – start BS antimicrobials (penicillin/gentamicin), flunixin meglumine 1.1 mg/kg
  - colic (see p. 59)
  - acute renal failure (see p. 179).

Prognosis

▶ Depends on initial severity, speed of intervention and response to treatment.
▶ Mild cases respond quickly with minimal treatment.
▶ More severe cases can be life-threatening – laminitis, skin sloughs and DIC can be seen several days afterwards.

KEY TIP

Ensure horses that will be working in conditions of extreme heat, humidity and/or altitude are sufficiently fit and allowed to acclimatise to the environment over at least 2–3 weeks.

Synchronous diaphragmatic flutter/thumps

Synchronous diaphragmatic flutter (SDF) can occur in horses with marked electrolyte alterations. These result in increased irritability of the phrenic nerve, causing spasmodic contraction of the diaphragm each time the heart beats. It is commonly seen after National Hunt or point-to-point racing and usually resolves within 15–20 min; these horses may have normal electrolyte parameters.

Clinical signs

▸ Rhythmic movement of the abdomen in time with the heart beat.
▸ ± An audible 'thump' (hence the name).

Diagnosis and treatment

▸ Clinical signs.
▸ Wait 15 min unless the horse is distressed, ataxic or showing other clinical signs (e.g. myopathy).
▸ Measurement of serum electrolytes (if possible):
  ▪ hypo-Ca^{2+} is most likely to be implicated
  ▪ ± hypo-Mg^{2+}.
▸ Administer 40% calcium borogloconate at 0.1–0.5 ml/kg by slow IV infusion over 2–3 h – monitor the heart/pulse and stop the infusion if any cardiac irregularities develop.
▸ As a guide for a 500-kg horse, add 250 ml of 40% calcium borogluconate diluted at least 1:4 in sterile saline/LRS and administer slowly to effect.
▸ If no response, base further electrolyte supplementation on results of electrolyte measurements (see texts).

Hyperthermia (heat stress/heat stroke)

This occurs where the heat load exceeds the ability of the horse's thermoregulatory system to dissipate it and the body temperature rises to a point above which normal cellular function fails and tissue destruction occurs. It is often seen in combination with severe dehydration, energy depletion and fatigue (exhaustion syndrome). Hyperthermia is most commonly seen in horses that are competing or working in hot, humid conditions, particularly in those that are less acclimatised to such conditions.

Clinical signs

▸ Pulls up during exercise or work/finishes distressed.
▸ Depressed, unwilling to move, ataxic ± signs of colic.
▸ Agitated, abnormal mentation.
▸ ↑ RR, rasping noise – if very hot get a reduction in RR but respiration becomes deep and desperate.
▸ ↑ HR, congested MM, weak pulses.
▸ Sweating – ranges from copious to very little ± may feel dry.
▸ ↑ T° ≥39°C (>102.2°F).
▸ Progression to collapse, convulsions, coma and death if untreated.

▶ History and clinical signs.
▶ Degree of hyperthermia important:
- ≥39°C (>102.2°F) – will benefit from cooling
- >40°C (>104°F) – heat stroke
- 41–42°C (105.8–107.6°F) – distress, unable to continue exercise
- >42°C (>107.6°F) – cell destruction, DIC and death.

Treatment

▶ Start aggressive cooling:
- apply cold water (4–10°C) over the horse, concentrating on the horse's hindquarters – owners are often concerned that this will cause muscle damage but there is no evidence for this
- apply water liberally (horse, tack and helpers will become soaked) and allow it to run off naturally/scrape the water off
- move the horse to a shady area with a breeze (or use large fans at competitions) and remove tack
- keep the horse walking slowly and continue to apply water at 30-s intervals.
▶ Check temperature at 5-min intervals – aggressive cooling can reduce the body temperature by 1°C in 10 min.
▶ Offer small quantities (4 L) of oral electrolyte solutions/water periodically during cooling.
▶ Continue cooling until the horse's temperature reduces to 38–39°C – the horse can be seen to become brighter and more alert, RR reduces and the skin feels cool to touch.
▶ Suspect exhaustion syndrome if after 30 min of cooling HR >56 beats/min, RR >25 breaths/min.
▶ If the horse is still distressed/dull/unwilling to eat or drink, assess as per exhaustion syndrome (see p. 211).
▶ Monitor for signs of colic/exertional rhabdomyolysis and treat as appropriate.
▶ Offer grass, water and hay if the horse remains bright.
▶ Keep rested.
▶ Avoid transport for 24 h.

> **KEY TIP**
> Do not apply ice packs directly to the skin (results in thermal damage to the skin) or apply wet towels or blankets (retains heat).

> **HANDY TIPS**
> Do not apply ice over the horse – the ice will quickly fall to the ground and will be wasted. Ice should instead be placed into large containers with water and jugs/small buckets used to pour water over the horse.

Hypothermia

This is uncommon in adult horses but can occur in debilitated individuals in extreme (cold) climates. It is more commonly seen in foals, horses following general anaesthesia or occasionally in donkeys.

Clinical signs

▶ Mild hypothermia 33.9–36.1°C (93–97°F):
  ▪ ↑ HR, cold extremities, shivering.
▶ Severe hypothermia <33.9°C (<93°F):
  ▪ loss of shivering reflex
  ▪ peripheral vasodilation – increasingly cold extremities
  ▪ ↓ HR, ↓ RR and ↓ respiratory effort
  ▪ ± neurological signs
  ▪ ⊥ clotting abnormalities
  ▪ ± frostbite lesions on the extremities
  ▪ coma and death.

Treatment

▶ Move inside to a warmer, draught-free environment.
▶ Passive rewarming– keep directly off the ground (on blankets/blankets on top of layer of bedding) and cover with blankets.
▶ Administer warmed IV fluids – correct fluid deficits (see p. 374).
▶ Active rewarming – be careful with use of direct heat sources near the extremities as they can cause peripheral vasodilation (worsening the ↓ in core temperature) and damage to the skin.
▶ Further investigation of any underlying cause/disease and ongoing treatment as appropriate.
▶ Administer NSAIDs once dehydration corrected.
▶ Administer BS antimicrobials.
▶ Nursing care as for recumbent horse (see p. 315).

References and further reading

• **Barton, M.H.,** 2010. Diseases of the liver. In: Reed, S.M., Bayly, W.M., Sellon, D.C. (Eds.), Equine Internal Medicine (third ed.). Elsevier, St. Louis, Missouri, pp. 939–975.

• **Becvarova, I., Thatcher, C.D.,** 2009. Nutritional management of the starved horse. In: Robinson, N.E., Sprayberry, K.A. (Eds.), Current Therapy in Equine Medicine (sixth ed.). Elsevier, St. Louis, Missouri, pp. 53–58.

• **Carr, E.A., Holcombe, S.J.,** 2009. Nutrition of critically ill horses. Vet. Clin. North Am. Equine Pract. 25, 93–108.

• **Conwell R.** 2009 The exhausted/dehydrated/hyperthermic horse. In: Proceedings of 48th British Veterinary Association Congress, Birmingham, September 9–12th, pp.186–187 (available via <http://www.ivis.org>)

• **Divers, T.J.,** 2008. Shock and temperature-related problems. In: Orsini, J.A., Divers, T.J. (Eds.), Equine Emergencies Treatment and Procedures (third ed.). Elsevier, St. Louis, Missouri, pp. 553–557.

• **Durham, A.E.,** 2006. Clinical application of parenteral nutrition in the treatment of five ponies and one donkey with hyperlipaemia. Vet. Rec. 158, 159–164.

• **Durham, A.,** 2008. Monitoring and treating the liver. In: Corley, K., Stephen, J. (Eds.), The Equine Hospital Manual. Blackwell Publishing, Chichester, W Sussex, UK, pp. 520–532.

• **Hammond, A.,** 2004. Management of hyperlipaemia. In Pract. 26, 548–552.

• **Hughes, K.J., Hodgson, D.R., Dart, A.J.,** 2004. Equine hyperlipaemia: a review. Aust. Vet. J. 82, 136–142.

• **Johns I.** 2010 Diagnosis and practical treatment of hepatic disease. In: Proceedings of the 49th British Veterinary Association Congress, Birmingham, UK 8–11th September, pp. 195–196 (available via <http://www.ivis.org)>

• **McGorum, B.C., Murphy, D., Love, S., Milne, E.M.,** 1999. Clinicopathological features of equine primary hepatic disease: a review of 50 cases. Vet. Rec. 145, 134–139.

• **McKenzie III, H.C.,** 2011. Equine hyperlipidemias. Vet. Clin. North Am. Equine Pract. 27, 59–72.

• **Peek, S.F.,** 2004. Cholangiohepatitis in the mature horse. Equine Vet. Educ. 16, 72–75.

• **Taylor, P.,** 1996. Heat stroke, exhaustion and synchronous diaphragmatic flutter. In: Dyson, S. (Ed.), A Guide to the Management of Emergencies at Equine Competitions. Equine Veterinary Journal Ltd, Newmarket, pp. 102–113.

• **Whiting, J.,** 2009. The exhausted horse. In: Robinson, N.E., Sprayberry, K.A. (Eds.), Current Therapy in Equine Medicine (sixth ed.). Elsevier, St. Louis, Missouri, pp. 926–929.

CHAPTER

12   Emergencies in foals

The basics

Like human and other animal neonates, disease progresses quickly and many equine neonatal illnesses are potentially fatal if left untreated. The early clinical signs are often subtle and it may not be possible to get a specific diagnosis before instituting treatment. It is better to start treatment while the foal is bright and standing rather than waiting for it to become recumbent. The routine postpartum check of the mare and foal are a good way of picking up abnormalities that may have not been noticed by the owner/carer. Supportive care can be provided on site but for the very sick foal this is often impractical. Intensive, critical care can be expensive (where facilities are available) and referral should be undertaken early. If unsure, discuss with the referral facility at an early stage.

Handling and clinical examination

▶ Neonates are very susceptible to infection, particularly via the oral route in the first 24 h of life – wear gloves when examining them and be as aseptic as possible when obtaining blood samples, administering IV medications or when placing IV catheters.
▶ Ensure the mare is properly restrained – serious injury to handlers can result where the mare cannot see the foal and panics or where the mare is overly protective and becomes aggressive.
▶ Minimise any stress to the foal – examination and treatment may be more easily performed by restraining the foal in lateral recumbency (Fig. 12.1).
▶ Do not lift the foal under the abdomen (increased risk of patent urachus).
▶ Normal clinical values are given in Table 12.1.

Medications

▶ Dosages of antimicrobial medications are different in the neonate due to inherent physiological differences compared to the adult (Table 12.2).
▶ Enrofloxacin is contraindicated in all skeletally immature individuals (cartilage damage).
▶ Other medications are used at the same dose rate as in adults, unless indicated otherwise.
▶ Responsible antimicrobial use must be considered when selecting the appropriate drug.

Sedation

<4 weeks old
▶ 0.1–0.25 mg/kg diazepam or midazolam IV ± 0.04 mg/kg butorphanol IV or
▶ 0.3–0.5 mg/kg midazolam IM
▶ Often results in recumbency for 15–30 min – keep the foal warm and monitor carefully

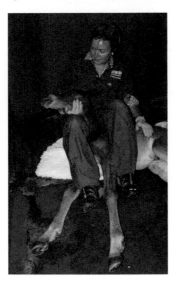

Figure 12.1 Restraint of a foal in lateral recumbency.

>4 weeks old

▸ Xylazine 0.25–0.5 mg/kg IV or
▸ Romifidine 0.02–0.08 mg/kg IV

Table 12.1 Normal clinical values in the neonatal foal

Parameter	Normal value
Length of gestation	335d (332–342d)
Time to sternal position	10 min (5–30 min)
Time to standing	60 min (15–105 min)
Time to nurse from mare	110 min (35–240 min)
Heart rate:	
Birth	60–80 beats/min
0–2 h	120–150 beats/min
Day 1–5	80–120 beats/min
Respiratory rate:	
Immediately post-foaling	60–80 breaths/min
1–48 h	30–40 breaths/min
Temperature	37.2–38.9°C (99.0–102.0°F)
Passage of meconium	<24 h
Urination	<6 h colt foals <10 h fillies
Urine specific gravity	More concentrated for first 48 h (up to 1.032) Then <1.012
Approximate weight (newborn)	Pony 30 kg TB 50 kg Draft breed 60–70 kg
Daily weight gain	1–1.5 kg (TB)
Milk volume intake/d (L)	25% body weight

Table 12.2 Dosages of antimicrobial medications that may be used in foals

Antimicrobial	Dose, route and frequency	Spectrum of activity	Main indications
Amikacin	30 mg/kg (neonate) or 20–25 mg/kg (older foal) IV q. 24 h	G −ve	Use with penicillin for BS use/sepsis
Ampicillin sodium	22 mg/kg IM q. 12 h or IV q. 6–8 h	G +ve	Combine with aminoglycoside for BS use
Azithromycin	10 mg/kg PO q. 24 h for 5 d then q. 48 h	G +ve and G −ve activity	*Rhodococcus equi* infection
Cefquinome	1–2.5 mg/kg q. 12 h IV or IM	Broad	Sepsis, pneumonia, joint/bone infections, meningitis
Ceftiofur	5–10 mg/kg IV or IM q. 12 h	Broad	Sepsis, pneumonia, joint/bone infections
Clarithromycin	7.5 mg/kg PO q. 12 h	G +ve, limited G −ve/anaerobes	*Rhodococcus equi* infections, umbilical/bone abscess, pneumonia
Doxycycline	10 mg/kg PO q. 12 h	Broad	Umbilical/other abscess
Erythromycin	20–30 mg/kg PO q. 6–8 h	Relatively broad	*Rhodococcus equi* infections, umbilical/bone abscess, pneumonia
Gentamicin	11–15 mg/kg IV q. 24 h	G −ve	Combine with penicillin for sepsis/BS use
Metronidazole	15 mg/kg PO or IV q. 8–12 h	Anaerobes	Clostridial/other anaerobic infection
Oxytetracycline	5–10 mg/kg IV q. 12 h	Broad	Bone infection/pneumonia
Penicillin (procaine)	22 000–44 000 IU/kg IM q. 12 h	G +ve, anaerobes	Combine with aminoglycoside for sepsis/BS use
Penicillin (sodium)	22 000 IU/kg IV q. 6 h	G +ve, anaerobes	Combine with aminoglycoside for sepsis/BS use

(Continued)

Table 12.2 Dosages of antimicrobial medications that may be used in foals (Continued)

Antimicrobial	Dose, route and frequency	Spectrum of activity	Main indications
Trimethoprim sulphonamide (TMPS)	30 mg/kg PO (IV/IM preparations also available)	G +ve, G −ve	Reasonable first-line antimicrobial (some bacterial resistance)
Rifampin	7.5 mg/kg PO q. 12 h	G +ve, anaerobes	Must be used in combination with other antimicrobial – *Rhodococcus equi* infections (plus macrolide), umbilical infection (plus TMPS)
Ticarcillin/clavulanic acid (Timentin®)	50 mg/kg IV q. 6 h	Broad	Sepsis

Emergency anaesthesia

▶ Sedation may induce recumbency in younger foals and it may be possible to perform minor procedures (e.g. radiography, cast application) without the need for GA.
▶ <4 weeks of age, liver function is immature but foals mature fast and >4 weeks of age are more like a young horse.
▶ Anaesthesia of sick neonatal foals and longer-duration anaesthesia of older foals should be performed in hospital facilities.

Resuscitation of the neonatal foal

Cardiac/respiratory arrest can occur in foals during parturition even where there may be no underlying cause. These foals are good candidates for resuscitation compared to critically ill foals/adults that arrest as a result of a disease process. This process can be started during prolonged vaginal delivery if it is possible to intubate and ventilate the foal (see EXIT technique, p. 156). Where a veterinary surgeon is not present at parturition, CPR may have to be initiated by stud staff. For less-experienced horse owners/carers, advice on how to perform mouth-to-nose resuscitation and chest compressions may need to be given over the telephone.

Foals that are more likely to require CPR

▶ Illness in the mare during pregnancy.
▶ Vaginal discharge during pregnancy.
▶ Identification of placental thickening.
▶ Early udder development.
▶ Delivery by Caesarean section.
▶ Prolonged vaginal delivery (stage 2 labour >20 min).

Indications for CPR

- No heart beat.
- No spontaneous breaths.
- Gasping/dyspnoeic/irregular respiratory pattern.
- HR <50 beats/min.

1. Make a note of the time and make sure the mare is properly restrained.
2. Place the foal in lateral recumbency on a clean, firm surface with the head on a towel (quickly check for any suspected fractured ribs – if so, place foal with the affected side nearest the ground).
3. Start the ABCD of resuscitation.

Airway

- **Intubate** via nares.
- If unsuccessful in 20s, intubate via the mouth.
- Check ET tube is in the trachea.

Breathing

- Connect resuscitation bag to ET tube.
- **Ventilate at 20 breaths/min** using supplemental oxygen if available – room air is fine.
- If no equipment is available, perform **mouth-to-nose resuscitation:**
  - cup the foal's chin and occlude the lower nostril with one hand
  - blow into the upper nostril
  - use the other free hand (or helper if available) to gently occlude to oesophagus on the LHS of the neck to minimise aerophagia.

Circulation

- **Start thoracic compressions immediately if no heart beat is detected (asystole) or if HR <50 beats/min.**
- Kneel on spine side of the foal.
- Place your hands on top of each other over the highest point of the chest immediately behind the triceps – make sure your shoulders are in line with your hands.
- Start chest compressions at 80–120 beats/min.

Drugs

- **If asystole/bradycardia (<40 beats/min) or HR is not increasing to >60 beats/min.**
- Administer **adrenaline IV** 0.01–0.02 mg/kg **(0.5–1.0 mL for 50-kg foal of 1:1000, 1 mg/mL preparation).**
- If IV access cannot be obtained, can give **intratracheally** (urinary catheter placed down ET tube at high dose rate 0.1–0.2 mg/kg (5–10 mL)).
- Alternatively, give **intraosseously** – 14G needle placed in proximal ⅓ tibia or radius.
- **Do not inject directly into the heart.**
- Other drugs should not be administered unless an ECG has been placed and specific therapy given, e.g. ventricular tachycardia.

4. Determine if resuscitation has been successful:

   a. assess PLRs at the same time – check for response

   b. stop chest compressions and check heart beat every 30 s.

5. If HR stable and >60 beats/min:

   a. stop respiration and check for spontaneous breathing (16 breaths/min) – if not, continue respiratory support

   b. **do not withdraw respiratory support too early** – can result in failure of CPR.

6. If there is no response to resuscitation:

   a. continue chest compressions and ventilation

   b. repeat adrenaline if no response every 3 min – increase dose to 0.1–0.2 mg/kg (5–10 mL)

   c. stop CPR if there is no development of spontaneous heart beat/respiration after 15 min (poor chance of survival).

7. If there is a HR but the pulse is weak or MM are pale/cyanotic, start fluid therapy:

   a. bolus given IV or intraosseously

   b. 10 mL/kg (500 mL) balanced electrolyte solution

   c. or 2 mL/kg (100 mL) hydroxyethyl starch (hetastarch 6%/pentastarch 10%).

HANDY TIP

To get an idea of the rate of compressions, the Bee Gees 'Stayin' Alive' has 104 beats/min (as recommended by the British Heart Foundation and American Heart Association as a guide to the rate at which chest compressions should be performed during CPR in humans).

What next?

▸ Move the foal and mare to a warm stable out of any draughts.

▸ Monitor closely for 30 min.

▸ Ideally, continue oxygen supplementation (facemask/nasal tube) and monitor with ECG (not practical in many situations outside hospital facilities).

▸ Discuss referral for hospitalisation and contact the referral centre – these foals are at high risk of developing complications, e.g. NMS, septicaemia.

▸ If this is not an option, monitor the foal closely.

The sick neonatal foal

Sick neonatal foals can deteriorate rapidly and are often more compromised than you might think. Sepsis is one of the most common causes of death in these foals and prompt, appropriate treatment is essential. Basic treatment, including administration of antimicrobials, fluid therapy and glucose supplementation, can be performed outside a hospital environment and can be life-saving if instituted early.

▶ Periparturient illness in the mare.
▶ Dystocia – any delay in stage 2 of foaling.
▶ Foals delivered by AVD/Caesarean section.
▶ Foals that have been resuscitated.
▶ Foaling in adverse environmental conditions.
▶ Poor-quality colostrum/milk supply.
▶ Orphan foal/maternal rejection.
▶ Any form of neonatal illness.

History

Obtain a full history – if the foal is collapsed this may need to be performed once the foal has been stabilised.

▶ Maternal history – previous foaling and any problems, health during most recent pregnancy, vaccination history, did mare run milk prior to foaling?
▶ Any on-farm problems, e.g. recent abortions, other sick foals?
▶ Gestation length – normal/abnormal?
▶ When was the foal born and did any problems occur (was foaling observed)?
▶ Placenta – normal/abnormal?
▶ Has the foal stood/nursed from the mare/urinated/passed meconium/routine umbilical care?
▶ Any other problems noted?

Initial clinical assessment

▶ Control any seizures (see p. 240).
▶ If the foal is collapsed, perform a brief initial examination to assess:
  ▪ general appearance and demeanour
  ▪ MM colour
  ▪ temperature of extremities
  ▪ RR and pattern
  ▪ HR – rate and rhythm
  ▪ ± measure systemic lactate and glucose.
▶ A full physical examination must be performed once the foal has been stabilised (Table 12.3).
▶ Rule out any congenital defects/other abnormalities that may have a bearing on prognosis (particularly if referral for more intensive care is likely to be required).

Initial treatment

Administer intranasal oxygen if required/available:

▶ Ideally oxygen should be administered intranasally following dystocia/resuscitation (5–10 L/min).
▶ Indicated if the foal is displaying the following signs:
  ▪ dyspnoea
  ▪ cyanotic MM
  ▪ evidence of meconium staining on the coat
  ▪ recumbency.
▶ This will be impractical to perform for prolonged periods outside hospital facilities.

Table 12.3 Checklist when examining the neonatal foal

	Normal	Requires further assessment/ treatment
General behaviour and mentation	Normal exaggerated response to sound and touch	Abnormal mentation/bizarre or unusual behaviour (consider NMS/ seizures)
General appearance and coat	Soft and evidence of foetal maturity	Dysmature/premature physical characteristics (see p. 230) Meconium staining – risk of aspiration pneumonia
Examination of the head and nares	No visual deformity or nasal discharge	Nasal discharge of milk – consider NMS, cleft palate or other congenital abnormality
Mucous membranes	Pink MM, CRT <2 s	Petechiation – septicaemia Jaundice – septicaemia, NI Pale – haemorrhage Congestion – birthing trauma Cyanosis – respiratory/cardiac compromise
Eyes	Pupillary light reflex present but slow Menace develops by 10–14 d Scleral bruising/ subconjunctival haemorrhage may be present for first few days	Painful/inflamed eye – do not miss corneal ulceration Evidence of entropion (correction by repeated manual eversion of eyelids/temporary sutures)
External assessment of the thorax	Check for evidence of wounds/swelling/crepitus over the ribs	Respiratory distress/flail chest (see p. 239)
Auscultation of the heart and lungs	Physiological flow murmur: left 3rd ICS, holosystolic, disappears by 3–7 d of age Closure of ductus arteriosus: continuous/machinery murmur – disappears <24 h Normal foals may have dysrhythmias for up to 15 min after birth – these usually resolve spontaneously	Murmur persists >7 d There is evidence of cyanosis/ exercise intolerance

(*Continued*)

Table 12.3 Checklist when examining the neonatal foal   (Continued)

	Normal	Requires further assessment/ treatment
Visual inspection and palpation of the umbilicus	Clean, dry and minimal/no swelling	Moisture, dribbling of urine (consider patent/persistent urachus) Heat/pain/swelling (consider umbilical abscess)
Scrotum/ perineum	Check for congenital abnormalities and testes descended	Scrotal enlargement (inguinal hernia) – conservative management involving manual reduction of hernia contents q. 8–12h indicated – most do not cause any problems and resolve over several weeks but strangulation of herniated intestine may be suspected if an affected foal develops colic and ↑ scrotal swelling
Legs and hooves	Epinicum on hoof ('foal slippers') – foal hasn't stood/ stood much Mild laxity and ALD common	Heat/pain/swelling around joint (consider joint sepsis) Severe deformities that prevent the foal standing
Rectum/anus	Yellow pasty faeces – confirm meconium (tarry black/brown) has been passed	No evidence of meconium passage within 24h
Check sucking and measure IgG (>18h) ± blood samples for laboratory assessment, e.g. SAA	Colostrum absorption ceases around 24h Normal IgG >8g/L (ideal) <4g/L increased sepsis risk	Failure of passive transfer if insufficient colostrum intake (should have at least 1 L in first 6h) Foals can become hypovolaemic in 4–6h if off suck

Administer IV fluids and glucose:

▸ If in doubt give! This is an easy way to potentially save a foal and you are likely to do more good than harm.
▸ Skin tent, PCV/TP are not reliable measures of hydration in the neonate – may need to rely on history of not nursing/other clinical signs.
▸ IV fluids should be administered if the foal:
  ▪ has not nursed in the last 4h (likely to be hypovolaemic)
  ▪ has weak pulses, cold extremities, tachypnoea.
  ▪ if systemic lactate >2.5mmol/L (definitely needed if ≥5mmol/L).
▸ How to give:
  ▪ via IV catheter in the jugular vein (16G, 8cm) – is easier and safer than doing 'off the needle'.

▶ Fluids to give:
   ▪ balanced electrolyte solution (Hartmann's/LRS/NaCl 0.9%):
      » 1 L for 50-kg foal, 500 mL pony foal/premature TB foal, 2 L for large draft breed foals
   ▪ can use colloids (theoretically better volume expansion, stay in circulation longer):
      » total daily dose not to exceed 10 mL/kg (hetastarch) or 15 mL/kg (pentastarch)
   ▪ plasma is impractical (may not be available/need to defrost) and there is the disadvantage of a possible immune reaction, which is not ideal in the acutely collapsed foal
▶ Can add 50% glucose or dextrose to resuscitation fluids (add 10–20 mL 50% solution per 1 L of fluids) to treat concurrent hypoglycaemia.
▶ How much to give – bolus method:
   ▪ 20 mL/kg Hartmann's solution (± 4–5 mL/kg colloid) + 20 mL 50% dextrose
   ▪ 1 L in a 50-kg foal (± 200–250 mL colloid)
   ▪ warm the fluids before administering
   ▪ auscultate the heart and lungs before starting fluid therapy
   ▪ give over 20 min
   ▪ reassess – if there is little improvement, repeat
   ▪ at least 2 boluses are usually needed (if no change, inotrope therapy required – see texts)
   ▪ if pulmonary oedema develops (unlikely), give furosemide 0.25–1.0 mg/kg IV.

Keep the foal clean, warm and dry:
▶ use blankets/rugs, leg bandages.
▶ keep in a warm, draught-free environment.

Perform full clinical examination, identify and treat any underlying illness (see Table 12.3):
▶ Take blood samples for IgG measurement, haematology and serum biochemistry.
▶ Perform sepsis scoring (Table 12.4).

Administer appropriate antimicrobial medication:
▶ If sepsis is suspected, start BS antimicrobial (Table 12.2) – if referral is likely, discuss with the referral centre first.

Monitoring and ongoing care

▶ Short-term mild illness – can be managed on site.
▶ Nursing care includes:
   ▪ if recumbent, ideally try to maintain in sternal recumbency or turn every 1–3 h
   ▪ encourage to stand to suckle every 2 h
   ▪ monitor carefully for corneal ulcers and decubital ulcers.
▶ If the foal is unable to stand and suckle, hospitalisation should be considered (ideally 24-h dedicated neonatal intensive care unit).
▶ Determine if oral nutrition can be instituted (no reflux/evidence of ileus and foal can maintain itself in sternal recumbency):
   ▪ encourage the foal to suckle from the mare q. 2 h (assist if required)
   ▪ if the foal will not suckle, obtain milk from the mare (or use a commercial milk replacer at 75% strength) and administer via a stomach tube.

Table 12.4 Sepsis scoring system for neonatal foals

Information collected	Factor	4	3	2	1	0	Score
Historical	High-risk foal (see p. 225)		Yes			No	
	Gestational age (days)		<300	301–310	311–330	>331	
Clinical examination	Petechiation/scleral injection (not 2° to eye disease or trauma)		+++	++	+	Normal	
	Pyrexia (°C)		>39	38–39		Normal	
	Hypotonia/coma/depression/convulsions			+++	+	None	
	Uveitis/diarrhoea/joint effusion/wounds	Yes				No	
Haematology	Neutrophil count (× 10⁹/L)	<2.0	2.0–4.0	4.0–8.0		Normal	
	Band neutrophils		>0.2	0.05–0.2		<0.05	
	Toxic neutrophils	+++	++	+		None	
	Fibrinogen (g/L) (or SAA)		>6.0	4.0–6.0	3.0–4.0	<3.0	
Serum biochemistry	Blood glucose (mmol/L)		2.0–4.0	<3.0	3.0–4.5	>4.5	
	IgG (g/L)	<2.0	2.0–4.0	4.0–6.0	6.0–8.0	>8.0	
						Total=	

Adapted from Knottenbelt, Holdstock and Madigan (2004) and the University of Florida.

A total score of ≥11 correctly predicts sepsis around 93% of the time and a score of ≤10 correctly predicts non-sepsis 88% of the time (+++ marked; ++ moderate; +slight).

▶ Seek advice/refer at an early stage (i.e. do not wait until the foal becomes comatose) – this gives the best chance of survival.

▶ Discuss costs, deposits and likely prognosis with the referral centre and relay this information to the owner for them to make an informed decision about referral – *costs of intensive care for neonates can be considerable.*

▶ Inform the insurance company (where appropriate).

▶ Discuss medications with the referral centre and send a copy of the clinical notes, medications administered and when, any blood results (including IgG status), placenta (if newborn, in leak-proof bag, tied securely) and colostrum/milk from the mare if the foal is initially being sent without the mare.

▶ If >90 min from referral centre, administer 1 L crystalloids – can be administered 'off the needle' using a 16 G needle (be as aseptic as possible).

▶ Organise transport asap – ensure that the mare cannot step on the foal (horse box better than trailer, sedate the mare if necessary), load the foal first and place the foal on vet bed/carpet.

▶ Bandage the foal's lower limbs, place padding under the foal and keep them warm.

▶ If there will be a delay with transport, transport the foal in a car (not in the boot/back of a pickup) and transport the mare later.

Prematurity/dysmaturity

▶ Prematurity = foal born <320 d that displays immature physical characteristics.

▶ Dysmaturity = foal born at term that displays immature physical characteristics.

▶ Low birth weight.

▶ Weak at birth and takes a long time to stand.

▶ Abnormally low or high respiratory rate/respiratory distress.

▶ Floppy ears and domed head.

▶ Short, silky hair coat.

▶ Flexor tendon laxity.

▶ Radiographic evidence of incomplete ossification of the carpal and tarsal bones.

▶ Usually require critical care:
  ▪ <305 d – most require intensive care
  ▪ <280 d – unlikely to survive despite intensive care (generally the prognosis is hopeless if there is incomplete ossification of cuboidal bones).

▶ Treatment – depends on findings on clinical examination.

Failure of passive transfer of immunity

This may be suspected where there has been insufficient colostrum intake in the first 24 h of life or where the colostrum is of poor quality (e.g. debilitated mares, mares that run milk before foaling and some maiden mares). Confirmation is provided by measurement of IgG status >12–18 h following birth.

Treatment

▶ If the mare has poor-quality colostrum, give 500 mL of good-quality donor colostrum (can be stored frozen for up to 18 months, do not microwave to defrost).
▶ If the foal doesn't suck, the mare can be milked (be hygienic, wear gloves) and colostrum can be administered by stomach tube.
▶ If neither of these options is possible, plasma can be given IV (or PO) or as a last option bovine colostrum can be given (poor alternative).
▶ Determine IgG level >18 h following birth:
  ▪ <4 g/L (<400 mg/dL) – increased risk of sepsis; plasma transfusion recommended
  ▪ 4–8 g/L (400–800 mg/dL) – not ideal but acceptable; monitor carefully, good management
  ▪ >8 g/L (>800 mg/dL) – ideal.
▶ If a plasma transfusion is required:
  ▪ ideal – commercial plasma (hyperimmune plasma – can be expensive)
  ▪ alternative – blood taken from mare or suitable donor (see p. 376), plasma separated and administered
  ▪ thaw plasma slowly to room temperature/in water <38°C – do not microwave
  ▪ place an IV catheter, administer via a giving set with a filter
  ▪ administer 25 mL in first 10–20 min to check for transfusion reaction
  ▪ can then administer up to 2 L/h
  ▪ septic foals require more plasma to increase IgG levels
    ▪ IgG 4–8 g/L: 1 L minimum (50-kg foal)
    ▪ IgG <4 g/L: 2–4 L minimum (50-kg foal).
▶ Repeat IgG in 12–24 h – if desired IgG not reached, can administer more plasma.
▶ If these options are not available, can do nothing but ensure the foal is monitored carefully.

Septicaemia

Septicaemia is common in neonatal foals and infection may occur in utero, by ingestion/inhalation or via the umbilicus. The prognosis is better if foals are treated early: so if septicaemia is suspected, initiate appropriate antimicrobial treatment early – do not wait until the foal becomes recumbent.

Clinical signs

▶ Depression, stop suckling.
▶ Hyperaemic and congested/jaundiced MM.
▶ Scleral injection.
▶ Hyperaemic coronary bands.
▶ Petechial haemorrhages (oral, nasal, vaginal mucosae, conjunctivae, within pinnae).
▶ Recumbency.
▶ Rectal T° often not reliable.
▶ ± Local infection – joints, umbilicus, lungs, eyes.

▶ Take blood samples for haematology, serum biochemistry (including fibrinogen/SAA), IgG status and culture (be sterile):
  ▪ WBC ↑/↓/ normal
  ▪ fibrinogen not always ↑
  ▪ SAA >100 mg/L increases suspicion
  ▪ −ve blood culture doesn't rule out sepsis.
▶ Determine the likelihood of sepsis based on the sepsis score (see Table 12.4).
▶ Start antimicrobial treatment (unless the foal is being referred and the hospital has requested that antimicrobials are not given until they have obtained blood for C&S).
▶ Administer bactericidal drugs IV initially.
▶ Usually G −ve organisms, so consider:
  ▪ gentamicin/amikacin and penicillin (only if well hydrated)
  ▪ ceftiofur
  ▪ cefquinome
  ▪ Trimethoprim sulphonamide (organisms may not be sensitive).
▶ Initiate fluid therapy ± plasma administration.
▶ Check and monitor for infection elsewhere – further investigations and treatment as required: (see relevant sections/texts)
  ▪ umbilical infection
  ▪ pneumonia
  ▪ septic arthritis
  ▪ enteritis – diarrhoea/colic
  ▪ meningitis (more common in foals compared to adults)
  ▪ can develop concurrent uveitis – ↓ survival in these cases.

Neonatal maladjustment syndrome (perinatal asphyxia syndrome)

This is a syndrome where behavioural/neurological abnormalities that are not related to a known cause are seen (also known as barker, wanderers or dummy foals). Neonatal maladjustment syndrome (NMS) is thought to be a sequel to hypoxia and ischaemia before, during or after parturition. Foals may be normal at birth and show no evidence of disease for hours to 4–5 d afterwards or they may exhibit violent CNS activity immediately following birth. This syndrome is also associated with systems other than the CNS – renal and vascular dysfunction and necrotising enterocolitis may also occur in affected foals.

Clinical signs

▶ Highly variable.

Mild

▶ Loss of affinity for the mare.
▶ Inappropriate suckle reflex/milk on forehead.
▶ Wandering, intermittent depression and stargazing.
▶ ± Facial spasms, lip curling/chomping, abnormal respiratory patterns.

More severe

▶ Unaware of environment.
▶ Blindness of central origin.
▶ Seizures – subtle, short duration (e.g. stretching activity) to violent tonic–clonic convulsions, opisthotonos, extensor rigidity.

Initial assessment and treatment

▶ Perform emergency resuscitation if respiratory arrest occurs (see Resuscitation, p. 223).
▶ Treat seizures if present (see Seizure, p. 240).
▶ Obtain a history. Specific questions that should be asked include:
  ▪ any history of prepartum problems
  ▪ problems at foaling – dystocia/Caesarean section.
▶ Perform a full clinical assessment.
▶ Take blood samples for haematology and serum biochemistry:
  ▪ rule out other possible causes, including metabolic or hepatic disease.
▶ Treatment is largely symptomatic.
▶ ± Oxygen therapy.
▶ BS antimicrobials (prevent secondary infection).
▶ Decide if IV fluids are required – use IV fluids judiciously as they can worsen cerebral oedema.
▶ If cerebral oedema is present can give:
  ▪ DMSO 0.5–1.0 g/kg IV as 10% solution
  ▪ mannitol 0.25–1 g/kg IV as 20% solution
  ▪ ± magnesium/thiamine (see texts).
▶ Decide how nutritional support is to be provided for the foal:
  ▪ if it won't suck, feed via an indwelling nasogastric tube – only if able to sit in sternal recumbency and has evidence of GI motility (check for presence of reflux first)
  ▪ if comatose, IV fluids/parenteral nutrition required.
▶ May have concurrent problems, e.g. uveitis, corneal ulcers.

Ongoing treatment and prognosis

▶ Depends on the severity of the initial insult and progression of oedema and cell damage.
▶ Determine if nursing care can be provided on site or if referral/hospitalisation is required.
▶ Can be difficult to differentiate vs meningitis/hydrocephalus – rule out if no improvement or deterioration.
▶ In many foals clinical signs are mild and they will recover over 1–2 d with no long-term effects.
▶ Seizures – if they can be controlled, the prognosis can be good with good nursing care and if secondary complications do not occur.
▶ Grave prognosis – fixed, dilated pupils.

Severe flexural limb deformities

These may be a cause of dystocia or may be severe enough to prevent the foal from standing and suckling. These foals should receive assistance to stand and suckle and prompt assessment and treatment is required for severe limb contractures (Fig. 12.2, Table 12.5).

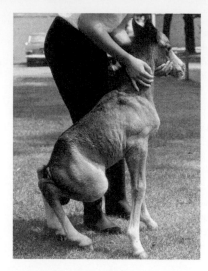

Figure 12.2　Bilateral patellar luxation in a foal.

Courtesy of Peter Clegg.

Table 12.5 Types of flexural limb deformities that may require immediate assessment and treatment

Deformity	Clinical signs	Initial treatment
Congenital carpal contracture	Carpi maintained in flexion 'praying mantis stance'	Limit exercise in mild cases Carpal splinting ± 3g/50kg oxytetracycline IV, repeat every 48h for 2 more doses (monitor renal function – urinalysis (casts) and serum creatinine) If severe, poor prognosis even with surgery
Congenital flexural deformity lower limbs	Distal limb (DIP/PIP and/or MCP/MTP joints) maintained in flexion	Bandage and apply splint ± Oxytetracycline (see above) Casting under sedation/GA if severe
Digital hyperextension deformity	Sunken fetlocks ± toe dorsally elevated Can develop skin abrasions	Light bandages (must not be too heavy or will exacerbate laxity) + light exercise If elevated toe – farriery required (heel extensions)
Lateral luxation of the patella	Crouched HL Relatively rare – more common in miniature breeds	Surgery required

Septic arthritis

This should always be suspected in cases of acute-onset lameness – owners/carers often wrongly assume that the foal has traumatised the limb or that it has been stepped on by the mare. In contrast to adults, infection is usually via the haematogenous route and concurrent osteomyelitis is common. Early diagnosis and appropriate treatment is essential in optimising prognosis.

Clinical signs

▶ Joint effusion – may be evident in multiple joints.
▶ Heat/pain/swelling/oedema around joint(s).
▶ Lameness.
▶ ± Pyrexia.

Diagnosis

▶ Synoviocentesis (see p. 346).
▶ Haematology and fibrinogen measurement.
▶ Radiography – check for concurrent osteomyelitis (can check contralateral limb if unsure whether normal/abnormal).
▶ US of joint(s) – US of the umbilicus should also be performed to determine if there is concurrent infection of the umbilical remnants (see texts/website).

Treatment

▶ Joint lavage – perform early, large volumes best.
▶ All affected joints must be treated.
▶ Optimal – arthroscopic lavage under GA (seek referral).
▶ Alternative – through-and-through needle lavage (see texts for further details):
  ▪ sedation/short GA, clip, sterile preparation and distend joint with 2% mepivacaine and leave for 5–10 min, LA around sites of needle placement
  ▪ 16–18G needles, 2–3 L sterile warmed balanced electrolyte solution flushed through joint.
▶ ± Umbilical resection (if infected umbilicus also present).
▶ Systemic antimicrobials:
  ▪ initially BS
  ▪ alter according to C&S results.
▶ ± Regional infusion of antimicrobials.

Prognosis

▶ Depends on the duration of synovial sepsis, severity (including bone involvement) and treatment performed.

Colic

Colic in the foal can be more challenging to investigate compared to the adult horse. Key points to consider in the foal with colic include:

▶ Their small size precludes rectal examination but US and radiography can be more useful than in the adult.

▶ Pain response is less reliable compared to the adult horse – severe pain may be exhibited in cases of impending enteritis and it can be challenging to differentiate between this and a lesion that requires surgical correction.

Possible causes

▶ Meconium retention.

▶ Congenital defects.

▶ Surgical disorders – SI volvulus/intussusception more common than in adults.

▶ Ileus – perinatal asphyxia syndrome, septicaemia.

▶ Enteritis.

▶ Ruptured bladder.

▶ Gastroduodenal ulceration.

Initial assessment

▶ Obtain a full history. Specific questions that should be asked include:
  ▪ if meconium has been passed (neonate)
  ▪ any previous/ongoing medication
  ▪ urination observed
  ▪ disease, e.g. enteritis in any other foals on the premises.

▶ Perform a general clinical examination:
  ▪ assess the foal from outside the stable – demeanour, posture, abdominal distension, signs of abdominal discomfort exhibited
  ▪ perform a general clinical examination (include percussion of the abdomen)
  ▪ check colt foals for inguinal herniation.

▶ Take blood samples for:
  ▪ haematology
  ▪ serum biochemistry and electrolytes
  ▪ IgG assessment (neonate).

▶ Pass a nasogastric tube – check for reflux (>500 mL significant).

▶ ± US examination of the abdomen:
  ▪ very useful – 5–7-MHz linear/microconvex transducer
  ▪ assess for ↑ abdominal fluid (consider ruptured bladder), evidence of SI distension (>3-cm diameter) or thickening (>5-mm thickness).

▶ ± Abdominocentesis:
  ▪ perform under US guidance
  ▪ teat cannula technique may be preferred (see p. 341) to minimise the risk of lacerating thin-walled intestine in neonates.

▶ ± Radiography (up to 250 kg):
  ▪ lateral radiographs
  ▪ ± contrast radiography – localise obstruction.

▶ ± Gastroscopy (if gastroduodenal ulceration suspected, ↑ hepatic enzymes or history of diarrhoea).

Assessment and plan

‣ Depends on underlying cause.
‣ Meconium retention – soapy water commercial (phosphate) or acetylcystine retention enema:
  ▪ 8 g N-acetylcysteine (or 40 mL 20% acetylcysteine) + 20 g bicarbonate of soda (baking powder)
  ▪ sedate the foal (see p. 219) and elevate the hindquarters
  ▪ administer using a Foley catheter and 50-mL syringe
  ▪ allow to flow in by gravity and try to keep the enema in for 30 min.
‣ Provide analgesia.
  ▪ NSAIDs – be careful regarding potential nephrotoxicity and ensure that the foal is well hydrated first
  ▪ butorphanol 0.01–0.04 mg/kg IV useful
  ▪ can administer hyoscine butylbromide 0.3 mg/kg IV.
‣ Initiate treatment as for sick foal (see p. 224).
‣ If no response to medical therapy – hospitalisation/referral required for further diagnostic evaluation and surgery or intensive medical care.

Diarrhoea

Diarrhoea is common in foals in the first 6 months of life and may range from mild, self-limiting disease of unknown aetiology to more severe enterocolitis and death. Cases of impending enterocolitis can also present with signs of severe colic. Hypovolaemia can occur rapidly in severe cases and these foals are at risk of septicaemia. Therefore early and aggressive treatment is important in these cases.

Initial treatment and diagnostic investigations

‣ Obtain a full history. Specific questions include:
  ▪ gestation length, problems during pregnancy/parturition, IgG status
  ▪ rate of progression and quantity/nature of diarrhoea
  ▪ whether other foals are/have been affected
  ▪ mare's vaccination status
  ▪ management change – new feed, mixing with older foals, access to grazing
  ▪ parasite control.
‣ Perform a full clinical examination:
  ▪ estimation of hydration status
  ▪ abdominal distension/signs of colic
  ▪ check for evidence of septic arthritis
  ▪ T°.
‣ Further diagnostic tests (see Table 12.6 for potential causes of diarrhoea):
  ▪ faecal samples for culture, rotavirus testing (do not take using latex gloves - false +ve results) and WEC
  ▪ blood sample – haematology and serum biochemistry ± IgG status
  ▪ toxin testing if clostridial disease suspected
  ▪ ± US/radiography.

Table 12.6 Common causes of diarrhoea in different ages of foals

<2 weeks	2–8 weeks	>8 weeks	All ages
NMS	Rotavirus*	*Strongyloides westeri**	*Salmonella* spp.*
Necrotising enterocolitis	*Crypto-sporidium parvum**	*Cyathostomum* spp.*	Nutrition (e.g. lactose intolerance)
Foal heat			
Rotavirus*	*Strongyloides westeri**	*Lawsonia intracellularis**	Luminal irritants
*Clostridium difficile**			
*Clostridium perfringens**			
*Cryptosporidium parvum**			

Adapted from Hepburn (2007).

*Denotes infectious conditions.

▶ Supportive care, including hydration and nutrition (see Sick foal, p. 224).
▶ Antimicrobial therapy if appropriate:
  ▪ indicated if pyrexic
  ▪ ceftiofur, cefquinome or penicillin/gentamicin (adjust according to C&S).
▶ NSAIDs:
  ▪ flunixin 0.5–1 mg/kg q. 12 h IV.
▶ Other therapies:
  ▪ Mild diarrhoea – bismuth subsalicylate 17–35 mg/kg (1–2 mL/kg Pepto-Bismol® q. 4–6 h PO) or di-tri-octahedral smectite (Bio-Sponge® – see manufacturer instructions)
  ▪ ± sucralfate 2–4 g PO q. 6–8 h
  ▪ ± omeprazole (controversial)
  ▪ >7 d old – probiotics/live yoghurt (*Saccharomyces boulardii* in particular).
▶ Nursing care:
  ▪ keep the perineal region clean – wash with baby shampoo, dry with a soft towel and apply Vaseline
  ▪ ± topical antimicrobial/steroid cream.
▶ Implement appropriate biosecurity measures, e.g. isolation if infectious disease suspected.

Ongoing treatment

▶ Severe cases – require hospitalisation, may require intensive care.
▶ Specific treatment – depends on the results of diagnostic tests (see texts).

Respiratory distress

Possible causes

▶ Fractured ribs ± pneumothorax.
▶ Pneumonia.
▶ DDSP (secondary to NMS or anatomic abnormality).

▶ Pharyngeal oedema (secondary to subepiglottic cyst, stenotic nares, tracheal collapse).
▶ Respiratory distress syndrome (associated with prematurity/dysmaturity).
▶ Choanal atresia/stenotic nares.
▶ Guttural pouch tympany.
▶ Congenital lung abnormalities.

Initial assessment and first aid treatment

▶ Check for nasal airflow, evidence of fractured ribs or obvious pharyngeal swelling.
▶ If URT obstruction is suspected, perform tracheotomy (see p. 356).
▶ Start oxygen therapy (if available 10 L/min).
▶ Specific treatment depends on underlying cause – see texts/seek specialist advice.
▶ Further assessment – endoscopy/radiography.

Rib fractures

Rib fractures are relatively common following a traumatic or rapid foaling and usually involves ribs 3–8. These fractures are often asymptomatic but in more severe cases can result in pneumothorax, haemothorax ± pericardial effusion and rapid death if a fractured rib lacerates the heart.

Clinical signs

▶ Often asymptomatic.
▶ Oedema around the fracture site.
▶ Clicking noise on auscultation.
▶ Dyspnoea/rapid breathing.

Diagnosis

▶ Palpation.
▶ US useful (best diagnostic test).

Treatment

▶ If respiratory distress is evident:
  ▪ administer intranasal oxygen
  ▪ perform thoracocentesis and drain chest (see texts/website/seek referral).
▶ BS antimicrobials if skin wound at the site/pneumothorax or haemothorax.
▶ NSAIDs.
▶ Surgical management indicated if displaced fractures/flail chest/haemothorax.
▶ ± Blood transfusion.
▶ Supportive care as required.

Guttural pouch tympany

▶ Clinical signs are related to the degree of GP distension.
▶ Perform emergency tracheotomy or percutaneous needle decompression of GP if severe respiratory distress.

▸ Initial conservative management – indwelling Foley catheters (see texts/seek referral).
▸ ± Surgical management may be required.

Seizures

Foals have a relatively low seizure threshold compared to adult horses and seizures most commonly occur as a consequence of NMS. Unobserved seizures may be suspected where unexplained traumatic injuries to the head have occurred, e.g. superficial abrasions or soil/grass impacted around the conjunctivae.

Clinical signs

Mild

▸ Facial grimacing.
▸ Twitching and jerky head movements.
▸ Repetitive blinking and eye movements.
▸ Chewing/jaw chomping.
▸ Repeated stretching/head and neck rigidity.

Severe

▸ Tonic–clonic convulsions.
▸ Dorsiflexion.
▸ Paddling.
▸ Coma and death.

Possible causes

▸ NMS/HIE.
▸ Hyponatraemia.
▸ Metabolic derangements (glucose, electrolytes, ammonia).
▸ Hepatic encephalopathy.
▸ Infection – EHV 1, septicaemia or meningitis.
▸ Trauma.
▸ Congenital abnormalities.
▸ Severe pneumonia causing hypoxia.
▸ Idiopathic – adolescent Arab foals.
▸ Persistent hyperammonaemia (older Morgan foals).

Control seizures

▸ Diazepam 0.1 mg/kg IV (5 mg in 50-kg foal) as required.
▸ If refractory, alternatives include:
  ▪ phenobarbital 8–20 mg/kg IV as loading dose diluted in saline given over 20–30 min to effect
  ▪ phenytoin 5–10 mg/kg IV, then 1–5 mg/kg IV, IM or PO q. 2–4 h
  ▪ pentobarbital 2–4 mg/kg IV slowly.

Table 12.7 Common causes of recumbency/collapse in the neonatal and older foal

Neonatal foal	1–6 months of age
Septicaemia	Trauma
Prematurity	Botulism
NMS/HIE	Pneumonia
Neonatal isoerythrolysis	White muscle disease
Septicaemia	HYPP (Quarter Horses)
Trauma	Congenital defects
Musculoskeletal disorders	
Congenital defects	

Treatment

▸ Supportive care as required (see Sick foal, p. 224).
▸ Investigation of the underlying cause and treatment as appropriate.

Prognosis

▸ Good – NMS without sepsis.
▸ Reduced – septicaemia.
▸ Poor – progressive loss of cranial nerve function, dilated, non-responsive pupils, coma >36 h.

Recumbency/collapse

Specific conditions should be considered in these cases depending on the age of the foal (see Table 12.7). Initial assessment is similar to the adult horse (see p. 313) and treatment will depend on the underlying cause (see relevant sections/texts).

Shaker foal syndrome (toxicoinfectious botulism)

This syndrome occurs in fast-growing foals between 1 week and 6 months of age, and is more common in certain geographic regions. Vaccination of mares and ensuring colostrum intake is adequate are important in high-risk regions.

Clinical signs

▸ Flaccid paralysis, weakness, muscle tremors.
▸ More pronounced with exertion.
▸ ↓ Eyelid, tail and tongue tone.
▸ Dysphagia.
▸ ± Colic.
▸ Can progress to paralysis and respiratory arrest.

Diagnosis

▶ Clinical signs in endemic area.
▶ Laboratory confirmation – low sensitivity.

Treatment

▶ Polyvalent antitoxin (antibodies vs types B and C) – 30 000 IU.
▶ Supportive therapy – intensive treatment often required (seek referral):
   ▪ respiratory support – oxygen, occasionally ventilation required
   ▪ administer BS antimicrobials if dysphagic:
      ▪ trimethoprim sulphonamides or ceftiofur
      ▪ do not administer aminoglycosides, tetracyclines or procaine penicillin – potentiate neuromuscular blockade
   ▪ nursing care as for the recumbent horse (see p. 315) – urinary catheterisation, try to keep in sternal recumbency or turn q. 2 h.

Uroperitoneum

Most commonly this occurs subsequent to a tear developing in the bladder at parturition. It can also occur secondary to infection and subsequent leakage of the bladder, urachus or ureters.

Clinical signs

▶ Initially healthy, nursing well for 24–48 h.
▶ Progressive lethargy, abdominal distension at 1–3 d of age.
▶ Straining to urinate, penile protrusion and frequent urine dribbling.
▶ DDx meconium impaction (usually tail waggling and elevation).

Diagnosis

▶ Peritoneal: serum creatinine >2:1.
▶ Free abdominal fluid evident on abdominal US/abdominal percussion.
▶ Hyper-K$^+$.
▶ Hypo-Na$^+$, hypo-Cl$^-$.
▶ Azotaemia.
▶ Metabolic and respiratory acidosis.

Treatment

▶ Referral for surgical repair – discuss fluid therapy/medication with referral centre prior to transport of the foal.
▶ Pre-operative stabilisation is critical.

Neonatal isoerythrolysis

This occurs as a result of immune-mediated destruction of the RBC of a newborn foal due to inherited incompatibilities in foetal and maternal RBC – most are associated with Qa and Aa blood groups. Clinical signs usually develop 12–48 h postpartum and will vary in severity from mild to severe.

Clinical signs

▶ Lethargy and depression.
▶ ↑ Time spent recumbent.
▶ ↑ HR, ↑ RR.
▶ Progressively stop suckling.
▶ Pale/jaundiced MM (Fig. 12.3).
▶ ± Haemoglobinuria.
▶ Severe – seizures, coma and death.

Assessment and diagnosis

▶ Obtain a full history. Specific questions that should be asked include:
  ▪ foaling history – more common in foals born to multiparous mares but can occur in primiparous mares
  ▪ age of foal and clinical signs seen.
▶ Perform a full clinical examination:
  ▪ assess concurrent dehydration.
▶ Further diagnostic tests:
  ▪ haematology – RBC $<4 \times 10^{12}$/L, Hb $</$ g/dL, PCV <20%
  ▪ ± evidence of haemolysis (haemoglobinaemia, PCV:Hb <3:1)
  ▪ ± jaundiced foal agglutination test/Coombs' test/saline agglutination cross-matching (see texts/website).

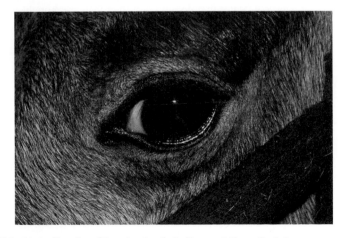

Figure 12.3 Marked jaundice of the sclera in a foal with neonatal isoerythrolysis.
Courtesy of Fernando Malalana.

Treatment

▶ Depends on the severity of clinical signs and degree of anaemia.
▶ If <36 h of age, prevent the foal from suckling from the mare, administer milk replacer or suitable donor mare colostrum (and strip colostrum from the dam's udder), then allow to suckle from the mare as normal >36 h of age.
▶ Mild cases:
   ▪ minimal handling and box rest
   ▪ monitor RBC parameters q. 12h for 48h.
▶ Blood transfusion is indicated if:
   ▪ PCV <12% and/or
   ▪ foal depressed/off suck/signs of hypoxaemia.
▶ Administration of washed RBC from mare (can calculate requirements (see p. 376) – 1–2 L packed RBC usually sufficient or 2–4 L whole blood).
▶ Wash RBC 3–5 times in saline and resuspend in an equal volume of saline.
▶ Alternatively blood can be given from cross-matched donor/gelding of the same breed (see p. 376).
▶ BS antimicrobials.
▶ Supportive treatment as required (see Sick foal, p. 224).
▶ If concurrent hypovolaemia, start fluid therapy (will ↓ haematocrit but will not ↓ number of circulating RBC and may improve tissue perfusion) and administer donor blood/washed mares RBC asap.
▶ Monitor the foal's T° and keep warm.
▶ Neurological signs and hepatic failure – poor prognosis.

Maternal rejection

This occurs in 1–5% of mares and is associated with around 6% mortality rate in rejected foals. Signs of potential rejection include avoiding, threatening, squealing at, chasing, biting and kicking their foal. Mares that do not reject their foals are more likely to lick, nicker at and defend their foal.

Factors that increase the risk of rejection

▶ Primiparous mares.
▶ Arabian mares.
▶ Multiparous mares with a history of rejection of ≥2 foals.
▶ Any mare separated from the foal for the first few hours of life.

Initial approach

▶ Ensure the safety of the foal.
▶ Restrain mare ± sedation if required (detomidine/acepromazine) or blindfolding/hobbling.
▶ Check that the mare is not painful, e.g. mastitis – analgesia/sedation.
▶ Induce/improve maternal behaviour (excessive owner observation and handling may be detrimental).
▶ Stimulate lactation (see p. 168).
▶ If these attempts are not successful, consider hand rearing/foster mare (next section).

Emergency management of the orphan foal

This may be needed if mare is dead, the mare has rejected the foal or has agalactia. Ideally the foal should be placed on a foster mare (can bottle feed whilst waiting for mare to arrive). Foals can be hand raised on mare milk replacer but this is very time consuming and owners/carers should be counselled regarding this (cute foals can turn into larger, difficult-to-handle horses). Common problems encountered with hand rearing include thermoregulation and feeding an appropriate level of nutrition.

▸ Ensure the foal has had colostrum (if newborn):
  ▪ ideally 1–2 L (minimum 500 mL) and best if fresh from mares in the same environment
  ▪ frozen colostrum can be given as an alternative (many studs store good-quality colostrum – can be stored at –20°C for 18 months and thawed at room temperature/water <38°C)
  ▪ can get artificial equine preparations (unreliable, not recommended)
  ▪ in an emergency can give equine plasma IV/PO or bovine colostrum.
▸ Keep in a warm, draught-free stable with access to fresh water at all times – rug and bandage legs/place under heat lamp if required.
▸ What milk to give:
  ▪ commercial mare milk replacers available – follow the instructions, warm to 38°C and for the first couple of feeds, give half the normal strength to avoid constipation
  ▪ alternatives in an emergency until mare milk replacer arrives: goat's milk, cow's milk or calf milk replacer.
▸ Decide how milk is going to be administered – take care to avoid aspiration of milk:
  ▪ tube feeding – needed in initial stages in foal's with poor/absent suck reflexes (ensure tube is placed in oesophagus and not in trachea)
  ▪ bottle feeding:
    » can use foal/lamb nipples and bottle – sterilised between feeds
    » get foal to stand, place hand over the foal's eye, position head under the handler's arm and hold the bottle at the normal feeding angle (do not keep too vertical)
    » try to get the foal to drink from a bucket over the next 2–3 d
  ▪ bucket feeding – do not try if planning to place foal on foster mare, as may refuse to nurse from the mare:
    » start with a shallow, clean bowl
    » hold a teat on the surface if reluctant to drink
    » be hygienic!
▸ Monitor the foal's weight if possible (check normal daily weight gain) and keep a daily diary of feeds.
▸ Can then discuss ongoing management, e.g. creep feed.
▸ Useful organisations and contacts for foster mares/milk replacer:
  ▪ local stud farms
  ▪ internet – online forums for horse clubs/equine magazines
  ▪ commercial foster mare services.

References and further reading

• **Annear, M.J., Furr, M.O., White, N.A.,** 2011. Septic arthritis in foals. Equine Vet. Educ. 23, 422–431.

• **Bernard, W.V.,** 2003. Jump starting the dummy foal In the Proceedings of the 49th AAEP Congress. Available via: <http://www.ivis.org>.

- Bernard, W., 2004. Colic in the foal. Equine Vet. Educ. 16, 319–323.

- Corley, K.T.T., Axon, J.E., 2005. Resuscitation and emergency management for neonatal foals. Vet. Clin. North Am. Equine Pract. 21, 431–455.

- Corley, K.T.T., Hollis, A.R., 2009. Antimicrobial therapy in neonatal foals. Equine Vet. Educ. 21, 436–448.

- Dugdale, A., 2010. Equine anaesthesia. In: Dugdale, A. (Ed.), Veterinary Anaesthesia: Principles to Practice. Wiley Blackwell, Chichester, UK, pp. 260–273.

- Gomez, J.H., Schumacher, J., Hunt, R.J., 2010. How to use a Foley catheter to treat foals for guttural pouch tympany. AAEP Proceedings, Baltimore, Maryland, pp. 173–175. Available via: <http://www.ivis.org>.

- Haggett, E., 2011. Antimicrobial use in the neonate. Br. Equine Vet. Assoc., 152–153.

- Hepburn, R., 2007. Management of diarrhoea in foals up to weaning. In Pract. 29, 334–341.

- Hollis, A., Corley, K., 2007. Practical guide to fluid therapy in neonatal foals. In Pract. 29, 130–137.

- Houpt, K.A., 2009. Foal rejection. In: Robinson, N.E., Sprayberry, K.A. (Eds.), Current Therapy in Equine Medicine (sixth ed.). Elsevier, St. Louis, Missouri, pp. 116–118.

- Knottenbelt, D.C., Holdstock, N., Madigan, J.E., 2004. Equine Neonatology: Medicine and Surgery. Saunders, Philadelphia, Pennsylvania, USA.

- Labelle, A.L., Hamor, R.E., Townsend, W.M., et al. 2011. Ophthalmic lesions in neonatal foals evaluated for non-ophthalmic disease at referral hospitals. J. Am. Vet. Med. Assoc. 239, 486–492.

- Marr, C., 2007. How to provide nutrition for sick foals. In: Proceedings of the 46th BEVA congress 12–15 September p 397–398.

- Palmer, J.E., 2007. Neonatal foal resuscitation. Vet. Clin. North Am. Equine Pract. 23, 159–182.

- Paradis, M.R., 2006. Equine Neonatal Medicine: A Case-Based Approach. Elsevier, Philadelphia, Pennsylvania, USA.

- Polkes, A.C., Giguere, S., Lester, G.D., et al. 2008. Factors associated with outcome in foals with neonatal isoerythrolysis (72 cases, 1988–2003). J. Vet. Intern. Med. 22, 1216–1222.

- Pusterla, N., Magdesian, K.G., Maleski, K., et al. 2004. Retrospective evaluation of the use of acetylcysteine enemas in the treatment of meconium retention in foals: 44 cases (1987–2002). Equine Vet. Educ. 16, 133–136.

- Richardson, D.W., Ahern, B.J., 2012. Synovial and osseous infections. In: Auer, J.A., Stick, J.A. (Eds.), Equine Surgery (fourth ed.). Elsevier, St. Louis, Missouri, pp. 1189–1201.

- Shepherd, C., 2010. Post-parturition examination of the newborn foal and mare. In Pract. 32, 97–101.

- Stoneham, S.J., 2008. Immunological conditions of the foal. In: Stoneham, S.J. (Ed.), Rossdale and Partners Foal Care Course. Lifelearn Ltd, Newmarket, UK, pp. 31–39.

Emergencies in donkeys and mules

Many emergency conditions are similar to those seen in horses. Donkeys and mules are more stoical in nature than horses and subtle signs of disease can be missed; therefore illness may be advanced by the time veterinary advice is sought. Any dull donkey or mule should always be examined and treated promptly, with particular effort made to prevent the development of hyperlipaemia.

The basics

General points

▶ In the developed world, most donkeys and mules are kept as pets or grazing companions and are more likely to develop obesity (e.g. laminitis) and age-related disorders (e.g. dental and neoplastic disease in geriatrics).

▶ Working donkeys and mules, particularly those in developing countries, are generally younger and colic, and lameness, respiratory tract infections, infectious diseases, wounds/abscesses and traumatic injuries are commonly seen problems in these populations.

▶ Education of donkey/mule-owning clients is important – they should be advised to seek veterinary advice even when minor signs of illness develop.

▶ Compared to horses, they are likely to be more physiologically compromised and in more pain than might be anticipated, e.g. signs of colic, response to application of hoof testers.

▶ Donkeys are physiologically and pharmacologically different from horses – mules have some features common to both but are physiologically more similar to horses.

▶ Donkeys have a particular tendency to develop hyperlipaemia when ill or stressed; any anorexic donkey must be monitored carefully and treated early.

▶ Companions should also be kept together at all times (irrespective of the species of the companion animal) and at times of severe stress (e.g. death of or separation from their companion, change of premises or other marked change in management routine); donkeys must be monitored carefully.

▶ Owners should be reminded of the importance of regular influenza and tetanus vaccination; infectious diseases such as influenza should be considered where outbreaks of disease occur in groups of donkeys or mules.

Useful sources of information
- The Donkey Sanctuary – http://www.thedonkeysanctuary.org.uk.
- WikiDonkey – http://www.wikivet.net.
- Veterinary Care of Donkeys, Matthews N.S. and Taylor T.S. (Eds.). International Veterinary Information Service, Ithaca, NY – http://www.ivis.org.
- UK Donkey Breed Society – http://www.donkeybreedsociety.com.
- British Mule Society – http://www.britishmulesociety.com.
- American Donkey and Mule Society – http://www.lovelongears.com.

Some useful facts

▶ Mule – offspring of a mare bred to donkey stallion (jack/jackass).
▶ Hinny – offspring of a female donkey (jenny) bred to a horse stallion.
▶ Gestation length – 365–376 d (can vary between 340 and 395 d).
▶ Lifespan – donkeys can live into their 30–40s.
▶ Energy requirements are approximately 75% of similar-sized pony requirements; hence the tendency for donkeys in UK to become obese.
▶ 1.3% DMI summer – 1.7% DMI winter (2.5–3.1 kg dry matter/d for a 180-kg donkey).

Normal clinical values (Table 13.1)

Table 13.1 Normal clinical values

	Average	Range
Heart rate (beats/min)	44	30–52
Respiratory rate (breaths/min)*	20	16–30
Temperature	37.1°C 98.8°F	36.2–37.8°C 97.2–100.0°F
Weight (kg)	160–180	Miniatures (100 kg) Mammoth (250 kg)

*Working donkeys may have resting respiratory rates up to 59 breaths/min to maintain a normal body temperature in hot climates.

Haematology and biochemistry

▶ PCV – donkeys do not haemoconcentrate until they are seriously (12–15%) dehydrated.
▶ There are some subtle differences in donkeys:
  ▪ ↑ compared to horses – alkaline phosphatase, GGT, TG, MCV, McHb, variable RBC
  ▪ ↓ compared to horses – creatinine, total bilirubin.
▶ Triglycerides should be routinely measured in all sick donkeys to monitor for development of hyperlipaemia.
▶ The Donkey Sanctuary will perform routine haematology and biochemistry on samples from the UK for a small donation.

Clinical examination and techniques

Handling

▶ Use a patient, calm approach – donkeys are not a flight animal so will tend to stand still when unsure of a situation and are usually easy to restrain once a headcollar has been fitted.
▶ Mules can be more challenging to deal with – consider use of personal protective equipment (hard hats, stocks) when dealing with them.
▶ Keep their companion close by – the additional stress of separation may make them more difficult to handle and make the effects of sedation less predictable.
▶ A nose twitch usually has relatively little effect – you can hold (but not twist or twitch) an ear.
▶ Even with a leg held up, they can still kick effectively.

Injections and blood sampling

▶ IM injections:
  ▪ use the neck or gluteal muscles but not the pectoral region (too little muscle mass)
  ▪ 18G 40-mm (1.5") needle – adults
  ▪ 19–21G 25-mm (1") needle – smaller donkeys/donkey foals
  ▪ donkey skin is thicker than that of the horse
  ▪ donkeys tolerate pushing the needle slowly through the skin and muscle better than the slap technique used in horses.
▶ IV injections and catheterisation:
  ▪ jugular vein – can be more difficult to see compared to horses especially if they are fat or well muscled
  ▪ easy to accidentally penetrate the carotid artery in very thin donkeys
  ▪ use 14G 8-cm (3.1") IV catheter
  ▪ due to thicker skin and fascia compared to horses – may need to angle the needle/catheter more steeply initially (60° vs 45° to the skin)

Nasogastric intubation

▶ Donkey nasal passages are relatively narrow for the size of the head compared to horses – use a small-diameter (13 mm), pony-sized stomach tube.

Rectal examination

▶ This can be performed safely – depends on size of the donkey.
▶ Rectal tears are rare if examination is performed carefully.

Table 13.2 Dosages of commonly used antimicrobials and NSAIDs based on specific pharmacological data obtained for donkeys

	Dose	Comments (use in donkeys)
Ampicillin	10 mg/kg IV q. 4–6 h	More frequent administration needed in donkeys
Carprofen	0.7 mg/kg IV or PO q. 24 h	Clearance time slower in the donkey – consider longer dosing interval
Flunixin meglumine	1.1 mg/kg IV q. 12–24 h	Metabolised more rapidly in the donkey
Gentamicin	2.2 mg/kg q. 8 h or 6.6 mg/kg q. 24 h IV	Mammoth donkeys may need lower doses and shorter dosing intervals
Meloxicam	0.6 mg/kg IV or PO q. 24 h	Metabolised more rapidly in donkeys
Oxytetracycline	10 mg/kg IV q. 24 h	Shorter dosing interval compared to horses
Penicillin G (sodium)	20 000 IU/kg IV q. 4–6 h	Shorter dosing interval compared to horses
Phenylbutazone	2.2–4.4 mg/kg IV or PO q. 12 h	Same dose q. 8 h for miniature donkeys (faster metabolism) 0.5 g (2.5–2.7 mg/kg for average-sized donkey) PO has been used for extended periods without problems

Unless otherwise stated, other NSAID and antimicrobial medications can be used at the same dose as horses. Taken from Grosenbaugh et al. 2011.

Medications

▶ Generally, most medications can be administered safely at similar dose rates compared to horses.
▶ Key differences are in the dosages of some sedative, anaesthetic and NSAID agents.
▶ Pharamacological data for donkeys is less extensive than in horses – Table 13.2 details differences in dose rates for certain NSAID and antimicrobial medications.

Sedation

▶ Similar to horses – usually α2 agonist/butorphanol combination.
▶ Constant rate infusions used in horses can also be used.

▸ The dose of α2 agonists usually needs to be higher to achieve the same level of sedation; mules may need a 50% higher dose compared to horses:
- xylazine 1.0–1.5 mg/kg IV *or*
- romifidine 0.1–0.15 mg/kg IV *or*
- detomidine 0.02–0.03 mg/kg IV
- combined with butorphanol 0.02–0.04 mg/kg IV.

Sedation of needle-shy/difficult-to-handle donkeys and mules

▸ Can administer IM sedation (2 × IV dose).

▸ Top up IV once sedated prior to performing further procedures.

▸ Detomidine oral gel is also useful for donkeys and mules that are difficult to inject – the label dose provides good sedation provided sufficient time is given (40 min) but mules might need a higher dose.

Epidural anaesthesia

▸ 1st intercoccygeal space in the donkey is narrower than second and there are no large tail muscles as in horses.

▸ Preferred site: between 2nd and 3rd intercoccygeal space introduced at 30° above horizontal.

General anaesthesia in emergency situations

General anaesthesia

▸ Donkeys metabolise ketamine more rapidly than horses and top-ups need to be given more frequently (e.g. every 10 min) compared to horses.

▸ Donkeys are more sensitive to guaifenesin (if using triple-combination IV infusions).

▸ Intubation can be more difficult due to anatomic differences between donkeys and horses – they have narrower nasal passages than horses, the trachea is relatively narrower than a similar-sized pony and the angle of epiglottis is slightly different:
- adults – 16- or 14-mm (internal diameter) endotracheal tube
- foals – 12-mm (internal diameter) endotracheal tube.

Emergency anaesthetic protocols

Protocols for short-duration emergency anaesthesia of donkeys and mules in the field (<40-min duration) are largely the same as for horses.

- Premedication:
  - detomidine (0.01–0.03 mg/kg) + butorphanol (0.02–0.04 mg/kg) IV *or*
  - romifidine (0.1–0.15 mg/kg) + butorphanol (0.02–0.04 mg/kg) IV.
- Wait 5 min.
- Induction:
  - ketamine 2.2 mg/kg IV (± diazepam 0.05 mg/kg) *or*
  - thiopental (thiopentone) 5 mg/kg IV.
- Top-ups:
  - ¼–½ the original dose of ketamine (every 10 min)/thiopental (as required) 1–2 mg/kg IV.

Overview of emergency conditions

Whilst there are variations in how donkeys and mules demonstrate clinical signs of disease compared to the horse, diagnosis and treatment of many conditions is largely the same. Key differences to be aware of when dealing with these in donkey and mules are outlined in Table 13.3.

Table 13.3 Overview of emergency conditions in donkeys and mules and key differences to be aware of compared to horses

Emergency type	Comments on emergency conditions in donkeys and mules
Wounds and integument	Bite wounds – consider rabies if they have been bitten by dogs/hyenas in endemic areas Injury to calcified fat pads can be extremely hard to treat successfully due to the poor blood supply to that region – treat seriously and promptly (can be extremely painful and require wide resection) Deep IM abscesses have been reported to precipitate hyperlipaemia – take care with injection technique
Musculoskeletal	Foot abscesses and laminitis are common causes of acute lameness Usually lameness is at a more advanced stage when clinical signs are seen due to their stoic nature If recumbent, they may have had reduced feed intake – check for evidence of hyperlipaemia and ensure good nursing care to make sure they are eating and drinking Hoof testers are less useful for detecting a response to foot pain compared to horses The radiographic anatomy of the donkey foot is slightly different to that in the horse (the differences are less marked in mules): – generally more upright anatomy – P3 is positioned more distally within the hoof capsule (average 10 mm) – the extensor process is not in line with the coronary band
Oral and gastrointestinal	Colic is common and is frequently associated with impactions Severe dental pathology is common – ensure that an oral examination is performed Gastric ulceration may be a concurrent problem in sick donkeys – treat with omeprazole as for horses Can develop diarrhoea readily with stress Intestinal parasites are an important cause of gastrointestinal problems and are treated in the same way as horses Cyathostominosis may present with ventral oedema prior to or without development of diarrhoea

(Continued)

Table 13.3 Overview of emergency conditions in donkeys and mules and key differences to be aware of compared to horses (Continued)

Emergency type	Comments on emergency conditions in donkeys and mules
Respiratory	Idiopathic pulmonary fibrosis (IPF) and tracheal collapse should be considered in geriatric donkeys presented with acute dyspnoea
	In non-working donkeys and mules, mild signs of respiratory disease may go unnoticed for some time and they may present as an emergency with respiratory disease that is at an advanced stage
	Many donkeys are not vaccinated against equine herpes viruses ± equine influenza and pet donkeys may not mix with others very often – disease outbreaks can occur in unvaccinated populations where donkeys mix (e.g. working populations in the developing world)
	Donkeys tend to be more severely affected than horses and are more likely to develop secondary bronchopneumonia (not so in mules) – early treatment with antimicrobials is important
	Avian influenza has been shown to develop in donkeys – consider as a potential cause of respiratory disease in groups of donkeys in affected areas during disease outbreaks
Ophthalmic	They are generally less prone to traumatic injuries (less 'flighty' than horses)
	In cases with an acutely painful eye – check for foreign bodies (donkeys often bury their heads in hay/straw and have a thick coat and hair face in the winter, increasing the risk of organic foreign bodies becoming lodged in and around the eye)
Neurological	Similar approach as in horses
	Donkeys can develop neurological signs secondary to EHV and AHV (asinine herpes virus) infection
	Senility can be seen in geriatric donkeys: aimless wandering, circling, loss of appetite but otherwise normal clinical parameters, haematology and serum biochemistry
Reproductive	Covering dates are often unknown so it is hard to assess readiness for birth and foal prematurity
	Foetal oversize can ↑ the risk of dystocia – more likely in miniature donkeys and where a jenny has been bred to a stallion
	↑ Risk of undetected twin pregnancies – check for second foetus
	Dystocia and late-term problems are often associated with hyperlipaemia

(Continued)

Table 13.3 Overview of emergency conditions in donkeys and mules and key differences to be aware of compared to horses (Continued)

Emergency type	Comments on emergency conditions in donkeys and mules
Reproductive (Continued)	Standing flank Caesarean sections have been performed in emergency situations overseas (see G. Kay – http://www.ivis.org) The cervical anatomy increases the risk of cervical injury with dystocia and makes uterine flushing difficult to perform (e.g. in cases of metritis) – it is longer and thinner and protudes into vagina, making catheterisation difficult
Urinary	Same approach as for horses
Cardiovascular	Blood transfusions – ideally use a donor donkey and cross-match as for horses but horse blood can be administered safely to donkeys (NB donkey/mule blood cannot be administered to horses due to presence of RBC antigens (donkey factor) that cause transfusion reactions in horses)
Hepatic, endocrine and metabolic	Hyperlipaemia is very common in donkeys – same approach to diagnosis and treatment as for horses (see p. 206) Acute pancreatitis has been reported (see References) Hepatic disease – similar approach as for horses Hyperthermia (heat stress) can occur in working donkeys in hot/humid climates pushed beyond their normal levels of fitness/or where underlying disease is present (see p. 214) Hypothermia is more likely to occur in donkeys compared to horses (larger body surface area relative to volume, allowing for greater heat loss) and this can develop in donkeys during periods of extreme cold (only seen during winter months in certain geographical regions)
Neonate	Neonatal isoerythrolysis is more common in mule than horse foals – same treatment as for foals (see p. 242) Failure of passive transfer – frozen horse plasma can be used successfully
Infectious diseases	See also Respiratory section, p. 253 Donkeys may exhibit less obvious clinical signs of disease, e.g. piroplasmosis, EIA, EVA, AHS It is important to determine if they may have originated from/travelled outside the UK when considering unusual disease presentations

The dull donkey

General dullness may be the presenting clinical sign for a variety of conditions and these cases should be seen urgently. Despite detailed clinical examination, a specific diagnosis may not be reached in many of these cases; however, colic and hyperlipaemia are common causes (Table 13.4).

History

Similar to obtaining a history in horses. Specific information that should be obtained includes:

▶ Age – geriatric donkeys are more likely to suffer from osteoarthritis/severe dental disease.
▶ Gender – whether pregnant if female.
▶ Vaccination status – they may not be routinely vaccinated.
▶ Routine dental care – dental disorders are common in aged donkeys.
▶ Normal diet.
▶ Stabling and turnout.
▶ Bedding type – impaction colic is more common in donkeys bedded on straw.
▶ Normal behaviour and any differences noted.
▶ History of previous disease – especially previous laminitis, renal/hepatic disease.
▶ Recent treatment – rule out oral pain following dental treatment.
▶ Recent separation from or death of a companion.
▶ Recent change of environment or management.

Table 13.4 Causes of dullness in a population of non-working donkeys in a UK donkey sanctuary

Disease	Percentage
Non-specific	38
Colic	19
Hyperlipaemia	15
Hepatic disease	5
Conditions of the foot	5
Respiratory disease	4
Renal disease	2
Pancreatitis	2
Other	10

Clinical examination

▶ Similar general approach as for horses.

▶ Determine body condition score – if they have a long winter coat it can be easy to miss the fact that they may be underweight.

▶ Check the oral cavity using a mouth speculum and head torch – important especially in older dull/inappetant donkeys.

▶ Careful observation of behaviour (normal or weak/mild abdominal pain/ataxia).

▶ Watch the donkey eating (donkeys can be good at putting their head in a bucket but not actually eating) – check they are masticating and swallowing food.

▶ They can deposit excessive fat in the crest either side on the mid-line and gluteals – do not mistakenly diagnose as tumours (with weight loss these deposits may calcify).

Initial treatment

▶ Identify and treat any underlying illness (see relevant sections).

▶ Triglycerides should be routinely measured to rule in/out hyperlipaemia.

▶ Good nursing care is essential to encourage them to eat, including:

- feeding by hand
- warming feed
- offering chopped forage together with crumbled ginger biscuits, carrots or apples (chopped/grated), unmolassed sugar beet, fruit juices (apple/cherry) or peppermint cordial, mint (dried/fresh), ginger (powdered/grated), yeast
- walking out to graze on grass and browse on hedgerows
- offering sloppy feeds of unmolassed sugar beet helps to encourage water intake and assist oral drug administration
- if hospitalised, offer the donkey its usual feed and ensure that it has physical/visual contact with its companion.

▶ Where there is no voluntary food intake but there is evidence of gastrointestinal motility, fibre pellets soaked to form a slurry can be administered by stomach tube or syringed into the mouth.

▶ Donkeys in stables with companions need regular checks of faecal output.

▶ Ensure adequate water intake ± IV fluid therapy required in more sick donkeys.

▶ Treat with gastric protectants if inappetant >24 h to reduce the risk of gastric ulceration developing.

Laminitis

▶ Common, same risk factors as for horses, including obesity (see p. 45).

▶ Clinical signs similar to that for the horse:

- these signs may go unrecognised – lying down, shuffly or slow gait
- donkeys may also hold alternate forelimbs high above the ground (not seen in horses).

▶ In chronic cases, muscle wastage of the shoulder region can occur.

▶ Radiographic signs of laminitis are similar to those in the horse:

- ↑ in angular deviation between dorsal aspect of P3 and the dorsum of the hoof wall
- ↑ distal displacement of P3

- radiographic measurements to determine likely prognosis based on these have not yet been determined in donkeys.
▶ Treatment is largely the same as for horses but frog supports are probably best avoided in donkeys – better to cover the entire sole with a thick soft dressing.
▶ Remove from pasture, put onto a high-fibre diet or short chopped fibre food with NSC <10%.
▶ Make sure they continue to eat – do not starve them!
▶ Check for PPID/EMS – there is often an underlying metabolic cause of disease.
▶ Ongoing restricted diet for energy needs may require supplementation with minerals/vitamins for adequate hoof quality in the repair phase.

Colic

▶ Clinical signs are less obvious and dramatic compared to the horse – they most frequently present with inappetance and anorexia.
▶ More severe signs such as recumbency and kicking at their abdomen are occasionally seen.
▶ Rule out non-gastrointestinal causes of colic, e.g. hyperlipaemia.

Epidemiology

▶ 55% of episodes of colic in an aged UK donkey population were due to suspected/confirmed impactions (most commonly at the pelvic flexure).
▶ Risk factors for colic: increasing age, previous history of colic, dental disease, being fed extra rations, bedding on paper/cardboard, limited/no access to pasture.
▶ Often those with poor teeth stabled to reduce weight will eat bedding and develop undiagnosed impaction colic especially if on NSAIDs and bedded on straw.
▶ High mortality rate (51%) – may have been due in part to the older age of this population and concurrent disease.
▶ Pedunculated lipomas are rare despite the donkey's propensity to become obese.

Clinical examination

▶ Similar as for the horse (see p. 60).
▶ PCV – more difficult to interpret changes compared to horses.
▶ Nasogastric intubation – if small-diameter tubes 9–11 mm have to be used, it can be difficult to assess for reflux.
▶ Rectal examination can be performed safely in larger donkeys/mules.
▶ Abdomiocentesis – they can have large quantities of retroperitoneal fat so may need to use a 19G 90-mm (3.5") spinal needle.
▶ Abdominal US is useful, particularly in donkeys that are too small to perform a rectal examination on safely.

Treatment

▶ Same as for horses (see p. 62).

Typhlocolitis

A syndrome of idiopathic typhlocolitis has been reported in aged donkeys.

Clinical signs

▸ Colic.
▸ Inappetance.
▸ ± Sudden death.
▸ Diarrhoea is not a feature.

Diagnostic features

▸ ↓ Albumin.
▸ ↓ WBC.
▸ Variable changes in PCV.
▸ ↑ Urea, ↑ creatinine.
▸ Bacterial/parasitic infections identified in some donkeys; no obvious cause found in others.
▸ US of colon wall – may demonstrate thickening of the ventral colon.

Prognosis

▸ Poor.
▸ Early identification and aggressive treatment may improve chances of survival.

Idiopathic pulmonary fibrosis

Where this occurs in sedentary donkeys, signs of mild disease may be missed by owners and affected donkeys may present in respiratory crisis with end-stage disease. The degree of fibrosis can vary from mild, focal disease to diffuse, severe changes.

Clinical signs

Mild

▸ ↑ RR, ↑ respiratory effort.
▸ Adventitious lung sounds.
▸ ± Inspiratory dyspnoea (differentiate from RAO where expiratory dyspnoea is more commonly seen).
▸ ± Pyrexia.
▸ ± Nasal discharge (secondary bacterial infection).
▸ Usually poor response to conventional treatment for RAO.

Acute, severe

▸ Severe inspiratory dyspnoea.
▸ Markedly ↑ RR and respiratory effort (particularly during inspiration).
▸ Stertorous noise – may have concurrent tracheal collapse.

Diagnosis

▸ Thoracic auscultation and percussion – absence of lung sounds surrounded by areas of hyperinflation and wheezes.

▸ Thoracic US – pleural thickening, evidence of subpleural fibrosis (comet tail lesions on the lung surface).

▸ Thoracic radiography – marked interstitial pattern.

Treatment

▸ Usually carries a poor prognosis due to the extent of irreversible, pathological changes in the lungs.

▸ Consider euthanasia in severe cases – absence of lung sounds and marked ↑ RR may be signs of an impending crisis.

▸ Palliative care – ↓ LRT inflammation:
  ▪ oral/inhaled steroids
  ▪ bronchodilators
  ▪ antimicrobials
  ▪ mucolytics.

Ongoing management

▸ Donkeys that are kept as pasture pets/companions can cope well with reduced lung function for years.

▸ Monitor respiratory rate and effort, body score, appetite and frequency of concurrent infections.

▸ Euthanasia is recommended where there is evidence of deterioration of clinical signs and before an acute dyspnoeic crisis occurs.

References and further reading

• **Abdel-Moneim, A.S., Abdel-Ghany, A.E., Shany, S.A.S.,** 2010. Isolation and characterization of highly pathogenic avian influenza virus subtype H5N1 from donkeys. J. Biomed. Sci. 17, 25.

• **Collins, S.N., Dyson, S.J., Murray, R.C., et al.** 2011. Radiological anatomy of the donkey's foot: objective characterisation of the normal and laminitic donkey foot. Equine Vet. J. 43, 478–486.

• **Cox, R., Proudman, C.J., Trawford, A.F., et al.** 2007. Epidemiology of impaction colic in donkeys in the UK. BMC Vet. Res. 3, 1.

• **Dey, S., Dwivedi, S.K., Malik, P., et al.** 2010. Mortality associated with heat stress in donkeys in India. Vet. Rec. 166, 143–145.

• **Doherty, T., Valverde, A.,** 2006. Anaesthesia of donkeys and mules. In: Doherty, T., Valverde, A. (Eds.), Manual of Equine Anaesthesia and Analgesia. Blackwell Publishing Ltd, Oxford, UK, pp. 234–237.

• **Du Toit, N., Burden, F.A., Getachew, M., et al.** 2010. Idiopathic typhlocolitis in 40 aged donkeys. Equine Vet. Educ. 22, 53–57.

- Grosenbaugh, D.A., Reinemeyer, C.R., Figueiredo, M.D., 2011. Pharmacology & therapeutics in donkeys. Equine Vet. Educ. 23, 523–530.

- Matthews, N., van Loon, J.P.A.M., 2013. Anaesthesia and analgesia of the donkey and the mule. Equine Vet. Educ. 25, 47–51.

- Matthews, N.S., Taylor, T.S., Hartsfield, S.M., 2005. Anaesthesia of donkeys and mules. Equine Vet. Educ. Man. 7, 102–107.

- Pritchard, J.C., Barr, A.R.S., Whay, H.R., 2006. Validity of a behavioural measure of heat stress and a skin tent test for dehydration in working horses and donkeys. Equine Vet. J. 38, 433–438.

- Stephen, J.O., Baptiste, K.E., Townsend, H.G.G., 2000. Clinical and pathologic findings in donkeys with hypothermia: 10 cases (1988–1998). J. Am. Vet. Med. Assoc. 216, 725–729.

- Svendsen, E.D., 2008.. In: Duncan, J., Handrill, D. (Eds.), Professional Handbook of the Donkey (fourth ed.). Whittet Books Ltd, Wiltshire, UK.

- Taylor, T.S., Matthews, N.S., 2002. Donkey and mule scenarios: When to stop, think, read or call. In: Proceedings of the 48th Annual Convention of the AAEP, Orlando, Florida, 4–8 December 2002, pp. 115–116. Available via <http://www.ivis.org>.

- Thiemann, A.K., 2012. Respiratory disease in the donkey. Equine Vet. Educ. 24, 469–478.

- WikiDonkey– <http://www.wikivet.net>.

Iatrogenic emergencies

General approach

These injuries/conditions are relatively common and may require emergency treatment. In most instances, these events are recognised risks associated with particular types of examination or treatment and are often not associated with negligence. However, when complications develop, it is common for owners to closely question the veterinary surgeon's actions both prior to and after the iatrogenic damage has been caused. Even if the iatrogenic damage was not associated with negligence on the part of the treating veterinary surgeon, failure to identify associated complications and deal with them appropriately may lead to a negligence claim. These situations may be extremely stressful and upsetting for all parties concerned, particularly where death of a horse occurs.

What to do if an iatrogenic injury/accident occurs

- Inform the owner what has happened, what needs to be done in terms of further investigation or treatment, associated costs and the likely prognosis (this may be based on advice given by a referral centre where appropriate).
- Say you are sorry for what has happened and empathise with their situation but do not accept liability for any consequential losses or costs.

- Make detailed notes about the date and time of events, treatment administered, advice given and other communications with the owner/agent (including the name of the person communicated to and any witnesses) as soon as possible.
- In the case of adverse drug reactions, contact the relevant agencies (see p. 267).
- Contact professional indemnity insurers (e.g. Veterinary Defence Society) for further advice even if it seems unlikely that owners/agents will pursue a claim for compensation (they can sometimes change their minds a few days later, particularly when they receive a bill).
- Determine whether there needs to be any change in costs (this should be discussed with indemnity insurers/practice principles or manager first).
- Reflect upon and discuss with other colleagues whether you could have done anything different in the circumstances or whether your clinical approach/practice policy should be revised in light of this episode.

Rectal tears

Identification of bright red (fresh) blood on the rectal sleeve following rectal examination is suspicious of a rectal tear having occurred (Fig. 14.1). These are a known risk associated with rectal examination and can have catastrophic consequences for the horse if appropriate action is not taken. Management of these cases also may be complicated by factors related to why the horse was having rectal examination performed in the first place (e.g. acute colic).

Initial assessment and first aid

▸ Inform the owner what has happened and what further assessment and treatment is required.

▸ Sedate the horse (e.g. xylazine/butorphanol).

▸ Administer butylscopolamine 0.3 mg/kg IV.

▸ ± Instil local anaesthetic directly into the rectum to stop straining.

▸ ± Perform epidural analgesia (see p. 362).

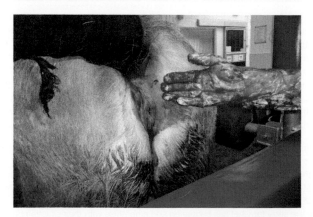

Figure 14.1 Fresh blood evident on the rectal sleeve following rectal examination in a horse that had sustained a large rectal tear a few hours previously.

▶ Evaluate the integrity of the rectal mucosa and deeper layers with a well-lubricated arm – it is often easier to perform this with bare hands/application of surgical gloves under a pair of rectal gloves with the fingertips cut off.
▶ Alternatively, if an endoscope is readily available, proctoscopy can be performed.
▶ Determine if a tear exists and its:
  ▪ location from anus (i.e. the retroperitoneal/peritoneal portions of the rectum)
  ▪ position on rectal wall (e.g. dorsal or ventral)
  ▪ approximate size
  ▪ thickness of tear (Table 14.1).
▶ Perform abdominocentesis:
  ▪ may take a few hours for changes in WBC and TP to be seen
  ▪ evidence of haemorrhage/free ingesta (ensure not due to inadvertent splenic puncture or enterocentesis) may be seen in grade 4 tears.

Further assessment and treatment

▶ This will be dependent on the grade of the rectal tear, its location (i.e. whether peritoneal portion involved), options for referral and owner factors, e.g. economics.

Table 14.1 Classifications of rectal tear, identification and prognosis

Grade	Layers of rectum affected	Findings on examination	Prognosis
1	Mucosa and submucosa	Shallow thin flap of tissue Usually located ventrally	Good
2	Muscularis	Thinner area of rectal wall ± outpouching palpable Usually located dorsally	Good
3a	Mucosa, submucosa and muscularis not on the dorsal midline	Enlarged cavity surrounded by thin, tough membrane Usually located dorsally (but not on midline)	Variable survival rates reported Generally guarded–poor
3b	Mucosa, submucosa and muscularis extending into the mesorectum on the dorsal midline	Enlarged cavity surrounded by thin, tough membrane Located on the dorsal midline	Variable survival rates reported Generally guarded–poor
4	All layers: mucosa, submucosa, muscularis, serosa	Enlarged cavity but a finger or hand can be entered into the abdominal cavity/perirectal tissues Usually located dorsally	Poor–hopeless

▶ The general approach to management of different grades of rectal tears includes:
  ▪ grade 1 – medical management/untreated
  ▪ grade 2 – medical management
  ▪ grade 3a & 3b – medical/surgical management
  ▪ grade 4 – surgical management (suture repair/colostomy/indwelling rectal liner).
▶ Contact the referral centre for further advice, including specific requests for treatment prior to transportation.
▶ Administer BS antimicrobials IV (penicillin/gentamicin).
▶ Administer flunixin 1.1 mg/kg IV.
▶ Check tetanus prophylaxis.
▶ Can administer epidural anaesthetic (see above), evacuate rectum and pack rectum with povidone iodine soaked cotton wool in stockingette.
▶ Where referral is not an option:
  ▪ grade 4 tears – euthanasia
  ▪ can attempt blind suturing for grade 3 tears – not recommended if tears >50% rectal circumference or in grade 4 tears (see specialist texts).
▶ Medical management (see texts for further details):
  ▪ antimicrobial therapy (at least 7 d)
  ▪ NSAIDs
  ▪ supportive therapy – IV fluids if required
  ▪ faecal softening – oral fluids, laxative diet
  ▪ serial monitoring of peritoneal fluid WBC, TP and lactate.

Complications following nasogastric intubation

The risk of complications can be minimised if this procedure is performed correctly (see p. 339), taking care to ensure that the horse is adequately restrained (including sedation in fractious horses), that excessive force is not used to pass the tube and checking that it is not positioned in the airway prior to administering fluids (particularly liquid paraffin).

Epistaxis

▶ Common – more likely to occur where repeated intubation has been performed or the patient is difficult to handle.
▶ Haemorrhage will usually subside within 5–10 min if the horse is left quietly in its stable.
▶ If haemorrhage does not stop within this time, consider a possible clotting disorder.
▶ Rarely is the degree of haemorrhage sufficient to warrant a blood transfusion; seek specialist advise if haemorrhage persists.

Inhalational pneumonia

▶ Occurs subsequent to inadvertent passage of the nasogastric tube into the airway instead of the stomach.
▶ Water inhalation:
  ▪ small quantities are usually not a problem but larger quantities may be associated with pulmonary oedema (see p. 91) or development of inhalational pneumonia (see p. 90).

▸ Liquid paraffin:
  ▪ associated with a severe lipoid pneumonia
  ▪ non-irritating but impairs mucociliary transport system and is poorly degraded by tissue enzymes
  ▪ prognosis is poor without appropriate, aggressive treatment (see p. 91).

Oesophageal perforation

▸ Rare complication.
▸ Most commonly associated with undue force being used to pass the tube or potentially could be associated with area of inherent weakness in the oesophagus, e.g. diverticulum.
▸ See p. 71 for further evaluation and treatment.

Complications following castration

Complications may be encountered in up to 25% of horses following castration. Most of these are mild and self-resolving but some complications are life-threatening or require immediate treatment.

Post-castration haemorrhage

▸ Assess the amount of blood lost (can be difficult where blood has soaked into the bedding):
  ▪ evaluate MM colour, pulse quality and HR for evidence of haemorrhagic shock (see p. 186).
▸ Administer sedation (α2 agonist/butorphanol) – ensure horse is sufficiently cardiovascularly stable for this:
  ▪ the horse must be sedated sufficiently to enable you to pack the scrotum, if required, so do not under-dose unless the horse is showing evidence of haemorrhagic shock (may not be required if the horse is lethargic and weak).
▸ ± Administer acepromazine 0.02 mg/kg IV if HR <60 beats/min – hypotensive effects can assist haemostasis.
▸ Aseptically prepare the scrotum and put on sterile gloves.
▸ If a source of haemorrhage can be identified, the offending vessel can be clamped and ligated/emasculated – it is relatively uncommon to be able to do this due to retraction of the spermatic cord into the inguinal canal.
▸ Pack the scrotum with:
  ▪ sterile gauze bandage (can tie with a reef knot if >1 length of bandage is needed)
  ▪ cotton wool within a stockingette sleeve
  ▪ do not insert individual swabs/cotton wool directly into the scrotum as these may remain in situ and act as a foreign body.
▸ Secure the packing with a pair of small towel clamps placed across the scrotal incision or place a large-diameter (4 metric) suture at the site and leave the ends long to facilitate their removal.
▸ Administer NSAIDs.
▸ Administer antimicrobials – procaine penicillin or trimethoprim sulphonamides.
▸ Remove the packing in 24–48 h.

▸ If there is evidence of continued haemorrhage, further investigation of the source of haemorrhage and ligation should be performed under GA.

▸ Check the emasculators to ensure they are working properly.

Evisceration

This may occur during, immediately after or several days following castration. Identification of small intestine herniated from the incision and/or signs of colic must be dealt with promptly and even if only a small portion of non-compromised intestine has herniated, immediate surgical management in a hospital environment with facilities to perform exploratory laparotomy is optimal.

Initial advice to the owner (Fig. 14.2)

▸ Keep the horse quiet.

▸ If possible sling prolapsed intestine (if a large quantity has prolapsed) to protect it until you arrive, e.g. using a clean, large plastic bag or a clean, moistened sheet.

Initial assessment and treatment

▸ Assess CV status – MM colour, heart rate.

▸ Administer sedation IV, e.g. α2 agonist/butorphanol.

▸ Lavage the intestine and scrotum with sterile saline/LRS.

▸ Assess the length of herniated intestine and intestinal viability.

▸ Administer BS antimicrobials (penicillin/gentamicin IV).

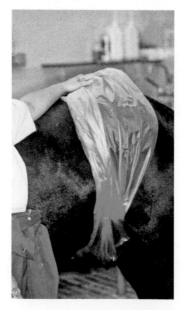

Figure 14.2 Use of a sterile, large plastic drape to protect and support herniated intestine following evisceration.

▶ Administer NSAIDs – flunixin 1.1 mg/kg IV.
▶ Determine whether referral is an option and, if so, contact the referral centre immediately.
▶ Euthanasia may be warranted if referral for surgical management is not an option or if the prognosis would be extremely poor even with surgery (e.g. large quantities of non-viable small intestine).
▶ Surgical management on site can be attempted as a last resort in cases of acute prolapse of small quantities of non-distended intestine where referral is not an option:
  ▪ be aware that failure to replace small intestine into the abdomen or ileus may result (the small intestine is usually wedged firmly in the inguinal ring)
  ▪ GA, aseptic preparation of scrotum and lavage of herniated intestine with sterile saline/LRS, push herniated small intestine back into the inguinal canal, twist the vaginal tunic and ligate
  ▪ ligate the contralateral vaginal tunic.

Where referral is an option
▶ Perform any other first aid treatment as requested, e.g. pass a nasogastric tube.
▶ If a small amount of non-distended small intestine has herniated (usually when identified at the time of castration), try to pack small intestine into scrotum/vaginal tunic and secure using sutures in the scrotal skin/vaginal tunic to prevent further trauma to eviscerated intestine (± under GA in the field – this should not unduly delay transport to the clinic and depends on the circumstances and distance from hospital/referral facility).
▶ If larger amounts of intestine have herniated, sling with sterile plastic drape (or similar) for transport (see Fig. 14.2).

Omental prolapse

This is generally not a life-threatening complication but it is important to attend the horse promptly to rule out potential evisceration. It is uncommon for evisceration to occur concurrently/subsequent to omental prolapse due to swelling of omentum in the inguinal ring and canal, reducing the space for small intestine to enter (Fig. 14.3).

▶ Sedate the horse and aseptically prepare the scrotum.
▶ Put on sterile gloves.
▶ Lavage herniated omentum with sterile saline/LRS.
▶ Apply gentle traction to the omentum to expose non-contaminated omentum.
▶ Emasculate/cut omentum proximal to site.
▶ Administer NSAIDs and antimicrobials.
▶ Monitor for signs of infection at the site (acute or chronic).

Adverse drug reactions

Emergencies due to ADRs are sometimes encountered in horses (Table 14.2). Certain drugs may be associated with particular toxicities (Table 14.3) and others have been associated with development of conditions such as corticosteroid-associated laminitis and phenothiazine-related priapism/paraphimosis. Owners should be warned of the potential risks when these drugs are administered or administration should be avoided in high-risk individuals.

Diagnosis and treatment

▶ Provide immediate first aid treatment in the case of anaphylaxis (see below)/seizures (see p. 144).

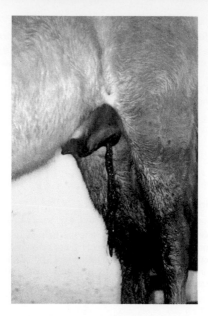

Figure 14.3 Omental prolapse following castration.

Table 14.2 Classifications of adverse drug reactions (ADRs)

Classification of ADRs	Examples and comments
Dose-related	Most common ADR, e.g. aminoglycoside-induced nephrotoxicosis Preventable and low mortality
Idiosyncratic (non-dose related)	Not related to pharmacology and not predictable, e.g. allergic reactions to penicillins More severe, higher mortality rate
Dose- and time-related (chronic)	Total cumulative dose, e.g. GIT ulceration and NSAID administration
Time related (delayed)	Teratogenic drugs
Withdrawal	Occurs shortly after discontinuation of drugs Uncommon in horses
Unexpected failure of therapy	Dose related, drug–drug interactions

Table 14.3 List of known drug toxicities

Adverse drug reaction	Drugs
Antimicrobial-associated colitis	Mild or infrequent: trimethoprim sulphonamides, penicillin, doxycycline Severe or frequent: clindamycin, lincomycin, oxytetracycline, erythromycin, moxifloxacin, florfenicol, tylosin
Other gastrointestinal toxicity	NSAIDs, misoprostol, digoxin, quinidine, erythromycin
Nephrotoxicity	NSAIDs, aminoglycosides, polymyxin B, tetracyclines, cephalosporins (rare), amphotericin B, imipenem, imidocarb
Hepatotoxicity	Glucocorticoids, isoniazid, fluphenazine, halothane, dantrolene
Cardiotoxicity	Doxycycline (IV), tetracycline (IV), tilmicosin, monensin, lasalocid sodium, digoxin, quinidine
Bone marrow suppression	Chloramphenicol, trimethoprim sulphonamides, pyrimethamine
Immune-mediated haemolytic anaemia	Penicillins, cephalosporins, trimethoprim-sulfamethoxazole, NSAIDs
Neuromuscular blocking agents	Aminoglycosides, tetracyclines
Central nervous system toxicity	Lidocaine, theophylline/aminophylline, metronidazole, fluphenazine, avermectins
Bone or cartilage damage in growing animals	Tetracyclines (not erythromycin), fluoroquinolones
Tetatogenic effects	Sulphonamides, griseofulvin, carbendazole, pyrimethamine
Skin reactions	Penicillins, sulphonamides, phenothiazine tranquilizers, NSAIDs, local anaesthetics, anticonvulsants

Modified from Davis (2009).

▶ Diagnosis of an ADR will be based on:
  ▪ clinical signs seen – are they consistent with an ADR?
  ▪ consideration of timing of administration, drug mechanism and known toxic side-effects (Table 14.3)
  ▪ likelihood that the drug has caused that effect based on circumstances surrounding the event.

▶ Inform the owner and document the situation.
▶ Ongoing investigation/treatment will be largely dependent on the likely and observed clinical effects.
▶ Report adverse drug reactions promptly to the relevant authorities, e.g. UK – Veterinary Medicines Directorate (http://www.vmd.defra.gov.uk – form MLA 252A), USA – FDA (http://www.fda.gov/cvm/adetoc.htm).
▶ Information to convey includes:
  ▪ name of person reporting ADR
  ▪ details of animal(s) – age, gender
  ▪ name of product, marketing authorisation number and batch number
  ▪ person who administered the product
  ▪ reason for treatment
  ▪ dose administered, route, site
  ▪ concurrent products administered
  ▪ time between treatment and reaction
  ▪ description of reaction
  ▪ number of animals with clinical signs (if >1)
  ▪ reaction to treatment and outcome.

Anaphylaxis

▶ Quickly assess CV system, respiratory system and neurological status.
▶ Administer adrenaline 0.01–0.02 mg/kg IV (if unresponsive, can give up to 0.2 mg/kg):
  ▪ using 1:1000 adrenaline = 1 mg/mL
  ▪ 0.01 mg/kg = 5 mL in a 500-kg horse.
▶ Administer dexamethasone 0.02–0.05 mg/kg IV.
▶ Follow as for resuscitation of the adult horse if cardiac/respiratory arrest occurs (see p. 185).
▶ Symptomatic treatment of subsequent clinical signs that develop (see relevant sections).

Intracarotid drug administration

This most commonly occurs when drugs are injected into the jugular vein in the distal third of the neck (due to the close proximity of jugular vein and carotid artery in this region). Reactions will be of variable severity depending on the drug administered, the volume injected into the carotid artery and inherent horse-related differences. These are usually less severe where water-soluble drugs (e.g. xylazine, butorphanol, acepromazine) have been administered. Administration of oil-based compounds, suspensions or viscous/irritant drugs are more likely to be associated with a worse outcome.

Clinical signs

▶ Usually seen immediately but can be delayed for a few minutes.
▶ Seizures.
▶ Collapse.

▶ ± Coma.
▶ ± Death.

Treatment

▶ Administer diazepam 0.1–0.2 mg/kg IV if seizures evident.
▶ Place in padded box/well-bedded stable if possible.
▶ Administer dexamethasone 0.02–0.05 mg/kg IV.
▶ Other symptomatic treatment based on clinical signs that develop subsequently (see relevant sections).
▶ Euthanasia may be required if the horse stabilises in an unsatisfactory condition, e.g. permanent bilateral blindness.

Perivascular injections

These can cause variable reactions from temporary, localised subcutaneous reactions to extensive skin sloughs and neuritis (including laryngeal neuropathy on the affected side). The degree of reaction depends on the drug and its acidity – the most severe reactions are seen following perivascular injection of hyoscine/metamizole and thiopental (thiopentone).

Treatment

▶ Immediately infiltrate sterile saline around the site to dilute the effects of the drug.
▶ Administer NSAIDs.
▶ Monitor the site closely.
▶ Further symptomatic treatment as required (e.g. wound management and healing by secondary intention if skin sloughs develop).

Injection site abscesses

These are uncommon but can occur following administration of IM injections and following perineural anaesthesia. Rarely do these present as an emergency situation but occasionally horses can develop clostridial infections that can be life-threatening if not identified and treated early. Where abscesses develop close to synovial structures (e.g. following abscess development at the site of perineural nerve blocks), horses should be monitored carefully for development of synovial sepsis.

Treatment

▶ Drainage (in severe cases may need to be performed under GA).
▶ Antimicrobial administration (ideally based on culture and sensitivity):
  ▪ usually staphylococcal reactions where abscesses develop secondary to perineural anaesthesia
  ▪ where clostridial infection is suspected, administer IV penicillin ± metronidazole PO.
▶ NSAIDs.
▶ Check tetanus status.
▶ Other symptomatic treatment as required.
▶ Hospitalisation/referral of severe or deteriorating cases, e.g. myonecrosis, synovial sepsis.

Iatrogenic synovial sepsis

Septic arthritis should be considered if acute lameness develops following intra-articular injection of any medication used for diagnostic/therapeutic reasons or following joint/tendon sheath surgery.

Clinical signs

▸ Marked synovial effusion.
▸ Severe/increasing lameness.

Diagnosis and treatment

▸ Similar clinical signs can be seen in cases of aseptic synovitis and it can be very difficult to differentiate between the two unless bacteria are identified in synovial fluid and/or bacterial growth occurs following culture.
▸ Treat as septic until proven otherwise.
▸ Obtain synovial fluid from the joint or tendon sheath and assess TP, WBC, submit for culture and sensitivity and cytology:
  ▪ usually fluid is turbid/mucopurulent
  ▪ ↑ TP (>35–40 g/L)
  ▪ ↑ WBC >20–30 × 10⁹/L
  ▪ >95% neutrophils.
▸ If equivocal results are obtained, serial monitoring of synovial WBC and TP may be helpful.
▸ Treatment of synovial sepsis – joint/tendon sheath lavage, systemic antimicrobials (see p. 47).

Broken needles

This is uncommon and the risks can be minimised by ensuring proper restraint of the patient and by using an appropriate-sized needle. High-risk situations include synoviocentesis/medication of the coxofemoral, scapulohumeral and femoropatellar joints. In these cases spinal needles should be used as they are more flexible and bend to accommodate stress rather than breaking.

What to do if a needle breaks

▸ If the needle is bent – remove the needle slowly following the curve of the bend.
▸ Breakage usually occurs at the level of the skin.
▸ If the shaft of the needle can be felt lying in a subcutaneous position:
  ▪ sedate or anaesthetise the horse for removal via a skin incision over the location of the needle shaft
  ▪ if sedating the horse, administer a regional nerve block (local administration of LA around the site increases swelling in the area, making it more difficult to feel and incise the skin over the site for removal).
▸ If the shaft of the needle cannot be felt – further investigations are required using US, radiography ± fluoroscopy.
▸ If in joint/tendon sheath – referral/hospitalisation for GA for better exploration of tissues and/or arthroscopic retrieval of the needle and lavage if required.

Broken intravenous catheters

This is relatively rare but can occur if the catheter is damaged during inappropriate insertion/removal or due to disruption by the horse. Care should be taken to insert and remove IV catheters properly (see p. 372) and where catheters are kept in place, ensure they are well secured and protected and that the horse is supervised on a regular basis (e.g. where a horse has to be placed on emergency IV fluids on the yard/farm).

What to do if a catheter breaks

▶ If this is identified immediately following breakage, raise the jugular vein distal to the site and attempt percutaneous retrieval if the catheter is just below the skin (e.g. administer local anaesthetic at the site and make a small skin incision).

▶ Where the fragment cannot be palpated, the catheter can become lodged in the pulmonary vessels or heart.

▶ Referral for assessment of position of the catheter using radiography and US is indicated in these cases.

▶ Leaving the catheter in situ may be elected as catheters rarely cause problems and retrieval can be problematic.

Air embolism

Catheters inserted down the jugular vein (i.e. with the tip directed towards the heart), if dislodged, can result in air being aspirated into the vein. Up to 4 L of air may be required to result in death but it is difficult to know how long a catheter may have been disconnected or how much air has been aspirated.

Clinical signs

▶ Restless, pacing the stable.
▶ Kicking out with hind limbs.
▶ ± Ataxia.
▶ ± Seizures.
▶ ± Blindness.
▶ Can develop pruritus at a later stage.

Treatment

▶ Symptomatic.
▶ Treatment of seizures (see p. 144).
▶ NSAIDs.
▶ Corticosteroids (see Anaphylaxis, p. 270).
▶ In severe cases where the patient is uncontrollable and a danger to itself/personnel, general anaesthesia and ventilation may be required.

Complications encountered during field anaesthesia

▶ Anaesthetic accidents are fortunately rare in field anaesthesia, as these procedures are normally performed on healthy horses for elective procedures of short duration, e.g. castration.

Table 14.4 Complications that may occur during field anaesthesia

Stage of anaesthesia	Complication
Induction	Intracarotid injection Under-dosage
Following induction/during anaesthesia	Apnoea Bradycardia Cyanosis Movement Limb rigidity Hypotension Cardiac dysrrhythmias Cardiac arrest Malignant hyperthermia
Post-anaesthesia	Post-extubation obstruction Myopathies and neuropathies

▶ Where pre-operative examination identifies factors that increase anaesthetic risk, consideration should be given to anaesthesia being performed in a hospital/referral environment.

▶ Occasionally anaesthesia will have to be performed in the field, as an emergency, in horses that may be sick/severely compromised.

▶ Anaesthesia is often undertaken as a last resort in these situations in order to save the horse's life but owners should be aware of the potential risks associated with anaesthesia should the horse die under GA or if complications associated with GA develop subsequently.

▶ Complications associated with general anaesthesia in a theatre environment are covered in specialist texts.

▶ In reality, where complications occur during field anaesthesia, there may be limited options for monitoring and treatment.

▶ Complications that may occur more commonly during field anaesthesia are listed in Table 14.4.

References and further reading

• **Bailey, S.R.,** 2010. Corticosteroid-associated laminitis. Vet. Clin. North Am. Equine Pract. 26, 277–285.

• **Bradbury, L.A., Archer, D.C., Dugdale, A.H., et al.** 2005. Suspected venous air embolism in a horse. Vet. Rec. 156, 109–111.

• **Caron, J.P.,** 2005. Intra-articular injections for joint disease in horses. Vet. Clin. North Am. Equine Pract. 21, 559–573.

- **Clegg, P.**, 2005. Is it just joint inflammation or is it septic? The nagging worry!. Equine Vet. Educ. 17, 210–211.

- **Clutton, R.E.**, 2011. Emergencies during field anaesthesia. In: Equine Field and Hospital Anaesthesia Course Notes, University of Liverpool, 15–16 June.

- **Davis, J.L.**, 2009. Adverse drug reactions. In: Robinson, N.E., Sprayberry, K.A. (Eds.), Current Therapy in Equine Medicine (sixth ed.). Elsevier, St. Louis, Missouri, pp. 1–6.

- **Driessen, B., Zarucco, L., Kalir, B., et al.** 2011. Contemporary use of acepromazine in the anaesthetic management of male horses and ponies: a retrospective study and opinion poll. Equine Vet. J. 43, 88–98.

- **Freeman, D.E.**, 2012. Rectum and anus. In: Auer, J.A., Stick, J.A. (Eds.), Equine Surgery (fourth ed.). Elsevier, St. Louis, Missouri, pp. 494–505.

- **Furr, M.**, 2008. Miscellaneous conditions. In: Furr, M., Reed, S. (Eds.), Equine Neurology. Wiley Blackwell, Chichester, W Sussex, pp. 403–405.

- **Henninger, R.W., Hass, G.F., Freshwater, A.**, 2006. Corticosteroid management of lipoid pneumonia in a horse. Equine Vet. Educ. 18, 205–209.

- **Lapointe, J.M , Laverty, S., Lavoie, J.P.**, 1992. Septic arthritis in 15 standardbred racehorses after intra-articular injection. Equine Vet. J. 24, 430–434.

- **Little, D., Keene, B.W., Bruton, C., et al.** 2002. Percutaneous retrieval of a jugular catheter fragment from the pulmonary artery of a foal. J. Am. Vet. Med. Assoc. 220, 212–214.

- **Mair, T.S.**, 2000. The medical management of eight horses with Grade 3 rectal tears. Equine Vet. J. 32 (Supplement 32), 104–107.

- **Moyer, W., Schumacher, J., Schumacher, J.**, 2011. Equine Joint Injection and Regional Anesthesia. Academic Veterinary Solutions, LLC, Pennsylvania.

- **O'Rourke, D.**, 2008. The practitioners role in SAR reporting. In Pract. 30, 398–402.

- **Peek, S.F., Semrad, S.D., Perkins, G.A.**, 2003. Clostridial myonecrosis in horses (37 cases 1985–2000). Equine Vet. J. 35, 86–92.

- **Scarratt, W.K., Moon, M.L., Sponenberg, D.P., et al.** 1998. Inappropriate administration of mineral oil resulting in lipoid pneumonia in three horses. Equine Vet. J. 30, 85–88.

- **Schumacher, J.**, 1996. Complications of castration. Equine Vet. Educ. 8, 254–259.

- **Sherlock, C., Peroni, J.F.**, 2009. Management of rectal tears. In: Robinson, N.E., Sprayberry, K.A. (Eds.), Current Therapy in Equine Medicine (sixth ed.). Elsevier, St. Louis, Missouri, pp. 451–455.

- **Singer, E.R.**, 2008. Clinical challenges of persistent articular sepsis. Equine Vet. Educ. 20, 353–356.

Infectious diseases

Overview

Many infectious diseases are not immediately life-threatening and may not present as equine emergencies. However, some may cause clinical disease that requires urgent veterinary attention and several may require prompt action to limit the spread of disease. This is of particular importance in highly contagious diseases, particularly those with high rates of morbidity and/or mortality. In addition, where a notifiable disease is suspected, relevant governmental bodies need to be informed.

General points to consider

▶ Most outbreaks of infectious diseases involve the pathogens *Streptococcus equi* subsp. *equi* (strangles), rotavirus, EHV, EI and *Salmonella* spp.
▶ Infectious disease occurrence varies between geographic areas – therefore it is important to be aware of the pathogens that are most commonly encountered in horses and other equids within a particular country or region (see Table 15.1).
▶ It is also important to be alert to the possibility of a new or unexpected pathogen.
▶ Outbreaks of emerging diseases or new variants of common pathogens should be considered with increased international/transboundary movement of horses and export of semen and embryos.
▶ Climate change may result in new vectors of disease becoming established in particular geographic regions.
▶ Veterinary surgeons should also be alert to the possibility of bioterrorism.

> **KEY TIP**
>
> 'Veterinary surgeons can become famous in two ways when a foreign animal disease hits: one way is to diagnose it; the other is to miss it.'
>
> (Brown, 2007)

Useful sources of information

Various websites have been set up to provide current, regularly updated information about disease notifications and outbreaks as the situation can change quickly.

Table 15.1 Websites providing useful sources of information about infectious diseases

Organisation	Description	Current website address and other contact details
OIE World Animal Health Information Database (WAHID)	Lists of new and emerging animal diseases and significant disease outbreaks	http://www.oie.int/wahis/public.php
Department for Environment, Food and Rural Affairs (DEFRA)	List of notifiable diseases, legislation and links to governmental organisations in Wales, Scotland, Northern Ireland and Republic of Ireland	http://www.defra.gov.uk/animal-diseases DEFRA Helpline Mon – Fri (08.00–18.00) 08459 335577
Horserace Betting Levy Board (HBLB)	Codes of practice on equine diseases	http://codes.hblb.org.uk
Animal Health Trust	Updates on equine diseases and diagnostic laboratory service	http://www.aht.org.uk Telephone: 01638 552993
University of Guelph	Blog discussing various current developments in infectious diseases	http://www.wormsandgermsblog.com/articles/equidblog
Queensland Government, Department of Agriculture, Fisheries and Forestry	Hendra virus information	http://www.daff.qld.gov.au/4790_2900.htm
American Association of Equine Practitioners (AAEP)	Guidelines on management of equine infectious disease outbreaks	http://www.aaep.org/control_guidelines_intro.htm
The American Veterinary Medical Association (AVMA)	Variety of articles on zoonotic diseases	http://www.avma.org
Health Protection Agency (HPA)	Details of clinical signs of infectious disease in humans including zoonoses	http://www.hpa.org.uk/topics/infectiousdiseases
The Center for Food Security and Public Health	Resources on animal diseases, infection control etc.	http://www.cfsph.iastate.edu

Notifiable diseases

Global coordination of equine infectious diseases – OIE

The World Organisation for Animal Health (Office International des Epizooties – OIE) is responsible for overall global co-ordination of animal health and has a wealth of resources available for veterinary surgeons worldwide. They should be notified about occurrence of any of the listed diseases as defined by the organisation (Table 15.2). Outside the listed diseases, the OIE should also be notified in the case of other infectious diseases:

▶ That have occurred in the country for the first time.
▶ That have recurred after the country had been declared free from a particular disease.
▶ Where a new strain of a pathogen is identified.
▶ Where there is a sudden/unexpected increase in morbidity or mortality.
▶ Where a new disease is identified which has significant morbidity/mortality.

National/regional regulations

Different countries have their own regulations regarding dealing with equine infectious diseases. In the UK, suspicion of any of the notifiable diseases that may occur in equids must be reported to the local animal health office.

Notifiable diseases in the UK

A list of the equine diseases that are notifiable in the UK together with the key body systems that are affected is given in Table 15.3.

Zoonotic diseases

Some zoonotic infections may cause mild and transient disease (e.g. dermatophytosis), whereas others are potentially life-threatening (e.g. salmonellosis, Hendra virus, anthrax and glanders) see website/texts for further details.

▶ Veterinary surgeons must consider ways in which they can protect their own health and that of employees/family.
▶ Horse owners/handlers must be informed of the potential risk to human health posed by certain equine diseases and ways in which the risk of disease transmission can be minimised.
▶ Appropriate precautions include good personal hygiene and wearing of suitable protective clothing (as a minimum wearing of examination gloves, coveralls and boots/foot covers).
▶ High-risk individuals include those who are immune-compromised and those in contact with very young, elderly or immune-compromised family members or friends.

List of zoonotic conditions that may be transmitted from equids to humans

- Anthrax
- Arboviral encephalitis (WNV, WEE, EEE and VEE)
- Brucellosis
- Enteric clostridiosis
- Campylobacteriosis

- Cryptosporidiosis
- Dermatophytosis
- Giardiasis
- Glanders/farcy
- Hendra virus
- Leptospirosis
- Listeriosis
- Lyme borreliosis
- MRSA
- Rabies
- Rotavirus
- Salmonellosis
- Vesicular stomatitis

Bioterrorism

This is defined as 'the use or threatened use of microorganisms or their toxins against humans, animals or plants by individuals or groups motivated by political, religious, ecological or other ideological objectives'.

▸ Animals act as sentinels for human disease after the release of a biological agent and veterinary surgeons may be the first to detect release of a biological agent – therefore it is important to report unusual and suspicious clinical signs of disease to relevant veterinary and public health agencies.

▸ Whilst there are only a few instances of acts of bioterrorism, this remains a potential and ongoing risk.

▸ Veterinary surgeons are considered to have expert knowledge regarding the effects of biological agents on animals – therefore it is important to be aware of the potential agents that may be used and the clinical signs that may be seen in affected animals.

▸ Based on various criteria (including economic and social impact and availability), agents that may be used in acts of bioterrorism have been classified by the Centers for Disease Control and Prevention (CDC) into categories A, B and C (Table 15.4).

Approach to management of an outbreak of suspected infectious disease

It is important to detect and respond early to animal disease outbreaks that arise due to natural, accidental or deliberate release of pathogens. Following introduction of an infectious disease, delay in diagnosis and implementation of appropriate control measures will have important implications in terms of equine welfare (mortality/morbidity) and economic cost.

> **KEY TIP**
> If in doubt isolate! It can be a big decision to stop movement on or off a premises but failure to do so can have serious welfare and financial implications.

Table 15.2 OIE listed notifiable diseases of equids and details of Hendra virus (as of 2011)

Disease/pathogen	Specific to equids	Key clinical signs in equids	Diagnosis
		Pulmonary form ('Dunkop')	Clinical signs consistent with AHS in endemic areas
		Pyrexia (up to 106°F/41°C)	
		Marked and rapidly progressive respiratory failure – ↑respiratory rate, respiratory distress, profuse sweating, paroxysmal coughing and frothy serofibrinous nasal discharge (Fig. 5.2 p. 94)	PM findings:
			– pulmonary form – severe oedema of lungs, froth and serous fluid in the trachea
		Mortality ~95%	
		Cardiac form ('Dikkop')	– cardiac form – yellow oedema in connective tissues, hydropericardium, petechiae/ ecchymoses on the ventral tongue, heart and GIT
		Pyrexia (102–106°F/39–41°C)	
		Oedema of supraorbital fossae, conjunctiva, spreading down rest of head and neck (Fig. 6.1 p. 106)	
		± Petechial haemorrhages on the conjunctiva and ventral tongue	
		± Severe colic	Virus isolation at an approved laboratory (lithium heparin blood sample, samples of tissues kept refrigerated)
		Mortality ~50%	
		Mixed form (most common)	
African horse sickness (*African horse sickness virus*)	Yes	Subclinical cardiac form followed by pulmonary form	
		Death 3–6d following pyrexia	
		Horse sickness fever	
		Donkeys, zebra and immune horses	
		Pyrexia (up to 104°C/40°C)	
		± Transient anorexia, congested conjunctiva, ↑RR, ↑HR	

Disease	Zoonotic/species affected	Clinical signs	Diagnosis
Anthrax (*Bacillus anthracis*)	No; most mammals susceptible (usually humans and ruminants)	*Peracute* Sudden death Classic hallmark of absence of rigor mortis Evidence of haemorrhage from body orifices *Acute form* Colic, acute enteritis Pyrexia Dyspnoea Subcutaneous oedema Usually rapidly fatal	Identification of organism from blood/splenic aspiration Fluorescent antibody testing/laboratory animal inoculation
Aujesky's disease	No; primarily pigs affected (infection rare in horses)	Anorexia, depression, ataxia, muscle tremors Intermittent blindness, head pressing, nystagmus, chewing, salivation Pyrexia (40°C) Very poor prognosis	Serology Virus isolation
Brucellosis (*Brucella abortus*, *B. melitensis*, *B. suis*)	No; multiple species including humans	*B. abortus* – predilection for tendons, muscles, bones and joints Often associated with septic bursitis of supraspinous bursa over dorsal spinous processes (fistulous withers) or supra-atlantal bursa over cervical vertebrae (poll evil) – heat, pain, swelling followed by purulent discharge Tenosynovitis, arthritis, osteomyelitis also reported Rarely – abortion	Bacterial culture – can be difficult to confirm Serology

(Continued)

Table 15.2 OIE-listed notifiable diseases and details of Hendra virus (as of 2011) (Continued)

Disease/pathogen	Specific to equids	Key clinical signs in equids	Diagnosis
Contagious equine metritis (*Taylorella equigenitalis*)	Yes	Copious purulent vaginal discharge up to 14 d post mating Temporary infertility in mares Abortion	Bacterial culture
Dourine (*Trypanosoma equiperdum*)	Yes	Pyrexia Genital oedema Abortion Cutaneous plaques, 'silver dollar plaques' Weight loss Anaemia, ocular lesions Neurological dysfunction – progressive weakness and ataxia, recumbency and death	Presumptive: clinical signs in endemic areas Identification of parasite in serum, EDTA blood or blood smears Serology
Eastern equine encephalomyelitis (*Eastern equine encephalitis virus*)	No; multiple species including humans	Pyrexia (39.1–40.3°C) Altered behaviour – depression/somnolence/mania/self-mutilation Inappetence Dysphagia, neuropathy of cranial nerves Head pressing, circling, blindness Seizures, coma, death 75–95% mortality	Serology CSF analysis PM examination – virus isolation, immunohistochemistry (NB zoonotic risk)

Echinococcosis/ hydatidosis (*Echinococcus* spp.)	No; multiple species including humans	Parasite may persist for years with no clinical signs being exhibited Clinical signs (if present) related to pressure of enlarging cyst on adjacent organs and tissues	Often incidental findings at PM/laparotomy or US examination of the abdomen/thorax
Equine infectious anaemia (*equine infectious anaemia virus*)	Yes	*Acute* Pyrexia, thrombocytopenia, lethargy, inappetance, occasional death Recurren: episodes of acute clinical disease lasting 3–5 d with variable lengths of time between episodes *Chronic* Vague, non-specific clinical signs, e.g. anaemia, thrombocytopenia, weight loss Occasional neurological signs *Inapparent carriers* Clinically normal, incidental discovery of virus during serological testing Reservoirs of infection	Serology Virus isolation Coggins' test
Equine influenza	Yes	Pyrexia Coughing Mucopurulent nasal discharge	Virus isolation PCR Serology
Equine piroplasmosis (*Babesia caballi* and *Theileria equi*)	Yes	*Peracute* Rare; collapse/sudden death *Acute (most common)* Pyrexia	Identification of parasites on blood smears

(Continued)

Table 15.2 OIE-listed notifiable diseases and details of Hendra virus (as of 2011) (Continued)

Disease/pathogen	Specific to equids	Key clinical signs in equids	Diagnosis
		↑HR, ↑RR, congested or jaundiced MM	Serology
		Colic, diarrhoea	
		Anorexia, anaemia, haematuria	
		Subacute	
		Weight loss, intermittent pyrexia	
		MM pale – icteric ± petechiae/ecchymoses	
		Mild colic, reduced GIT motility	
		Chronic	
		Mild inappetance, weight loss, poor performance	
Equine rhinopneumonitis (*equine herpes virus-1 and -4*)	Yes	Pyrexia	Virus isolation
		Respiratory disease (EHV-1 and -4)	Serology
		Coughing, nasal discharge	PCR
		Abortion (usually EHV-1, occasionally -4)	
		Disease in neonatal foals (EHV-1)	
		Weakness, jaundice, respiratory distress, death	
		Neurological signs (EHV-1 myeloencephalitis)	
		± Preceded by pyrexia	
		HL ataxia	
		Urine retention/dribbling, bladder atony	
		Recumbency	

Equine viral arteritis	Yes	Pyrexia, depression, anorexia Oedema – legs, ventrum, periorbital region, scrotum/prepuce or mammary glands (see Fig. 10.5, p. 200) Urticaria Conjunctivitis Rhinitis Abortion Mortality rare	Virus isolation Serology
Glanders/farcy (*Burkholderia mallei*)	No; multiple species including humans can be infected	*Nasal and pulmonary forms (glanders)* Sticky nasal discharge Progressive debility, coughing, ± diarrhoea *Cutaneous form (farcy)* Enlarged lymph vessels, nodular abscesses, ulceration and discharge of yellow purulent material	Presumptive: clinical signs Confirmed: OIE-approved laboratory Zoonosis
Hendra virus	No; primarily horses but other species including humans can be infected	Rapid-onset illness, including colic, pyrexia, ↑HR, discomfort/weight shifting, depression Rapid deterioration with development of respiratory and/or neurological signs Respiratory signs: respiratory distress, ↑RR, nasal discharge at death (clear progressing to white/blood-stained frothy nasal discharge) Neurological signs: ataxia, loss of vision, altered mentation, head tilt, circling, muscle twitching, urinary incontinence and recumbency	Presumptive – high-risk area, clinical signs and PM findings (only perform with adequate protective wear) Laboratory confirmation (highest level of biosecurity – level 4 pathogen) Zoonosis

(Continued)

Table 15.2 OIE-listed notifiable diseases and details of Hendra virus (as of 2011) (Continued)

Disease/pathogen	Specific to equids	Key clinical signs in equids	Diagnosis
Japanese encephalitis (*Japanese encephalitis virus*)	No; primarily equids and pigs but humans can be infected	*Transitory type syndrome* Pyrexia 2–4 d, inappetance, congested/jaundiced MM, recovery 2–3 d *Lethargic type syndrome* Pyrexic episodes, stupor, reduced vision, bruxism and chewing motions, dysphagia, ataxia, neck rigidity, paresis/paralysis – recovery around 7 d *Hyperexcitable type syndrome* Pyrexia, profuse sweating, muscle fasciculations, altered mentation, blindness, collapse, coma, death (mortality around 5–30%)	Presumptive based upon clinical signs in affected area (encephalitis, pyrexia) Serology Virus isolation
Leptospirosis	No; multiple species can be infected	Pyrexia, icterus, periodic uveitis, abortion Septicaemia, pyrexia, leptospiruria and haematuria in the neonate Can cause renal disease	Bacterial culture (difficult) Serological tests Zoonosis
New and old world screwworm (*Cochliomyia hominivorax* and *Chrysomya bezziana*)	No; multiple species including humans can be infected	Evidence of egg masses/larvae around wounds Secondary bacterial infection, death if infestation severe and untreated	Identification of larvae, eggs or flies (80% ethanol or isopropyl alcohol, not in formalin)

Disease	Zoonotic	Clinical signs	Diagnosis
Rabies (*rabies virus*)	No; multiple species including humans can be infected	*Spinal form (most common)* Localised hyperaesthesia, self-mutilation (Fig. 7.2 p. 147) Progressive ascending ataxia and weakness *Dumb form (uncommon)* Depression, anorexia Paralysis of facial nerves – dysphagia, head tilt, ataxia, blindness Tail/penis/bladder paralysis Progressive paralysis *Furious form (rare)* Aggression, bizarre behaviour, anxious Hyperaesthesia Muscle tremors and weakness, incoordination Seizures **Death occurs in all forms**	No definitive ante-mortem test – presumptive based on history of bite, endemic region, clinical signs Definitive: virus confirmation in brain performed at approved laboratory (NB significant zoonotic risk when performing PM)
Surra (*Trypanosoma evansi*)	No; multiple animal species can be infected	Pyrexia (can be intermittent and recurrent) Progressive anaemia Weight loss despite good appetite Urticarial lesions, distal limb oedema, petechial haemorrhages Neurological signs – progressive weakness and ataxia progressing to death Abortion	Clinical signs in endemic areas Visualisation of parasite on blood smear Serological methods

(Continued)

Table 15.2 OIE-listed notifiable diseases and details of Hendra virus (as of 2011) (Continued)

Disease/pathogen	Specific to equids	Key clinical signs in equids	Diagnosis
Vesicular stomatitis (*vesicular stomatitis virus*)	No; equids, cattle, pigs, camelids (south American) and humans can be infected	Similar to foot and mouth disease (which horses are resistant to) Excessive salivation Blanched raised/broken vesicles on gums, upper surface of tongue, surface of lips, around nares and corners of mouth	Virus isolation Serology Zoonosis
Venezuelan equine encephalomyelitis	No; can infect multiple species	See clinical signs for Eastern equine encephalomyelitis ± Diarrhoea/colic Mortality 40–90%	See Diagnosis of Eastern equine encephalomyelitis, p. 282
West Nile fever (*West Nile virus*)	No; multiple species including humans can become infected	Variable – disease may occur in any part of the CNS Initially: pyrexia, anorexia, depression ± colic Altered mentation and behaviour, cranial nerve deficits, ataxia, paresis (Fig. 7.3, p. 147) Muscle fasciculations (face, neck, can affect limbs and trunk) – more common in WNV encephalomyelitis compared to other adult CNS disorders Can make full recovery/have residual CNS deficits	Clinical signs, biochemistry, haematology, CSF analysis Serology Virus detection in PM tissues
Western equine encephalitis	No; multiple species including humans can become infected	See Clinical signs for Eastern equine encephalomyelitis Mortality 20–40%	See diagnosis of Eastern equine encephalomyelitis, p. 282

Disease	Central nervous system	Respiratory system	Skin/integument	Ocular	Cardio-vascular system	Reproductive system	Gastrointestinal system	Sudden death
African horse sickness (see Figs 5.2, 6.1 p. 94 & 106)*		✓			✓		(✓)	
Anthrax	✓	✓	✓		✓		✓	✓
Aujesky's disease	✓							
Contagious equine metritis						✓		
Dourine	✓		✓	✓	✓	✓		
Epizootic lymphangitis (Fig. 2.12 see p. 32)			✓		✓			
Equine infectious anaemia				✓	✓	✓		
Equine viral arteritis (Fig 10.5 p. 200)	✓	✓	✓	✓				
Equine viral encephalomyelitis	✓							
Glanders (farcy)		✓	✓					
Rabies (see Fig. 7.2 p.147)	✓							
Vesicular stomatitis*			✓					
Warble fly			✓					
West Nile fever	✓						(✓)	

Key body systems that are affected and conditions that may result in sudden death are denoted by a ✓. (✓) which denotes that clinical signs related to that body system may be inconsistently seen.
*Specified diseases are subject to compulsory slaughter, and imposition of protection and surveillance zones (distance dependent on pathogen) around the premises.

Table 15.4 Bioterrorism agents as classified by the Centers for Disease Control and Prevention (CDC)

Category	Disease	Pathogen
A	Anthrax*	*Bacillus anthracis*
	Botulism*	*Clostridium botulinum* (toxin)
	Plague	*Yersinia pestis*
	Smallpox	*Variola major*
	Tularaemia	*Francisella tularensis*
	Viral haemorrhagic fever	Ebola and Lassa viruses
B	Brucellosis*	*Brucella* spp.
	Glanders*	*Burkholderia mallei*
	Melioidosis	*Burkholderia pseudomallei*
	Psittacosis	*Chlamydophila psittaci*
	Q fever	*Coxiella burnetti*
	Epidemic typhus fever	*Rickettsia prowazekii*
	Encephalitis*	Western, Eastern and Venezuelan equine viruses
	Toxic syndromes*	Ricin
	Food safety*	*Salmonella* spp., *Escherichia coli*
	Water safety*	*Cryptosporidium* spp.
C	Emerging threats	Nipah virus
		Hanta virus

*Agents that have the potential to cause disease in equids.
From Davis (2004).

Approach to dealing with an outbreak of a suspected infectious disease
- Identify the problem and potential pathogens that may be involved.
- Implement immediate steps to manage the problem.
- Confirm the diagnosis.
- Implement ongoing management and disease investigation.

Identify the problem and potential pathogens that may be involved

▶ Following initial contact, review possible diagnoses before the visit, e.g. biology, epidemiology, clinical signs, diagnosis, treatment and control:
  ▪ consider the geographical region of horses and season
  ▪ be aware of diseases most likely to occur in that region/at that time of year
  ▪ be alert to recent disease outbreaks in that region

- consider most likely diagnosis based on these but keep an open mind to the possibility of something different, particularly in the case of recent importation/long-distance travel of a horse or in-contacts.

▶ Take a full history. Specific questions that should be asked include:
  - duration of clinical signs and progression of disease
  - contact with other horses and whether clinical signs have been seen in those in-contacts
  - recent importation of that horse/in-contacts
  - recent travel of that horse/in-contacts, including long-distance travel and attendance at shows/transport to stud farm.

▶ Consider patterns that may be relevant, e.g. age of horses, affected groups (location on yard, in-contacts):
  - determine the possible disease source and how disease is being spread.

▶ Before examining the horse, consider:
  - potential risks to human safety, e.g. rabies, injury by ataxic, seizing or aggressive horse
  - what protective clothing is required
  - disinfection of equipment between horses.

▶ Perform a thorough clinical examination of affected horses, taking appropriate biosecurity measures.

▶ Make an initial diagnosis or list of most likely diagnoses.

▶ Take initial samples (see Table 15.5):
  - if unsure what samples may be required, contact the laboratory directly
  - consider the logistics of sample submission to avoid delay in samples sitting in the post over weekends and bank holidays (keep refrigerated).

▶ Administer appropriate treatment and make a treatment plan for individual horses.

Implement immediate steps to manage the problem

▶ Decide what measures are appropriate to that situation based on likely diagnosis, numbers and groups of horses affected and individual premises – there needs to be a balance between over-reaction and not doing anything at all.

▶ If a notifiable or reportable disease is suspected, contact the relevant veterinary agencies (this will vary depending on country/region) – in these cases, these agencies may take over the following steps.

▶ If the suspected pathogen is zoonotic, consider the risk to yourself and to other human in-contacts, be aware of clinical signs associated with disease and steps to take.

▶ Communication is critical and as a veterinary surgeon, leadership (i.e. taking control of the situation), education (i.e. informing lay personnel of the likely risk to horses and personnel and importance of preventive measures) and professionalism (i.e. informing relevant veterinary and health agencies and other veterinary professionals) is essential.

▶ Discuss findings with owner/stable manager:
  - most likely diagnosis and how long it will take to confirm this
  - treatment required for affected horses and clinical signs to monitor for in other horses on the yard
  - what biosecurity measures need to be implemented and why
  - what information needs to be conveyed to yard staff/other horse owners and how this will be done.

Table 15.5 Diagnosis of contagious, infectious respiratory, diarrhoeal and neurological conditions

	Infectious respiratory disease	Infectious diarrhoeal disease	Infectious neurological disease
Pathogens to rule in/out (based on likelihood according to geographic region)	*Streptococcus equi* var *equi* Equine influenza Equine herpes virus-1 (EHV-1) Equine herpes virus-4 (EHV-4) Equine viral arteritis (EVA)	*Salmonella* spp. Clostridial enteritis Potomac horse fever Rotavirus	Equine herpes virus-1 (EHV-1) Botulism EEE/WEE/VEE WNV Rabies
Samples and laboratory tests	Nasopharyngeal swabs for virus isolation/PCR/ bacterial culture Heparin sample – virus isolation Serum sample – serology Keep refrigerated	Bacterial culture of faeces (3–5 g faeces/2–3 rectal swabs) – keep refrigerated and send cooled Sensitivity testing PCR – PHF Serum sample – serology	Nasal swab for virus isolation/ immunoassay/PCR Blood sample (EDTA) – PCR, IgM detection Serum sample – serology ± CSF – cytology, virus isolation, PCR ± PM tissue samples (NB zoonotic risks)

▶ Establish necessary biosecurity procedures and ensure these are communicated to all relevant parties, including yard/farm staff:
  - group horses into affected, exposed/in-contact and non-exposed groups (see Table 15.6)
  - isolate horses (see p. 387)
  - personal hygiene – protective clothing, hand washing
  - area separation – separate physical regions on the yard, equipment and staff
  - cleaning and disinfection – affected stables, vehicles, horse trailers, pasture management
  - waste disposal of manure
  - pasture management
  - visitors to/foot traffic on the yard
  - insects, rodents and other animals.
▶ Communicate with other veterinary surgeons (if relevant):
  - this will vary with the suspected disease and each situation
  - where veterinary surgeons from the same or other practices attend horses on that yard, they should be informed of the current situation and ideally should co-operate and agree upon a unified plan.

Table 15.6 Initial management of horses on premises where a disease outbreak is suspected

Affected horses	Exposed/in contact with horses	Non-contact horses
Move to separate isolation area or confine to stables	Confine within current area	Determine risk to these horses and whether movement restriction of horses on/off premises is required – if in any doubt, stop movements until results of tests are known
Implement biosecurity measures and determine which personnel should manage these horses	Determine appropriate biosecurity measures and personnel who should have contact with these horses	
Institute appropriate medical therapy	Monitor horses for clinical signs of disease and record rectal temperatures twice daily	Monitor twice daily for clinical signs of disease

Confirm the diagnosis

▶ Co-ordinate with the laboratory and maintain communication with owners/stable manager, i.e. keep them informed of progress.

▶ Discuss the results with the laboratory (where relevant) and communicate the results of the tests to relevant people as soon as these are available:

  ▪ check that the clinical signs and results of the laboratory tests are consistent with the diagnosis

  ▪ be alert to different strains of pathogens, i.e. where the clinical signs/morbidity and mortality rates seem different in this disease outbreak

  ▪ review the biology of the disease, treatment and control if required and contact other veterinary professionals if necessary (e.g. in the case of limited experience of managing a disease outbreak associated with that pathogen).

▶ If a notifiable disease is confirmed, contact the relevant agencies; where there is potential risk to human health, health agencies should be contacted.

▶ Report the findings to the relevant horse owner/yard manager and other relevant lay people and veterinary colleagues.

Implement ongoing management and disease investigation

▶ Implement necessary disease controls – these will be individual for that pathogen. For the most common infectious diseases, see the HBLB Codes of Practice (http://www.hblb.org.uk). AAEP contingency plans (www.aaep.org) or ACVIM codes of practice (www.acvim.org).

▶ Make changes to biosecurity procedures and treatment plans based on these results:

  ▪ determine whether isolation procedures are still required or if movements on and off premises can be changed

  ▪ review whether current biosecurity measures are effective for that pathogen, e.g. type of disinfectants used

  ▪ make any relevant changes to treatment plans for affected horses and, if certain pathogens have been ruled out, determine whether further diagnostic tests are required

- consider prevention in other horses, e.g. antimicrobial treatment, vaccination, screening tests.
▸ If test results are inconclusive or the cause for the disease outbreak cannot be determined, decide what further investigations need to be performed:
  - specify the clinical signs and test results seen in affected horses
  - define the magnitude of the problem, i.e. how many horses are affected, mortality and morbidity rates
  - contact veterinary specialists in epidemiology/infectious diseases for further advice.
▸ Once the disease outbreak has been controlled, do not forget to review biosecurity on the premises with the yard/farm to avoid a similar situation occurring again – formulate an agreed biosecurity and outbreak control plan:
  - isolation of new arrivals on the yard for at least 14 d – ask about recent diarrhoea, respiratory infections and check for signs of disease on arrival. This is especially important in the case of imported horses/horses that have travelled abroad
  - protection of resident horses/those that travel on a regular basis
  - vaccination – depends on area, disease risks.

References and further reading

- **Anon.,** 2011. American Association of Equine Practitioners, Infectious Disease Control <http://www.aaep.org/control_guidelines_intro.htm>.

- **Anon.,** 2012. OIE World Organisation for Animal Health Listed Diseases <http://www.oie.int/animal-health-in-the-world/oie-listed-diseases-2012>.

- **Anon.,** 2013. Animal Disease Information, the Centre for Food Security & Public Health <http://www.cfsph.iastate.edu/diseaseinfo>.

- **Banks, M.,** 1996. Aujesky's disease in the horse. Equine Vet. Educ. 8, 219–220.

- **Bender, J.B., Tsukayama, D.T.,** 2004. Horses and the risk of zoonotic infections. Vet. Clin. North Am. Equine Pract. 20, 643–653.

- **Bernard, W.,** 2009. Clinical commentary: leptospirosis. Equine Vet. Educ. 21, 485–486.

- **Brown, C.C.,** 2007. Recognition of foreign animal diseases. In: Stellon, D.C., Long, M.T. (Eds.), Equine Infectious Diseases. Elsevier, St. Louis, Missouri, pp. 546–549.

- **Dwyer, R.M.,** 2007. Control of infectious disease outbreaks. In: Stellon, D.C., Long, M.T. (Eds.), Equine Infectious Diseases. Elsevier, St. Louis, Missouri, pp. 539–545.

- **Davis, R.G.,** 2004. The ABCs of bioterrorism for veterinarians, focusing on Category A agents. J. Am. Vet. Med. Assoc. 224, 1084–1095.

- **Guthrie, A.J.,** 2007. African horse sickness. In: Stellon, D.C., Long, M.T. (Eds.), Equine Infectious Diseases. Elsevier, St. Louis, Missouri, pp. 164–171.

- **Irby J.R.,** 2002. Anthrax, screwworms, and equine piroplasmosis – subdued but not eradicated. In: Proceedings of the American Association of Equine Practitioners Annual Convention 48, 12–15 <http://www.ivis.org>.

- **Long, M.T.,** 2007. Flavivirus infections. In: Stellon, D.C., Long, M.T. (Eds.), Equine Infectious Diseases. Elsevier, St. Louis, Missouri, pp. 198–206.

- **Weese, J.S.,** 2002. A review of equine zoonotic diseases: risks in veterinary medicine. In: Proceedings of the American Association of Equine Practitioners Annual Convention 48, 362–369 <http://www.ivis.org>.

Poisoning, bites and stings

CHAPTER
16

General approach to suspected poisoning

Dealing with suspected acute poisoning (toxicoses) can present a diagnostic and therapeutic challenge, especially if multiple horses are involved. General points to consider include:

▶ In an emergency situation, the priority is to prevent other animals and humans being affected:
  ▪ removal of horses from the pasture
  ▪ bathing of horses where there has been cutaneous exposure to a toxic agent – take precautions to prevent exposure in humans during this process.
▶ Treatment often has to be started before the aetiological agent is known – this is usually symptomatic, based on the clinical signs seen (which usually involve multiple organs) and the suspected/potential toxic agent.
▶ Any list of toxins is likely to be incomplete and any substance has the potential to be toxic in large enough quantities (Table 16.1).
▶ Certain toxins are more likely to occur in different geographical areas (particularly plants known to be toxic to horses).
▶ It is important to be aware of those that occur most commonly and the presenting clinical signs of toxicity and treatment.
▶ Deliberate poisoning is relatively uncommon.

Situations that may increase suspicion of potential poisoning

▶ Sudden death of unknown cause.
▶ Multiple horses sick where there is no known infectious disease – especially if on similar feedstuffs and in the same environment.
▶ History of potential exposure to toxin:
  ▪ pesticide spraying close to horse pasture
  ▪ change premises/pasture
  ▪ change of feed
  ▪ inadequate pasture
  ▪ soil disturbance/other construction work.
▶ Uncommon clinical signs (do not forget about potential infectious diseases).

Useful sources of information

- Veterinary Poisons Information Service (UK) – http://www.vpis.co.uk (helpline: 020 7188 0200).
- ASPCA National Animal Poison Control Center (USA) – http://www.napcc.aspca.org.

General approach to treatment

- Identify the potential source of poisoning and the likelihood of exposure.
- Prevent continued and repeat exposure to the toxin.
- Stabilise the patient.
- Enhance toxin removal.
- ± Administration of antidote (if available).
- Start supportive treatment.
- Observation and additional treatment as required.

Initial advice to owner/carer

▸ Find out what the suspected poison is – ask the owner to look at labels on containers/bags.

▸ Take the horse away from a known hazard.

▸ If relevant, warn about potential human hazards, e.g. handling a sick horse, exposure to toxins.

Initial assessment and first aid

▸ Perform immediate assessment of collapsed horses or those showing severe signs of colic, respiratory distress or neurological signs (see relevant sections).

▸ Triage if multiple horses involved to determine which horses are most severely affected.

▸ Check for respiratory, cardiovascular and neurological abnormalities:

- oxygen ± tracheotomy if URT swelling
- ± intubation and ventilation (if equipment available)
- sedate if neccessary – avoid phenothiazines, e.g. acepromazine (reduce seizure threshold)
- control seizures if present (see p. 144)
- consider stringhalt (equine reflex hypertonia) if classic locomotor signs are evident (see p. 138).

▸ Assess heart rate, rhythm and check for dysrrhythmias.

▸ Check body temperature:

- hyperthermia can occur in chlorophenol poisoning (e.g. in wood preservatives) (see p. 214)
- can develop hypothermia – use blankets and heat lamps to warm the horse (as the metabolic rate slows, the rate of poison degradation slows too).

▶ Obtain blood samples for:
- haematology
- serum biochemistry
- electrolytes
- ± clotting profiles

▶ Start supportive therapy, e.g. IV fluids.

Further investigation

▶ Obtain a full history. Specific questions that should be asked include:
- known or high level of suspicion about exposure to potentially toxic agent, e.g. grazing in field with large quantities of ragwort
- recent change of pasture/premises/feed
- recent pasture treatment, e.g. application of herbicides or pest control
- known contact with paints/solvents or recent excavation/building work.

▶ Perform a through clinical examination of the affected horse(s) and horses in the same environment:
- consider possible differential diagnoses based on clinical signs observed (Table 16.1).

▶ Examine the environment (Fig. 16.1):
- feed
- pasture – plants
- water source.

Table 16.1 List of toxicoses to consider based upon the predominant organ system affected**

	Toxic agent
Signs predominantly related to the GIT	
Plants	Black locust (*Robinia pseudoacacia*)
	Buttercups (*Ranunculus* spp.)
	Castor bean (*Ricinus communis*)
	Deadly nightshade (*Atropa belladona*)
	Horse chestnut (*Aesculus hippocastanum*)
	Jimsonweed, thornapple (*Datura* spp.)
	Leyland cypress (*Cupressocyparis leylandii*)
	Nightshade (*Solanum* spp.)
	Oak (*Quercus* spp.)
	Pokeweed (*Phytolacca americana*)
	Privet hedge (*Ligustrum* spp.)
	Tobacco (*Nicotiana* spp.)

(Continued)

Table 16.1 List of toxicoses to consider based upon predominant organ system affected** (Continued)

	Toxic agent
Signs predominantly related to the GIT (continued)	
Other	Aluminium
	Amitraz
	Arsenic (inorganic)
	Atropine
	Blister beetle (cantharidin)
	Carbamate insecticides
	Chlorates
	Dioctyl sodium sulphosuccinate
	Mercury poisoning
	Organophosphate insecticides
	Pentachlorophenol
	Petroleum distillates
	Phosphorus (red/white forms)
	Pyriminil
	Salt poisoning
	Slaframine (mycotoxin)
	Tetrachlorodibenzodioxin
	Thallium
Signs predominantly related to CNS stimulation	
Plants	Locoweed (*Astralagus and Oxytropis* spp.)
Other	4-Aminopyridine
	Ammonia
	Blue-green algae (Cyanobacteria)
	Carbamate pesticides
	Carbon disulphide
	Chlorinated hydrocarbons
	Levamisole
	Metaldehyde
	Methiocarb
	Nervous ergotism – mycotoxin
	Nicotine
	Organophosphates
	Strychnine
	Urea/non-protein nitrogen

Table 16.1 List of toxicoses to consider based upon predominant organ system affected** (Continued)

	Toxic agent
Signs predominantly related to CNS depression	
Plants	Black locust (*Robinia psuedoacacia*)
	Bracken fern (*Pteridium aquilinum*)
	Horsetail (*Equisetum* spp.)
	Milkvetch (*Astragalus* spp.)
	Milkweed (*Asclepias* spp.)
	Russian knapweed (*Acroptilon repens*)
	Yellow starthistle (*Centaurea solstitialis*)
Other	Fumonisin B1 mycotoxin
	Lead
	Propylene glycol
	Triclopyr
Signs predominantly related to hepatic dysfunction	
Plants containing pyrrolizidine alkaloids	Common groundsel (*Senecio vulgaris*)
	Groundsel (*Senecio longilobus*)
	Houndstongue (*Cynoglossum officinale*)
	Ragwort (*Senecio jacobaea*)
Other plants	Alskie clover (*Trifolium hybridum*)
Other	Alfatoxins
	Iron
Signs predominantly related to the cardiovascular system	
Plants	Foxglove (*Digitalis* spp.)
	Yew tress (*Taxus* spp.)
	Maple (*Acer* spp.)
	Oleander (*Nerium oleander*)
	Onion (*Allium* spp.)
	Rayless goldenrod (*Isocoma wrightii*)
	Rhododendron (*Rhododendron* spp.)
	White snakeroot (*Eupatorium rugosum*)

(*Continued*)

Table 16.1 List of toxicoses to consider based upon predominant organ system affected** (Continued)

	Toxic agent
Signs predominantly related to the cardiovascular system (continued)	
Other	Bicarbonate
	Coumarin derivatives
	Cyanide
	Dimethyl sulphoxide
	Ionophore antimicrobials
	Lasalocid
	Monensin
	Nitrates/nitrites
	Organophosphate or carbamate insecticides
	Sodium fluoroacetate (1080)
	Salinomycin
Signs predominantly related to the urinary tract	
Plants containing oxalates	Beet/mangold (*Beta vulgaris*)
	Black greasewood (*Sarcobatus vermiculatus*)
	Halogeton (*Glomeratus* spp.)
	Lambsquarters (*Chenopodium* album)
	Pigweed (*Amaranthus* spp.)
	Purslane (*Portulaca oleracea*)
	Rhubarb (*Rheum rhubarbarum*)
	Russian thistle (*Salsola* spp.)
	Sorrel/dock (*Rumex* spp.)
Other plants	Sorghum (*Sorghum* spp.)
Other	Mercury/cadmium
	Vitamins D_2/D_3
	Vitamin K_3
*Signs predominantly related to musculoskeletal system/integument excluding photosensitisation**	
Plants	Black walnut (*Juglans nigra*)
	Hairy vetch (*Vicia villosa*)
	Hoary alyssum (*Berteroa incana*)
	Tall fescue (*Festuca arundinacea*)
	Wild jasmine (*Cestrum diurnum*)

Table 16.1 List of toxicoses to consider based upon predominant organ system affected** (Continued)

	Toxic agent
Signs predominantly related to musculoskeletal system/integument excluding photosensitisation (continued)	
Other	Fluoride
	Gangrenous ergotism (*Claviceps purpurea* mycotoxin)
	Iodine
	Selenium/zinc
	Snake venom (see p. 304)

*A long list of plants may cause photosensitisation – as these do not usually present as emergencies, refer to other texts if this is suspected.

**Material taken from Poppenger and Puschner (2008), Talcott (2010) and the Veterinary Poisons Information Service (www.vpisuk.co.uk).

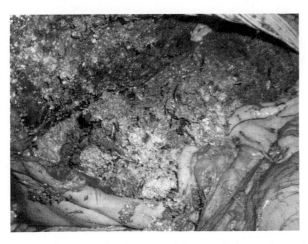

Figure 16.1 PM examination and opening of the stomach in a horse that was euthanased due to severe abdominal pain; large quantities of crushed acorns were found within the stomach, consistent with the clinical signs of acorn oak toxicosis.

Courtesy of Gavinder Panesar.

▶ Perform a PM examination if death occurs and collect samples.
▶ Ideally consult a veterinary toxicologist first:
  ▪ check sample requirements and preservation (Table 16.2)
  ▪ if known or high suspicion of involvement of a particular toxin, determine if an antidote is available.

Table 16.2 Samples required for toxicological analysis. Ideally check with the laboratory first regarding sample quantities, timing and storage

	Sample type and amount	Storage/preservation
Environmental samples	Feedstuffs – >500 g of representative feed	In sealed paper/plastic bag or glass containers
	Plants (whole)	Pressed and dried or frozen
	Fungus (whole mushroom/ toadstool)	Keep cool and dry in paper bag
	Horse drinking water (1 L)	Secure, clean, airtight container that will not leak
	Herbicide/agents for vermin or insect control	Freeze in bag and send with any packaging
Ante-mortem samples	Whole blood (10 mL)	EDTA tube
	Serum (10 mL)	Plain tube and remove clot; if testing for zinc, sample must not have contact with rubber
	Urine (50 mL)	Plastic, screw top container
	Stomach contents (gastric lavage) 500 mL	Secure container that will not leak
	Faeces (100 g)	Freeze – may be worth collecting several samples at different time points
	Biopsy specimins (e.g. liver biopsy)	Freeze
PM samples	GI contents from multiple sites (stomach, small intestine, caecum, large colon) – 500 mL from each in separate containers	Freeze
	Samples from organs (100 g) – liver, kidney, fat, spleen, lung, brain (put into separate containers)	Freeze and put small representative samples into formalin
	Tissue samples from specific area e.g. injection site (100 g)	Freeze
	Eye (ocular contents)	Freeze

Adapted from Poppenga and Puschner (2008).

Treatment plan

Where contact poisoning has occurred

▶ Beware human exposure – wear protective clothing, including gloves, masks, goggles, long sleeves, aprons.

▶ If dry/powdered toxin – brush or vacuum the horse's coat but don't wet the coat (increases toxin absorption).

▶ If wet toxin, remove with mild detergent (e.g. washing-up liquid) in warm water until the smell of toxin has gone.

Ingested toxins

▶ ± Gastric lavage:
   - only useful if the horse is presented shortly after toxin ingestion
   - unlikely to get coarse plant material back
   - use a large-bore tube, copious quantities of water and save some of the gastric contents for toxicology.

▶ Administer activated charcoal (AC):
   - very adsorptive for a number of toxins, except metals and alcohols
   - give asap after ingestion and do not administer at same time as mineral oil (reduces absorptive capacity)
   - 1–3 g/kg BW PO – powdered charcoal better than tablets
   - make up as a slurry and administer via stomach tube.

▶ ± Kaolin pectin/bismuth compounds:
   - demulcents with weak adsorbent properties (AC is better choice)
   - kaolin pectin 2–4 L/450 kg PO
   - bismuth salicylate 1–2 L/450 kg PO.

▶ ± Administer cathartics to accelerate clearance from GIT:
   - only beneficial if given soon after ingestion, e.g. magnesium sulphate (Epsom salts) 0.2–1 g/kg in 4 L warm water PO
   - oily cathartics – generally best avoided and AC given instead
   - mineral oil – less effective than AC but good if lipid-soluble toxicants.

Increase toxin elimination

▶ Administer oral or IV fluids to promote diuresis as most toxins are excreted via the kidneys:
   - check renal and pulmonary function first
   - ideally monitor PCV/TP and urine production (>2 mL/kg/h)
   - ± administer diuretics, e.g. furosemide 0.5–1.0 mg/kg IV.

Antidotes

▶ These are only available for certain drugs (consult toxicology service).

▶ Can be toxic themselves.

Ongoing supportive care and treatment

▶ Monitor carefully for any change in clinical parameters.

▶ Most toxins affect multiple organs – determine organ function based on results of serum biochemistry (including serial samples).

▸ Determine whether hospitalisation is warranted.
▸ ± ECG if dysrhythmia/persistent tachycardia:
  ▪ generally dysrhythmias associated with poisoning should not be treated with anti-arrythmic drugs (can act syngergistically and can be proarrythmic and negatively inotropic)
  ▪ treat underlying fluid and electrolyte disturbances first – often cardiac abnormalities disappear once these are corrected (see specialist texts).

Snake bites

Snake bites in the horse are usually by members of the viper family and the likelihood of this will be largely dependent on geographic region. Most information about snake bites has been obtained from the USA where rattlesnakes are responsible for most snake bites. In Australia, brown, tiger and red-belly snakes are commonly involved, whereas in Europe, snake bites are most likely to be due to the common adder.

General points about snake bites

▸ The constituents of snake venom will differ between species.
▸ These can have a variety of local (oedema, haemorrhage, skin necrosis, myonecrosis) and systemic effects, including neurotoxicity, myotoxicity, coagulation disorders, haemolysis, cardiotoxicity, renal toxicity and other CV effects (usually hypotension).
▸ Subsequent sequelae may be responsible for mortality in affected horses, e.g. laminitis, myocardial failure.
▸ Not all snake bites will result in evenomation.
▸ Where this has occurred, clinical signs can vary considerably between affected horses, depending on the concentration of toxins injected, the site of bite and the rate at which toxins diffuse into circulation.
▸ Inherent snake related factors may also play a role in the clinical effects seen, including species, time since their last meal and seasonal influences in feeding patterns or hibernation.

Clinical signs

▸ Acute, severe swelling and oedema (Fig. 16.2).
▸ ± Evidence of fang marks at the site of the bite.
▸ Pain ± local haemorrhage.
▸ Respiratory distress if swelling around the nasal passages/URT.
▸ Bites most common on the nose, head, neck and distal limbs.

Immediate first aid

▸ If severe nasal swelling is developing and the horse may take some time to be reached, the owner/carer may need to place some form of tubing into the nasal passages until you arrive (making sure this tubing can be retrieved again).
▸ Establish and maintain a patent airway if severe nasal swelling has developed:
  ▪ pass a nasal tube (e.g. small endotracheal tube or shortened piece of stomach tube) and secure in position or
  ▪ perform a tracheotomy if severe nasal swelling/dyspnoea is evident (see p. 356).

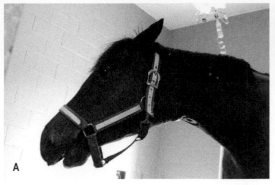
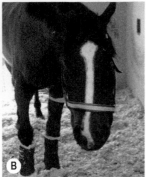

Figure 16.2 (A,B) Severe facial oedema that developed following a snake bite (and envenomation) to the face of a horse.

Courtesy of Barbara Schmidt.

▸ Keep the horse calm and limit its movement.
▸ Do not interfere with the site of the bite wound.

KEY TIP

Do not apply a tourniquet, apply suction to or incise over the site or perform cryotherapy –
this increases the risk of infection and promotes tissue necrosis.

Further assessment and treatment

▸ Obtain a full history. Specific questions that should be asked include:
  ▪ if a snake was seen in the vicinity at the time and the type of snake seen.
▸ Perform a full clinical examination;
  ▪ where there is minimal tissue reaction in an area with fang marks, the horse may
    have been bitten by a non-venomous snake or little/no venom was produced by a
    venomous snake.
▸ Take blood samples for:
  ▪ haematology
  ▪ serum biochemistry, including cardiac enzymes
  ▪ electrolytes
  ▪ coagulation profile.
▸ Check tetanus status (see p. 23).
▸ Perform ECG examination if cardiac dysrhythmias/tachycardia are evident:
  ▪ atrial fibrillation and ventricular tachycardia are the most common abnormalities
    identified in these cases (see texts/website).
▸ NSAIDs – take care with their use especially if coagulopathies are evident.
▸ Corticosteroids – controversial and only indicated if allergic complications occur.
▸ IV fluids (see p. 374).

▸ Enteral/parenteral nutrition depending on severity of clinical signs.
▸ Plasma transfusion if prolonged clotting times/thrombocytopenia (see p. 376).
▸ Blood transfusion if spontaneous haemorrhage/signs of haemolysis (see p. 376).
▸ BS antimicrobials if development of cellulitis/infection at the site.
▸ Keep quiet.
▸ Monitor for signs of colic/development of other clinical signs, e.g. facial nerve paralysis.

Antivenin treatment

▸ Lack of information and evidence.
▸ Monovalent (if snake type known)/polyvalent.
▸ May be available commercially in some geographic regions.
▸ Optimal dose and duration of treatment are unknown.
▸ May be economically non-viable (very expensive) and too late (in humans ideally given <4 h following bite).
▸ Indicated in cases that have severe systemic clinical signs or rapidly spreading local signs and are deteriorating despite treatment.

Prognosis

▸ Rattlesnakes – 10–30% of snake bites in horses are fatal.
▸ Adders – 9–43% mortality (few case reports).

Insect bites

▸ Rarely present as emergencies – most effects are related to localised dermatological reaction, delayed hypersensitivity reaction and clinical disease that develops following transmission of infectious diseases.
▸ Occasionally anaphylactic reactions will be seen and death has been reported following attacks by swarms of biting and stinging insects.
▸ Clinical signs seen following bites by venomous insects are shown in Table 16.3.
▸ Treatment – largely symptomatic:
  ▪ remove sting (if left in situ)
  ▪ bathe site with mild alkaline solution in bee stings (2% bicarbonate of soda) or mildly acidic solution (diluted vinegar) in the case of wasp stings and spider bites
  ▪ topical/systemic anti-inflammatories – dexamathasone 0.02–0.1 mg/kg IV if anaphylaxis or severe, extensive reaction
  ▪ ± apply ice packs over the affected region
  ▪ ± adrenaline 0.01–0.02 mg/kg IV (up to 0.2 mg/kg) if anaphylaxis
  ▪ ± flunixin 1.1 mg/kg IV
  ▪ ± fluid therapy.

Stinging nettles

▸ Physical contact with stinging nettles (*Urtica dioica*) most commonly causes an urticarial skin reaction.
▸ Ataxia and behavioural signs of distress have been reported in horses with known or suspected contact with stinging nettles based on exclusion of other causes.

Table 16.3 Clinical signs related to bites and stings by venomous insect

Venomous insect	Clinical signs
Wasps	Each wasp may sting several times Several bites may occur in close proximity Attacks by swarms can result in death
Bees	Oedematous wheals and plaques Usually a single sting – potency of venom differs between individual bees and different subspecies Death may occur when attacked by a swarm
Spiders	Bites by black, brown and red widow (*Latrodectus* spp.), brown recluse (*Loxosceles reclusa*) and black house (*Ixeuticus* spp.) spiders result in an acute, painful oedematous swelling – usually a single bite Can result in skin necrosis and sloughing

▶ Clinical signs resolve within 4 h, with no residual problems or recurrence.

▶ Treatment with sedatives and analgesics to reduce pain and self-trauma.

▶ Perform a full clinical and neurological examination to exclude other potential causes, particularly where there is no evidence of concurrent urticaria.

References and further reading

• **Anlen, K.G.,** 2008. Effects of bites by the European adder (*Vipera berus*) in seven Swedish horses. Vet. Rec. 162, 652–656.

• **Bathe, A.P.,** 1994. An unusual manifestation of nettle rash in three horses. Vet. Rec. 134, 11–12.

• **Fielding, C.L.,** 2011. Rattlesnake envenomation in horses: 58 cases (1992–2009). J. Am. Vet. Med. Assoc. 238, 631–635.

• **Knottenbelt, D.C.,** 2009. Metazoan/parasitic diseases. In: Knottenbelt, D.C. (Ed.), Pascoe's Principles and Practice of Equine Dermatology. Elsiever, St. Louis, Missouri, pp. 191–227.

• **Landolt, G.A.,** 2007. Management of equine poisoning and envenomation. Vet. Clin. North Am. Equine Pract. 23, 31–47.

• **Poppenga, R.H., Puschner, B.,** 2008. Toxicology. In: Orsini, J.A., Divers, T.J. (Eds.), Equine Emergencies Treatment and Procedures (third ed.). Elsevier, St. Louis, Missouri, pp. 593–623.

• **Talcott, P.,** 2010. Toxicologic problems. In: Reed, S.R., Bayly, W.M., Sellon, D.C. (Eds.), Equine Internal Medicine (third ed.). Elsevier, St. Louis, Missouri, pp. 1364–1412.

CHAPTER

17

Other specific emergency situations

Trapped horses

These situations can vary from those where a horse can be freed easily to more challenging ones such as a road traffic accident that may involve human casualties and an injured horse stuck in an overturned trailer. A number of challenges may be faced, including dealing with a large, frightened and unpredictable horse, a distressed owner (who may behave irrationally and display a variety of emotions, including guilt, anger and fear) and other 'assistants' who may help or hinder your efforts. In addition, owners and bystanders may put themselves in danger and expect rescuers to do the same, posing a threat to your own safety.

Useful organisations/information

- British Equine Veterinary Association Safer Horse Rescues – http://www.beva.org.uk.

- British Animal Rescue and Trauma Care Association – http://www.bartacic.org.

- Technical Large Animal Emergency Rescue – http://www.tlaer.org.

A few golden rules of horse rescues

- Remember that trapped horses will not always react in a predictable way and the presence of unfamiliar humans, including vets and rescue services, will act as additional stressors.

- Be aware of the kicking and head-butt zones – you should always work from the 'safer working area' on the spine side of the horse (Fig. 17.1).

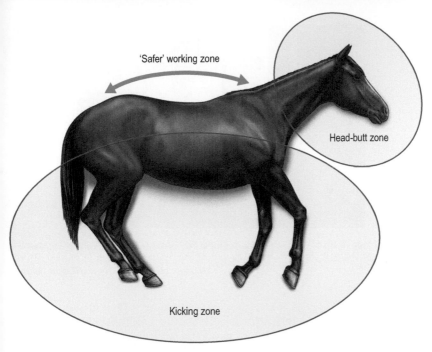

Figure 17.1 When dealing with a recumbent horse, it is safest to work from the spinal side of the horse. The kicking and head butt zones must be avoided to reduce the risk of human injury.

- Ensure you have control of the horse's head – a headcollar or halter must be placed.
- Be prepared to sedate/anaesthetise horses to assist rescue efforts.
- Never release the horse unless it has somewhere safe to go – if being released on a motorway, wait until another vehicle is ready for the horse to be loaded onto before freeing it.
- Always plan an exit route to prevent yourself and other people becoming trapped or crushed.

Prior to arriving at the scene

▸ Ensure you have been given full details of how the horse has become trapped and a clear description of its location together with mobile telephone contact number should it be difficult to locate the scene.

▸ Check that any human casualties are being dealt with and that the Fire and Rescue Service has been called if their services are likely to be required (call 999 in the UK) (Fig. 17.2).

▸ Ensure that you have necessary medication and equipment with you to sedate and possibly anaesthetise the horse.

▸ Have suitable personal protection – sturdy boots (± steel toe caps), hard hat (Fire and Rescue Service will also have these) ± reflective tabard with VET written on it.

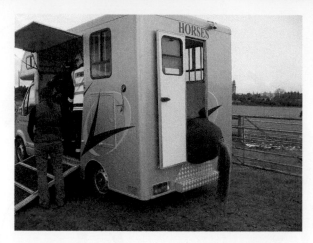

Figure 17.2 Liaison with the Fire and Rescue Service is frequently required when dealing with horses that have become trapped.

Courtesy of Hampshire Fire and Rescue Service.

On arrival at the scene

▸ If Fire and Rescue and other emergency services are already in attendance, identify yourself to the Incident Commander/other relevant person in charge and ask them to give you a summary of the situation.

▸ Dealing with human casualties is a priority; this may cause some delay in dealing with any horses involved.

▸ Assess the situation for potential hazards; this will include the horse itself (which may be distressed), other animals nearby, people present and the actual environment (e.g. water, traffic in close proximity).

▸ Ensure that the horse has been secured (unless it is unsafe to do so at this stage) by placing a headcollar/halter.

▸ A bridle and reins should not be relied upon, as the leather can easily snap – this should be replaced if it is safe to do so at this stage.

▸ Keep the horse calm – this may include keeping another horse close by, feeding small quantities of food ± keeping the owner with the horse (depending on the horse's demeanour/safety) or placing a blindfold in certain circumstances. Emphasise the need for quiet at the scene and avoid movement of machinery and people if possible.

▸ If the horse is recumbent and it is safe to do so, a competent person can kneel on the horse's neck from the spine side to prevent the horse from struggling (undertake this only if necessary); appropriate padding should also be placed under the horse's head to protect its eyes and between the headcollar and face to prevent facial nerve trauma.

▸ Approach the horse calmly and perform a quick initial assessment – basic evaluation of cardiovascular (MM colour, pulse quality, HR, skin tent), respiratory (RR and effort) and musculoskeletal systems (obvious wounds/limb deformities) may be all that you can safely perform at this stage.

▸ Determine whether rescue is feasible – there may be clear-cut situations where euthanasia at this stage is the only viable/most humane approach (see p. 328). Seek a second opinion if you are in any doubt.

- Make an initial plan with other rescue personnel involved and discuss with the owner how the rescue team intends to implement this.
- It is often better for the owner to be kept away from the scene once the rescue begins to avoid additional distractions to the team.
- Some preparation may be required first, e.g. getting appropriate equipment or additional personnel to help, cutting back vegetation or lowering banks.
- Determine if sedation is required – in most situations this will greatly facilitate rescue but in occasional situations, e.g. horse stuck in deep water, heavy sedation may not be appropriate.
- Key points regarding sedation include:
  - use a combination of drugs that you are familiar with
  - IV administration is best but IM or PO may be the only routes available (and can be followed up with IV administration)
  - be aware of the effects of adrenaline in stressed horses – you may have to administer a relatively higher dose to have the same effect compared to more routine situations requiring sedation
  - provided the horse is cardiovascularly stable, in general it is better to slightly overestimate rather than underestimate the dose required
  - make sure people around the horse are aware that, despite sedation, the horse may be able to kick and bite accurately (and less predictably).
- General anaesthesia may be required in certain situations, e.g. fractious horses or at certain points during a rescue such as use of cutting equipment and hoisting of horses (see p. 361).
- For more prolonged rescues, consider the use of continuous infusion sedative protocols (see p. 360) and administration of IV fluids via a jugular catheter.
- Keep the owner updated regarding progress and any changes to the plan, including deterioration of the horse's condition/identification of previously unidentified injuries.

Techniques for freeing trapped horses

- A variety of techniques can be used to move recumbent horses, utilising wide pieces of webbing ('strops') – these are approximately 3" in width.
- Avoid use of ropes or other thin material.
- Techniques for sideways, forward and backwards skids are outlined in Figures 17.3–17.5.
- See website for details about how to perform a controlled rollover manoeuvre.

> **KEY TIP**
> Simply placing a rope around a horse's neck and applying traction is not appropriate when trying to free a live horse.

Following freeing of the horse

- Perform a thorough clinical examination.
- Some injuries may have been identified prior to or during rescue, whereas others may only become apparent once the horse has been freed.
- More common injuries/medical problems include:
  - limb fractures (see p. 53)

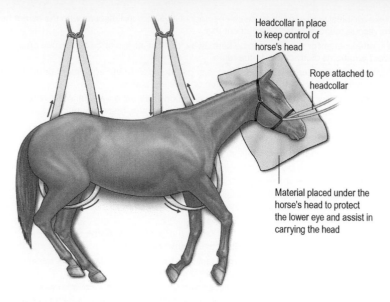

Headcollar in place
to keep control of
horse's head

Rope attached to
headcollar

Material placed under the
horse's head to protect
the lower eye and assist in
carrying the head

Figure 17.3 Demonstration of placement of strops in order to perform a sideways skid manoeuvre in a recumbent horse.

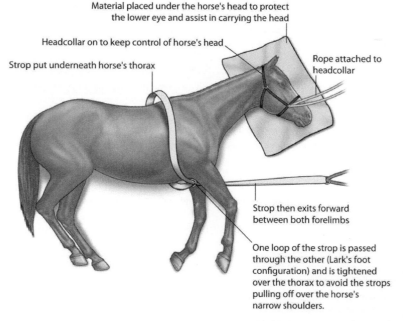

Material placed under the horse's head to protect
the lower eye and assist in carrying the head

Headcollar on to keep control of horse's head

Strop put underneath horse's thorax

Rope attached to
headcollar

Strop then exits forward
between both forelimbs

One loop of the strop is passed
through the other (Lark's foot
configuration) and is tightened
over the thorax to avoid the strops
pulling off over the horse's
narrow shoulders.

Figure 17.4 Placement of strops in order to perform a forwards skid. This places a lot of strain on the horse's thorax, so, wherever possible, a sideways skid should be undertaken in preference.

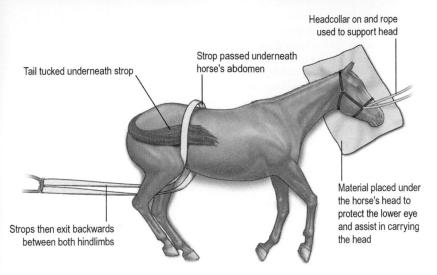

Headcollar on and rope used to support head

Strop passed underneath horse's abdomen

Tail tucked underneath strop

Material placed under the horse's head to protect the lower eye and assist in carrying the head

Strops then exit backwards between both hindlimbs

Figure 17.5 Placement of strops in order to perform a backwards skid manoeuvre in a recumbent horse.

- penetrating injuries into synovial structures, the thoracic or abdominal cavities (see pp. 47, 68 and 93)
- ocular injuries (see Ch. 6)
- head injuries (see relevant sections)
- hypothermia (see p. 216)
- dehydration (see p. 375)
- acute haemorrhage (see p. 186)
- URT inflammation/infection due to water aspiration (see p. 90).

▸ Discuss the treatment of any injuries with the owner/rider and administer medication and other first aid measures as appropriate.

▸ In some instances, e.g. suspected limb factures, further assessment and treatment may be best performed at hospital facilities with necessary equipment and expertise. Discuss this with the owner/rider and contact a referral centre if relevant (see p. 7).

▸ If you are not the horse's usual veterinary practice and the horse will be going back home, provide a brief written summary of your clinical findings, treatment administered and recommendations for ongoing veterinary care together with your contact details; in some instances it may be appropriate to contact their practice directly.

▸ Liaise with emergency services for debriefing, including a discussion of what worked/did not work so well.

Collapsed/recumbent horse

Horses may be found recumbent in the field/stable or may collapse during or immediately after exercise. These situations can be distressing for the owner/rider and members of the general public (particularly when they occur during competitions) and it can be difficult to determine the underlying cause.

▶ Determine whether the horse is trapped.
▶ Ensure safety of the horse and maintain control of the head – place a headcollar/halter or keep the bridle on as a temporary measure.
▶ If seizuring, administer sedatives/anticonvulsants (see p. 144).
▶ Administer immediate first aid treatment as required, e.g. secure airway, control haemorrhage.
▶ Concurrently obtain a succinct relevant history, including the circumstances in which this occurred, known aetiology or previous episodes of collapse seen.

Further clinical assessment

Obtain a full history. Specific questions that should be asked include:

▶ Circumstances leading up to recumbency/collapse – whether this occurred at exercise or not and if associated with known trauma.
▶ If collapse occurred at exercise, whether the horse was normal prior to this point.
▶ Any loss of consciousness/change in behaviour immediately before or after.
▶ Duration of recumbency (acute/gradual) and progression.
▶ If duration unknown, when the horse was LSN.
▶ General signalment and medical history.
▶ Prior history of recumbency/collapse.
▶ Recent illness/trauma.
▶ Vaccination status.
▶ Health of in-contacts.
▶ Potential exposure to toxins.

Perform an initial visual assessment

▶ Surroundings.
▶ Evidence of trauma/struggling/efforts to stand.
▶ Mentation.
▶ Ability to eat, drink and evidence of urination/defecation.

Perform a full clinical examination

▶ Body condition.
▶ MM, CRT, hydration status and T°.
▶ Auscultation of thorax – HR, RR and effort, dysrhythmias, murmurs.
▶ Palpation of limbs/vertebral region, check feet.
▶ External examination: urogenital tract (female).
▶ Rectal examination.
▶ ± Roll horse onto opposite side and repeat evaluation of contralateral side.

Perform a neurological assessment – determine if neurologically normal or not (see p. 132 for neurological assessment of a recumbent horse)

▶ Check cranial nerves.
▶ Neck, limb and tail tone.
▶ Reflexes – triceps, nociceptive flexor, patellar.

Take relevant samples for further analysis, including:

▸ Haematology.

▸ Serum biochemistry.

▸ Electrolytes.

▸ ± Blood gas analysis.

▸ ± Serology/virus isolation.

HANDY TIP

Rolling a horse onto the other side may enable the horse to be able to get back up or may enable the problem, e.g. fracture on the previously downward side, to be identified. This should be performed carefully to prevent further injury to the horse/injury to handlers if

the horse struggles (see website for controlled rollover details).

Make an assessment and initial treatment plan

▸ Decide on the most likely cause for recumbency or rule out possible causes (see Table 17.1).

▸ Discuss the findings with the owner/agent.

▸ Administer relevant medication based on the most likely diagnosis.

▸ Discuss euthanasia if appropriate (see p. 328).

▸ Move the horse if appropriate, e.g. to a stable/field shelter.

▸ Decide if transportation to hospital/referral facilities for further assessment and treatment is indicated and discuss this with owner/carer and referral centre.

▸ If the horse remains recumbent, whilst waiting to determine response to treatment, appropriate medical and nursing care is essential.

▸ Administer BS antimicrobials – inhalation pneumonia.

▸ Hydration:
  - if voluntary intake is possible, ensure that the horse can access oral fluids if able to support itself in sternal recumbency
  - ± repeated fluid administration via nasogastric intubation (only if in sternal recumbency)
  - IV fluids.

▸ Nutrition:
  - voluntary intake
  - gruel or liquid diet
  - parenteral nutrition.

▸ Physical protection:
  - non-abrasive, absorbent, comfortable bedding
  - ± blanket between bedding and the horse
  - protection of the eyes if the horse is recumbent.

▸ Physiotherapy:
  - keep in sternal position ideally – will still need to be turned
  - if head trauma and lateral recumbency, keep the head elevated 30°
  - turn onto the other side q. 2–6 h
  - ± assist to stand with a sling
  - manual extension and flexion of joints and muscle massage.

Table 17.1 Possible causes of collapse and recumbency in horses

Musculoskeletal	Fracture
	Laminitis
	Exertional rhabdomyolysis
	Atypical myopathy
	Severe arthritis/degenerative joint disease
	Clostridial myonecrosis
Neurological	Trauma
	EHV-1
	Botulism
	Tetanus
	Encephalitis/CNS inflammation
	CVM
	Rabies
	Seizures
	Sleep disorders
Cardiovascular	Acute internal/external haemorrhage
	Hypovolaemic shock
	Cardiac dysrhythmias
	Acute cardiac failure
	Sepsis
Hepatic/metabolic	Exhaustion/hyperthermia
	Hyperlipaemia
	Malnutrition
	Hypothermia
	Hepatoencephalopathy
	Electrolyte abnormalities
	Hypoglycaemia
	Hyperkalaemic periodic paralysis (HYPP)
Gastrointestinal	Colic
	Endotoxic shock
	Acute diarrhoea
Respiratory	Winded after a fall
	URT obstruction
	Severe pulmonary disease
Urogenital	Dystocia
Toxicoses	Various (see Ch. 16)
Miscellaneous	Anaphylaxis, e.g. ADR
	Intracarotid injection

▶ Monitoring:
  ▪ faecal output ± rectal evacuation of faeces q. 12h
  ▪ urine output ± repeat catheterisation q. 6–8h
  ▪ corneal ulceration
  ▪ pressure sores
  ▪ compressive neuropathy/myopathy.

Further investigations and treatment/prognosis

▶ Determine whether further diagnostic tests are required:
  ▪ ± radiographs, CSF sampling (see specialist texts/seek specialist advice).
▶ Perform repeated clinical re-evaluation.
▶ Response to therapy, progression of clinical signs over time and the result of additional tests will aid further treatment and diagnosis.

Electrocution

Mild electric shocks felt by humans when in contact with horses may lead to suspicion of electrocution where collapse or recumbency has occurred, particularly where multiple horses have been affected. Contact with electric currents, e.g. faulty underground cables, have more serious effects in horses (and other 4-legged animals such as cattle) compared to humans. This is due to the greater distance between the points where voltage is applied (i.e. feet), the fact that horses may have metal shoes and that current flows through the limbs in contact with the ground. This results in current flowing through the trunk (compared to up and down the legs of humans), which can have adverse and potentially fatal effects on the heart and respiratory muscles.

Clinical signs

▶ Intense excitement.
▶ Muscular spasms.
▶ Collapse.
▶ ± Death.

Treatment

▶ Remove from the electrical field if death has not already occurred – they can make a rapid recovery (ensure safety of handlers).
▶ Symptomatic treatment of any residual clinical signs or acquired injuries (see relevant sections).

Lightning strikes

There occur relatively infrequently in horses but may be a cause of sudden death or recumbency.

Clinical signs

▶ Respiratory distress.
▶ Rhabdomyolysis.

- Skin burns.
- Pain.
- ↑ HR.
- Vestibular disease.
- Sudden death.

Treatment

- Symptomatic based on clinical findings (see relevant sections).

Fires and smoke inhalation injury

Horses may have become trapped within a burning stable/barn or have been caught in the path of a wildfire. Injuries can range from mild to life-threatening, horrific injuries due to:

- Thermal injury to the skin (Fig. 17.6).
- Respiratory tract injuries.
- Systemic 'burn shock'.

Initial assessment and first aid treatment

- Triage horses (where multiple horses involved) to determine the severity of injuries and initiate first aid using helpers as necessary.

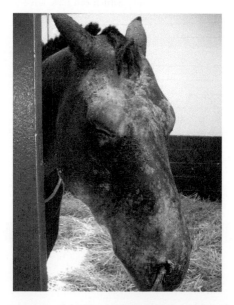

Figure 17.6 Facial burns injuries sustained in a horse that been involved in a barn fire.
Courtesy of Thijs de Bont.

- Stop the burning process – cool affected areas with lukewarm water (do not use ice or very cold water as this will cause acute vasoconstriction, further compromising poorly perfused tissues).
- Remove any blankets or other materials on the horse as these will hold heat.
- Administer sedatives/anxiolytics if the horse is distressed.
- Administer flunixin meglumine 1.1 mg/kg IV.
- Place an IV catheter in severely affected horses at an early stage (i.e. in horses likely to need ongoing intensive care) – once oedema develops, it can be very difficult to obtain IV access.
- ± Administer oxygen.
- Perform a tracheotomy if severe URT swelling is suspected (see p. 356).
- Euthanasia is indicated in:
  - horses that have sustained severe, deep/partial- to full-thickness burns involving 30–50% of the total body surface area
  - horses that present in severe shock and that are close to death.

Further assessment and ongoing care

- Obtain a general history, including a more detailed history about the circumstances of the fire (if not present at the time of the fire).
- Perform a full clinical examination.
- Determine whether any cardiovascular compromise is apparent – 'burn shock':
  - in these cases, hospitalisation/referral is recommended to enable monitoring of the cardiovascular system and provision of appropriate fluid therapy (including serial PCV/ TP, lactate, urine production and blood pressure measurement and, monitoring for organ dysfunction).
- Assess the horse's respiratory rate and effort for evidence of pulmonary oedema or smoke inhalation injury (see p. 91):
  - further assessment and treatment of the respiratory tract, including endoscopy, thoracic radiography, blood gas analysis, haematology, ongoing oxygen therapy ± tracheotomy, bronchodilators and diuretics, may be indicated.
- Assess burn severity and initiate appropriate wound management and ongoing supportive care (see p. 32).
- Check the eyes for any burn injuries; gently remove any carbonated fragments from the conjunctiva using lavage with sterile saline/LRS and initiate ocular treatment as required.
- Determine where the horse can be managed – alternative stabling at another site may be required in horses with minor injuries (if there is no stabling left on site) or admission to hospital facilities with necessary equipment and expertise may be required in more severely affected horses.

Flood injuries and near drowning

Flooding is common in some geographical regions and preparations can be made in advance to reduce the risk of injury/death to horses in high-risk areas (see p. 334).

Initial first aid and assessment

- Assess systemic status – HR, RR, T°, MM, hydration.
- Initiate emergency treatment if the horse is in severe shock/near to collapse, e.g. administer IV fluids.

▶ If the horse's condition is stable, decontaminate it first (if required) to remove any toxins, debris and microorganisms (this will also assist assessment of other injuries) – use human/animal shampoos without additives.

Further evaluation

▶ Perform further full clinical assessment – for specific injuries and diseases that should be checked for and treated in these horses see Table 17.2.

Table 17.2 Checklist of common conditions that may require treatment following flood injury in horses

Musculoskeletal system	As for normal assessment of musculoskeletal system – check for traumatic injuries
	Pick out feet and check for thrush due to prolonged soaking of hooves
Integument	Dermatitis and cellulitis are common due to exposure to chemicals/salt water/sewage
	Bacterial (clostridial) infection – treat with penicillin/gentamicin ± metronidazole
	Fungal infections (e.g. *Pythium*) – rule out if no response to antimicrobials
Ophthalmic	Check for traumatic injuries, including corneal ulcers and uveitis – can be missed easily
Gastrointestinal	Colitis/colic due to ingestion of contaminated feed/water – treat accordingly (see Ch. 4)
Neurological	Trauma to the head and neck is common
	Increased risk of tetanus, botulism, clostridial disease, viral encephalitis (in affected regions); administer tetanus toxoid/antitoxin if vaccination status unknown
	Salt poisoning (hypernatraemia) due to ingestion of salt water
Respiratory disease	Check for evidence of aspiration pneumonia/pleuritis (see p. 88–90)
	Can develop upper respiratory tract inflammation (pharyngitis/laryngitis/chondritis) and obstruction causing respiratory distress (see p. 85)
Infectious disease	High risk, particularly where mixing of horses has occurred; monitor for carefully if horses are being kept at a holding centre (e.g. influenza, rhinopneumonitis, *Streptococcus equi* var *equi*)
	Vaccination is contraindicated at this stage due to severe stress in affected individuals – their immune response is less likely to be effective and may increase the risk of adverse reactions

Dealing with the emergency welfare case

Cases of suspected neglect, abuse or cruelty may require emergency veterinary assessment to prevent vital evidence being lost. The actions of the assessing veterinary surgeon have a critical role in subsequent legal action and, even if performed in emergency circumstances, it is essential that the correct procedures are followed ensuring that clear, irrefutable clinical evidence can be presented in a court of law. In the UK, veterinary attendance at suspected welfare cases will be requested by the RSPCA/SSPCA or local authority and/or police and this section outlines the procedures required in the UK.

Key points to consider

▶ This should be performed by veterinary surgeons with sufficient experience in equine work to act as a credible witness in court (e.g. a more experienced colleague may need to be contacted).

▶ Ensure that sufficient time is taken to perform a full clinical examination – this may involve more than one horse.

▶ In cases with large numbers of horses involved, a range of ages, uncastrated males and sometimes unhandled horses may be encountered.

Equipment

- As per basic equipment for performing a complete physical examination.
- Notepad for recording findings.
- Microchip scanner.
- Camera – useful to act as an aide to recording findings (NB in the UK there are strict guidelines that must be followed in order for these to be used as legal evidence and police/welfare agencies are usually responsible for obtaining these).
- Identification of horses – spray paint/board and writing material.

> **HANDY TIP**
>
> It is useful to have a checklist of findings that need to be recorded in these cases (see p. 322).

Initial assessment

▶ Liaise with RSPCA/SSPCA or local authority officials.

▶ Be aware that in the UK, the police and a limited number of public servants, e.g. local authority inspectors, are the only people with the power to enter premises without permission and they may assist collection of evidence and taking witness statements.

▶ Record the place, date and time.

▶ Record the names and relevant numbers (e.g. police officers) of people present at the time of examination or who are on the premises.

▶ Find out the owner/carer's usual veterinary surgeon or practice.

▶ Obtain a history, including details of previous veterinary treatment, provided by owner/carer of the horse (if known).

▶ Identify each horse:
  - check for a microchip if present

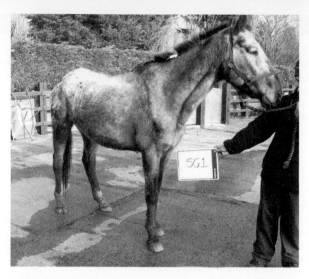

Figure 17.7 Collection of photographic evidence in a welfare investigation is vital. Individual horses must be properly identified in any images obtained.

Courtesy of Redwings Horse Sanctuary.

- record their age, gender, colour, markings (similar to recording horse identification on vaccination records/passport)
- ensure that a photographic record of each horse is taken, including any identifying features and their teeth (this is usually undertaken by the RSPCA officer).
▶ Make a detailed description of the premises (unless the horse has already been moved to a sanctuary or clinic):
- useful to make a graphic outline of premises and take photographs
- make a note of other horses/livestock present
- detail findings on inspection of the premises – provision of food, water and bedding, feed storage, worming treatment details.

Photographic records

▶ It is usually better for these to be taken by the inspector/police to ensure that they are of suitable forensic quality.
▶ Horses must be properly identified, e.g. number on cardboard/small whiteboard, tag on the headcollar or spray marker on the horse (Fig. 17.7).
▶ Where dead horses are present, pictures must be taken prior to movement of the body.

Further assessment

Perform a full clinical examination (if more than one horse, take separate notes for each).
▶ Performed at rest and then at walk and trot (if appropriate).
▶ Any limitations in the examination, e.g. horse cannot be handled, must be noted.
▶ Record the following findings (these are covered on the pro-forma for the veterinary examination of RSPCA equine welfare cases):

- body condition score – use a validated body scoring system (see National Equine Welfare Council compendium – http://www.newc.co.uk)
- record gender (including whether entire/castrated male)
- assess age – record the basis on which this assessment is made (photography useful)
- basic physical parameters – TPR
- mentation
- ability to stand/walk
- evidence of weakness/lameness
- ability and willingness to eat
- condition of hooves/shoeing
- lesions/abrasions of skin
- full clinical examination of body systems (see p. 11)
- faecal consistency (including evidence of diarrhoea)
- evidence of external/internal parasites
- description of a particular lesion/clinical abnormality
- full and accurate description and assessment of injury/problem(s)
- take photos – close-up with identification number.

Take any relevant samples

▸ Appropriate samples must be taken prior to any treatment being performed – at a minimum this should include blood and faecal samples that are screened and stored for subsequent analysis if required.
▸ Samples of blood/faeces/hair plucks/swabs must be placed in appropriate containers and labelled fully in the presence of a witness – faeces must either be collected from the rectum or from an observed, freshly passed sample to ensure they are from that particular horse.
▸ Duplicate samples must be taken and one set offered to the owner/carer for independent analysis – details on how these samples should be stored must be provided.
▸ These must be analysed at a suitable veterinary laboratory (i.e. 'in-house' testing is not appropriate for legal cases).

Decide on next course of action

▸ Contact the horse's usual veterinary surgeon if currently under veterinary care and check that the owner/carer is acting according to veterinary advice.
▸ Decide which of the following is most appropriate based on clinical examination and the circumstances.

Ongoing care of the horse/horses

▸ Make a provisional diagnosis and treatment plan.
▸ In the case of starvation, a detailed nutrition plan should be made (see p. 210). In these cases it is important to be aware of the 'refeeding syndrome' in which excessive food offered too soon can result in death.
▸ Care of the case should be handed over to another veterinary surgeon (if relevant).
▸ The treatment plan may change, based on laboratory results.

Removal (seizure) of horses

▸ This should only be performed where the life or welfare of the horse would be jeopardised by leaving the horse on the premises or where more intensive treatment/nursing care is required (seek appropriate advice if unsure).

Euthanasia

▶ This may be undertaken if the prognosis for the affected horse is deemed to be hopeless, the individual is suffering and where removal from the premises for further treatment would not save the horse.

▶ If permission cannot be given by the owner/carer, the horse can be euthanased provided a police officer is present and authorises euthanasia on the basis of veterinary advice (ideally a statement should be provided by the veterinary surgeon and police officer).

▶ Samples must be taken prior to euthanasia and arrangements made for an independent PM examination to take place.

Post-mortem examination

▶ In the case of dead horses or where immediate euthanasia is required, PM examination should take place at an appropriate centre with equine pathology expertise.

Actions to be taken following examination

▶ Send the samples to an appropriate veterinary laboratory:
- the laboratory should be experienced in the analysis of equine samples
- samples should be sent by courier and signed on receipt or delivered by hand – do not send by normal post
- provide relevant details to the laboratory, e.g. age, horse/donkey, breed of horse and requests for specific tests/storage
- inform the laboratory that the results of these tests may be used as proceedings in court.

▶ Perform interpretation of laboratory samples/other tests.

▶ Make a provisional diagnosis and make any relevant changes to the treatment plan.

▶ Prepare a statement/report on practice-headed notepaper – this must be factual, accurate and unbiased and should contain:
- details about case, including personnel present
- full description of the horse
- findings on initial clinical examination
- justification for decisions made
- description of results of laboratory analysis
- final diagnosis
- progress of case.

▶ Date and sign the report.

References and further reading

• **Bedenice, D., Hoffman, A.M., Parrott, B.,** et al. 2001. Vestibular signs associated with suspected lightning strike in two horses. Vet. Rec. 149, 519–522.

• British Equine Veterinary Association. Rescue and emergency medicine training for equine vets <http://www.beva.org.uk>.

• **Chandler, K.,** 2000. Clinical approach to the recumbent adult horse. In Pract. 22, 308–314.

• **Green P.** 2011 The role of the attending veterinary surgeon in equine welfare cases. Proceedings of the 50th BEVA Congress, Liverpool, UK, pp. 259–260.

• **Green, P., Tong, J.M.J.,** 2004. The role of the veterinary surgeon in equine welfare cases. Equine Vet. Educ. 16, 46–56.

- **McConnico, R.S.,** 2007. Flood injury in horses. Vet. Clin. North Am. Equine Pract. 23, 1–17.

- **Marsh, P.S.,** 2007. Fire and smoke inhalation injury in horses. Vet. Clin. North Am. Equine Pract. 23, 19–30.

- **Miller, J.L.,** 2009. Nursing care of the recumbent horse. In: Robinson, N.E., Sprayberry, K.A. (Eds.), Current Therapy in Equine Medicine (sixth ed.). Elsevier, St. Louis, Missouri, pp. 922–925.

- **Nout, Y.S., Reed, S.M.,** 2005. Management and treatment of the recumbent horse. Equine Vet. Educ. 17, 324–336.

- **Novales, M., Hernandez, E., Lucena, R.,** 1998. Electrocution in the horse. Vet. Rec. 142, 68.

- **Piercy, R.J., Marr, C.M.,** 2010. Collapse and syncope. In: Marr, C.M., Bowen, I.M. (Eds.), Equine Cardiology (second ed.). Elsevier, St. Louis, Missouri, pp. 227–237.

- **Williams, J.B.,** 2001. Survival of lightning strike and its sequelae in a native pony. Equine Vet. Educ. 13, 25–28.

Sudden death

This is relatively rare in horses and the term should be applied only when death occurs in a closely observed and previously apparently healthy animal. Investigation of the cause of death in these circumstances can be difficult, time consuming and unsuccessful; even with extensive PM investigations, the cause remains unknown in approximately 30% of these horses (Table 18.1).

Approach to investigation

▶ Find out about the circumstances surrounding the event:
  - be aware that owners may be reluctant to tell the truth
  - keep an open mind and do not jump to conclusions
  - be aware of potential conflicts of interest, e.g. in the case of sudden death due to potential iatrogenic causes and the possibility of foul play.
▶ Take full and detailed notes and keep these stored safely should legal issues arise.
▶ Examine the environment in which the horse died and obtain photographic evidence of the horse in situ, prior to it being moved (Fig. 18.1).
▶ Obtain a detailed history about the circumstances surrounding the horse's death – specific questions that should be asked include:
  - general medical history, including any recent illness/injury
  - health of any in-contact horses
  - recent long-distance travel in that horse/in-contacts.
▶ Determine if PM examination is required by the insurance company/relevant sporting regulatory body or if this has been requested by the owner. A PM may not be required in all cases but any relevant body parts should be kept, e.g. fractured limb.
▶ Check whether the horse needs to be transported to a particular centre for PM examination or if this has been requested by the owner:
  - if so, speak to the relevant centre and organise transport of the body

Table 18.1 Possible causes of sudden death in horses

Cardiovascular	Pulmonary haemorrhage
	Extrapulmonary haemorrhage
	Severe haemorrhage from other location (internal/external)
	Cardiac/cardiopulmonary failure, e.g. gross cardiac lesions, acute dysrhythmias
Respiratory	Acute respiratory obstruction
	Severe pneumonia
Gastrointestinal	Acute colitis
	Ruptured viscus
CNS	CNS haemorrhage
	Vertebral fracture
	Brain trauma secondary to skull fracture
	Spinal cord trauma – vertebral instability
Toxic	Ingestion of certain plants, e.g. yew (*Taxus baccata*), water hemlock (*Cicuta virosa*) or water dropwort (*Oenanthe* spp.)
	Monensin ingestion
Musculoskeletal	Atypical myopathy
Trauma	Electrocution/lightning strike
	Gunshot wounds
	Fractured vertebrae/skull following collisions with fixed objects
	Severe abdominal/thoracic or other soft tissue trauma
Iatrogenic	Adverse drug reactions (including anaesthesia)
	Intracarotid administration of medication
	Air embolism

- if the horse cannot be transported immediately, discuss storage of the body (better to be refrigerated)
- check whether blood/CSF samples are requested.

▶ Perform a PM if requested/required by the insurance company (if not required to be performed elsewhere or where there is no potential conflict of interest) (see p. 395).

▶ If poisoning is suspected, take samples of relevant feedstuffs or take appropriate samples at PM examination (see p. 302).

▶ Keep the owner/agent and any other relevant organisations, e.g. insurance company and regulatory body informed of the results, ideally as a written report. Consider risks to other horses on the premises and advise accordingly (where appropriate).

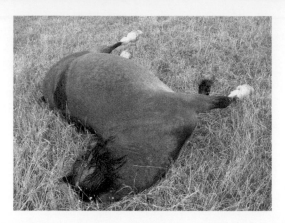

Fig. 18.1   Sudden death in a pony suspected to have died as a result of a lightning strike.
Courtesy of Fernando Malalana.

Euthanasia and insurance issues

The decision on whether to advise an owner to euthanase a horse on humane grounds in an emergency situation should be based upon clinical assessment, regardless of whether it is insured or not. The main responsibility of the veterinary surgeon is to ensure that the welfare of the horse takes priority.

General points

▸ Determine whether the horse is insured before euthanasia is performed. Compliance with insurance policy conditions is a matter for the owner/agent – however, it is reasonable for them to discuss insurance implications with the attending veterinary surgeon who should be aware of common issues that may arise in these situations.

▸ Should the insurance company/adjuster be uncontactable, the veterinary surgeon and owner/agent should document attempts to notify the insurance company prior to euthanasia.

▸ In an emergency situation, there are guidelines as to what constitutes grounds for equine euthanasia under an insurance policy (see Table 18.2).

▸ If in any doubt as to whether immediate euthanasia is required and the insurance company is not contactable, always seek an opinion from a second veterinary surgeon.

▸ Obtain relevant photographs/videos/radiographs that can be provided as evidence on which the decision was based.

Guidelines issued for euthanasia

BEVA Guidelines for the destruction of horses under an All Risks of Mortality Insurance Policy (1996) states

'that the insured horse sustains an injury or manifests an illness or disease that is so severe as to warrant immediate destruction to relieve incurable and excessive pain and that no other options of treatment are available to that horse at that time'.

Table 18.2 List of conditions that may constitute immediate destruction of a horse on humane grounds

Musculoskeletal	P2 fracture – comminuted, no intact strut
	Comminuted long bone fractures
	Displaced fractures of the humerus/radius/tibia/femur in adult horses
	Pelvic fracture resulting in recumbency
	Unilateral rupture of the SDFT at the musculotendinous junction
	Bilateral rupture of the SDFT at the musculotendinous junction/ distal to the carpus
	Complete laceration of the SDFT, DDFT and SL
	Laminitis with solar prolapse of the tip of the distal phalanx
Gastrointestinal	Colic where there is evidence of terminal shock with no/little likelihood of survival following surgical intervention
Neurological	Continual seizures following trauma/infection
	Severe ataxia (CVM grade 5)
	HL paralysis/paresis following suspected/confirmed spinal fractures
	Recumbent and non-responsive post trauma
Urogenital	Mare that is unable to rise post foaling (obturator paralysis ± fracture)
	Non-reducible uterine prolapse
Other severe general illness	If the horse is likely to die imminently and all treatment options have been exhausted
	Where a horse poses a significant and immediate danger to handlers/members of the general public and it is impossible to control the horse with sedation/analgesia, immediate euthanasia may be justified

Modified from House and Collins (2008).

AAEP grounds for euthanasia

- Inhumane suffering.
- Incurable diseases with a grave prognosis.
- Clinical conditions in which the horse is deemed a hazard to itself or its handlers.
- Conditions necessitating lifelong medication for relief of pain.

American Association of Equine Practitioners (AAEP) – http://www.aaep.org. N.B. It should be noted that these appear more lenient than the UK guidelines due to the fact that most insurance policies in the USA do not have permanent loss of use sections.

What to do when performing euthanasia in the insured horse

These are based upon guidelines issued by BEVA (2008) – this may vary in different countries depending on relevant legislation (see Table 18.3).

▶ Check the identity of the horse.
▶ Confirm who is the owner of the horse and who the insurance policy is under (e.g. in the situations of a horse on loan).
▶ Carry out a complete clinical examination and record the details of this.
▶ Obtain written consent for euthanasia.
▶ Following euthanasia an independent PM should be performed or sufficient evidence should be obtained to justify the claim where a full/independent PM is not required or performed.

Preparation for dealing with emergencies at competitions

Veterinary cover is an essential part of competitive events, ranging from the local agricultural show through to a high-profile equestrian international event. It is essential that veterinary surgeons providing cover at these events have the necessary experience (e.g. certain requirements have to be fulfilled for veterinary surgeons working on the racecourse or at FEI-regulated events) and are prepared on the day to deal with all eventualities.

Dealing with emergencies at equine competition brings a few additional pressures

▶ Dealing with the general public and media.
▶ Actions taken are potentially more greatly scrutinised and the general public may video what it is going on and distribute this on the internet – this is not usually welcome fame!
▶ The economic value of competition horses and pressures of competition places additional pressures on owners, trainers, riders and treating veterinary surgeons.
▶ Decisions may be delayed where various connections need to be contacted and informed of any injuries or treatment required.
▶ It is important to be well versed and up to date with the rules set out by different regulatory bodies, including procedures: e.g. relevant paperwork to be completed, prohibited substances, drug detection times.

Initial arrangements

▶ Determine the type of event and level:
  ▪ establish the level of veterinary cover required
  ▪ on call but not on site
  ▪ if on site, whether required to be present on the course or a treating vet at the stables
  ▪ how many veterinary surgeons will be present and their role
▶ Check whether you fulfil the necessary requirements (e.g. FEI regulations regarding treating veterinary surgeons) or have the necessary experience or back-up (e.g. working alongside a more experienced veterinary colleague at the event).
▶ Ensure that the organisers have confirmed the details in writing, including the date and times you are required, expenses and subsistence payments provided.
▶ Check whether a vehicle is required (e.g. if covering the course), whether it needs to be a four-wheel drive and if one will be provided by the organisers.

Table 18.3 Decision making when faced with request for euthanasia to be performed in an insured horse

Situation	Procedure
Definite grounds for immediate euthanasia	If there is a clear-cut case for immediate euthanasia on humane grounds, delay should be avoided
	Ideally a second opinion should be sought from another veterinary surgeon but welfare is the priority and this should not unduly delay euthanasia
	PM examination may be required or suitable evidence should be collected (e.g. photographs/videos/radiographs) to corroborate any decision made
Suspected but not definite grounds for immediate euthanasia	It is advisable to seek a second opinion before proceeding
	The insurance company should ideally be contacted and they may require a nominated veterinary surgeon to examine the horse/ provide advice
	Appropriate first aid treatment and stabilisation should be performed until a second opinion has been obtained ± transport to a clinic for further investigation if required
Cases where injured/ill horses require urgent surgical/ specialist medical intervention to save the horse's life	Keep the insurance company notified
	Without specific advice to the contrary (e.g. out-of-hours when the insurer cannot be contacted), economic constraints are unlikely to be accepted by an insurer as grounds for foregoing the need to meet BEVA guidelines – if an owner is unwilling to fund appropriate available treatment, and as a result euthanasia is required, the veterinary surgeon should advise the owner that an 'All Risks Mortality Insurance' claim is not likely to succeed
	If the cost of treatment may not be economic based on the horses value, this requires negotiation directly between the insured and the insurance company
No grounds for immediate euthanasia in the opinion of the attending veterinary surgeon	Inform the insured that they need to contact the insurance company as soon as possible for guidance
	If difficulties are encountered, seek a second opinion from another veterinary surgeon to corroborate your own view
	If the insured still insists on euthanasia, inform them that this may invalidate their insurance claim and that an independent PM examination may need to be performed if they still wish to proceed
Cases where the insured requests euthanasia of a horse for other reasons	Where request for euthanasia has been made for reasons other than on humane grounds, check that the insured understands they have no recourse to the insurance company following euthanasia
	If they wish to proceed, ensure that you document your findings and that they have signed a euthanasia consent form indicating that the horse has been destroyed at their request

Modified from House and Collins (2008).

▶ Determine what facilities will be available (e.g. treatment in car park or at stables area) and whether a horse ambulance and farrier will be on site.

▶ Check that the organisers have the necessary equipment for dealing with any emergencies: e.g. screens, ropes, access to water, access to ice/fans or shade (if there is a risk of hyperthermia occurring in competing horses).

Preparation prior to the event

▶ Check relevant indemnity cover is in place (and the level of this cover, particularly when working with high-value horses).

▶ Ensure any necessary passes have been sent prior to the day.

▶ Have the contact details for the following, and ideally contact each prior to the event:
   ▪ regional equine referral centres
   ▪ local small animal veterinary surgeries
   ▪ local horse ambulances (if one will not be on site)
   ▪ local horse disposal companies.

▶ Be aware of the types of injuries/medical conditions most commonly encountered in that discipline, how to treat these problems and check that you have the relevant equipment for emergency treatment.

Equipment

See also equipment listed on p. 2–4. Specific items that may be useful at competitions include:

• Rules of the event (if relevant).

• Relevant treatment/costing forms.

• In addition to routine splinting material, ± commercial equine splints/casting material (application of cast bandages).

• Binoculars.

• Temperature/humidity gauge.

• 40% Calcium borogluconate and 50% dextrose solutions (IV preparations).

• ± Portable haematology/electrolyte analysers (e.g. endurance horses where metabolic emergencies are common).

On the day

▶ Ensure you are properly attired and equipped; it is useful to have a change of clothes with you, e.g. where original clothing has become covered in blood.

▶ Arrive within plenty of time prior to the event starting (at least 1 h) and introduce yourself at the secretary's tent.

▶ Collect radio and vehicle (if relevant).

▶ Make sure the organisers have your mobile telephone number and that you have the contact numbers of relevant people that you may need to contact directly (e.g. event organiser, other veterinary surgeons, horse ambulance driver).

▶ Check that you have a programme and map of the course (if relevant).

▶ Liaise with other veterinary surgeons (if more than one vet in attendance) and co-ordinate who is doing what.

▶ Ensure that you have paperwork for recording details of clinical examination and treatment and costing sheets.

▶ Introduce yourself to the doctor/medical team and course repair team.

▶ Ensure you are familiar with the course and access, check for areas where horses are not in direct field of view and make plans for how to extract any horses that become stuck (where relevant).

▶ Also ensure that the driver of the horse ambulance is familiar with the course and access to each site.

▶ Ask for any non-urgent requests for veterinary treatment to be made via the secretary's tent.

▶ Plan for the worst-case scenario – what to do if there is a horse fatality, how to move the body, where a body can be stored until it is collected.

During the event

▶ Provide relevant first aid and determine whether the horse needs further evaluation/ stabilisation or potential referral to appropriate hospital facilities.

▶ Maintain clinical records for all horses that are examined or treated.

▶ Do not make any hasty decisions.

▶ Remember that it can be difficult to assess horses fully when they are under the influence of adrenaline.

▶ If in any doubt, transport a horse off the course rather than walking it back.

▶ Inform other relevant veterinary surgeons about the horse, including initial injuries, treatment and suspected problems.

> **KEY TIP**
>
> Be aware that people will be listening into conversations on radios and never communicate about emergencies over a general radio channel or a public address system.

At the end of the event

▶ Hand in any radios and debrief with other veterinary surgeons (if relevant) and the organisers.

▶ Make any suggestions for future events if problems have been encountered or potential for this has been identified.

▶ Submit invoice for veterinary services performed (as agreed prior to the event).

> **KEY TIP**
>
> Where horses are injured, a statement to the effect of 'the horse has been taken away for further assessment and treatment' is sufficient for the purposes of updating the general public/media. Where a horse fatality has occurred, refer to the event organisers and do not communicate directly to the media.

Disaster preparedness/dealing with adverse weather conditions

Most response and rescue efforts go towards saving human life but prior planning can help to reduce the loss of animal life (horses and other domestic/livestock animals) and reduce the heath problems in affected animals. It is essential that preparations are put into place in situations where an impending natural disaster is known or in an area where there is a high likelihood of these occurring. Whilst this handbook provides advice on emergency treatment of the consequences of natural disasters on affected equids, it is impossible to cover disaster preparedness in detail. There are a variety of governmental and veterinary organisations and specific texts that provide specific advice in these situations to which readers are directed.

Useful organisations and websites

- AAEP Emergency and Disaster Preparedness Guidelines – http://www.aaep.org.
- Wildfire readiness – http://emilms.fema.gov/IS10A/AID0105270text.htm.
- Information for livestock owners – http://www.fema.gov/plan/prepare/livestock.shtm.

Adverse weather conditions can occur in geographic locations where natural disasters are less frequently encountered. Some general advice on ways in which the risk of injury to horses can be minimised in these situations includes:

Extreme floods/high winds

▸ If horses cannot be evacuated, turn them out onto large open pastures – do not confine to barns/stables where they cannot exit and may drown.

Wildfires – if there is a known, impending risk

▸ Consult the local fire department regarding fire safety on the premises, including equipment and firebreaks, and take preventive measures to reduce the risk of fires.
▸ Keep fire tools in the stable/barn, including garden hoses, fire extinguishers, shovels, rakes, buckets and water pumps.
▸ Ensure barn/stable staff or owners know where fire extinguishers are kept, how to use them and the procedure for evacuation.
▸ Purchase leather/cotton rope halters or headcollars (nylon ones can melt and cause deep burns).

Where a wildfire is close-by

▸ Wet down roofs and other surfaces (NB this must not affect the water supply/pressure needed by fire-fighters in the area).
▸ Leave immediately when officials evacuate the area – determine whether safe enough or appropriate to transport horses.
▸ If horses are being left, remove any blankets and wet their manes and tails.
▸ Let them out of the barn/stable into a paddock and close the barn/stable doors to stop horses running back in.
▸ Turn off the power and gas and disconnect any electric fences.

Extreme cold weather

▸ Ensure horses have shelter, windbreaks and plenty of dry bedding if they cannot be housed.
▸ Ensure horses have plenty of food and water and are checked regularly – ice that develops in buckets/water baths must be broken at least twice daily.

References and further reading

- **Anon,** 2011. Hurricane equine evacuation – <http://www.aaep.org/emergency_prep.htm>.

- **Anon,** 2011. Wildfire readiness – <http://emilms.fema.gov/IS10A/AID0105270text.htm>.

- **Anon,** 2011. Information for livestock owners – <http://www.fema.gov/plan/prepare/live-stock.shtm>.

- **Anon,** 2011. AAEP Emergency & Disaster Preparedness Guidelines – <http://www.aaep.org>.

- **Brown, C.M., Kaneene, J.B., Taylor, R.F.,** 1988. Sudden and unexpected death in horses and ponies: an analysis of 200 cases. Equine. Vet. J. 20, 99–103.

- **Dyson, S.,** 1996. Arrangements prior to the event and on the day. In: Dyson, S. (Ed.), British Veterinary Association Manual: a guide to the management of emergencies at equine competitions. Equine Veterinary Journal Ltd, Newmarket, UK, pp. 1–6.

- **House C., Collins J.** 2008 A guide to best practice for veterinary surgeons when considering euthanasia on humane grounds: where horses are insured under an All Risks of Mortality Insurance Policy – <http://www.beva.org.uk>.

- **Kirk, R.K., Byars, T.D.,** 2009. Equine insurance. In: Robinson, N.E., Sprayberry, K.A. (Eds.), Current Therapy in Equine Medicine (sixth ed.). Elsevier, St. Louis, Missouri, pp. 37–38.

- **Lucke, V.M.,** 1987. Sudden death. Equine. Vet. J. 19, 85–91.

- **Lyle, C.H., Uzal, F.A., McGorum, B.C.,** et al. 2011. Sudden death in racing Thoroughbred horses: an international multicentre study of post mortem findings. Equine. Vet. J. 43, 324–331.

- **McConnico, R.S., French, D.D., Clark, B.,** et al. 2007. Equine rescue and response activities in Lousiana in the aftermath of hurricanes Katrina and Rita. J. Am. Vet. Med. Assoc. 231, 384–392.

How to...

Perform injections/blood sampling

Locations for IM injections

▶ Gluteal muscles.
▶ Cervical muscles.
▶ Pectoral muscles.
▶ Semimembranosus/tendinosus muscles (foals, occasionally adults).

Equipment for IM injections

▶ Needle – 18–20G, 38–40-mm (1.5") adult horses; 20G, 25-mm (1") needles in foals/small ponies (also depends on viscosity of the drug).

Technique for IM injections

1. Insert needle into the musculature in a single, swift action.
2. Check there is no blood in the hub – if so redirect/start again.
3. Connect the syringe, making sure the needle remains fixed in place.
4. Draw back a final time to check for blood and steadily inject the medication.
5. Maximum volume depends on patient size (~20 mL per site in an adult horse).

Location for IV injections

▶ Jugular vein most frequently used.
▶ Alternative sites of venous access in an emergency:
  ▪ cephalic vein
  ▪ lateral thoracic vein
  ▪ saphenous vein (recumbent/anaesthetised).

Equipment for IV injections

▶ Needle size – 19G (range: 18–21G, depending on viscosity of the medication), 40 mm (1.5") adult horses; 20G, 25 mm (1") needles in foals/small ponies.

Technique for IV injections

1. Clip hair over the site if the horse has long hair or the vein is difficult to see/palpate.
2. Wipe the site with alcohol-based disinfectant if the area is grossly contaminated.
3. Raise the jugular vein midway down the neck with one hand – observe/palpate distended vein.
4. Insert the needle into the vein at 30–45° using the other hand.
5. Observe venous blood dripping from the hub of the needle, reduce the angle of the needle and advance up the vein to the needle hub.
6. If bright red (arterial) blood streams out, it is likely that the needle has punctured the carotid artery – remove the needle and start again.
7. Discontinue raising the vein – use this free hand to connect the syringe to the needle, keeping the needle fixed in position.
8. Draw blood back into the syringe, inject the medication slowly (over 10–60 s, depending on the drug, viscosity and volume), drawing back intermittently to ensure the needle is still in the vein.

> **KEY TIP**
>
> Do not inject in the lower half of the jugular vein – the carotid artery is much closer to the jugular vein at this location and is easier to accidentally puncture (see p. 270).

Blood sampling

▶ Blood obtained should be placed into appropriate tubes (Table 19.1).
▶ If repeated samples are required/jugular vein is not accessible – can take a sample from the facial venous sinus (just below the facial crest at level of the middle of the eye)
  ▪ insert 20–23G 16–25-mm (5/8–1") needle at 90° to the skin, 1 cm below the facial crest
  ▪ push until it reaches the bone, then withdraw slightly; allow blood to drip into a collection tube or connect a syringe and slowly aspirate blood (Fig. 19.1).

Table 19.1 Suitable blood sample collecting tubes for various tests that may be required in an emergency

Test	Suitable blood containers
Haematology	EDTA (lilac Vacutainer®/blue Monovette®)
Clotting profiles, fibrinogen*, platelet counts* (if agglutination of the sample has occurred, this type of container would be required to measure fibrinogen and platelet counts)	Sodium citrate (blue Vacutainer®/green Monovette®) – ensure filled exactly to the line
Serum biochemistry/serology/ electrolytes	Plain (red Vacutainer®/brown Monovette®) 5–10 mL whole blood/5 mL serum
Plasma glucose	Fluoride/oxalate (grey Vacutainer®/yellow Monovette®)
Ammonium	Lithium heparin (green Vacutainer®/orange Monovette® – check with laboratory first)
Blood lead	Lithium heparin (green Vacutainer®/orange Monovette®)
Virus isolation	Lithium heparin (green Vacutainer®/orange Monovette®) 3 × 10 mL

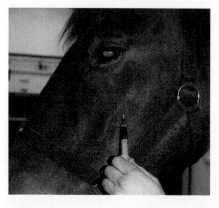

Figure 19.1 Blood sampling from the facial venous sinus. This is located just below the facial crest at the level of the middle of the eye.

Pass a nasogastric tube

Equipment

▶ Stomach tube of suitable diameter and length that does not have any roughened areas/sharp edges:
  - adult horse: 18–19 mm (outer diameter)
  - pony: 13–16 mm
  - foal: 8–9.5 mm.
▶ Lubricant.
▶ Twitch ± sedatives.
▶ Funnel + measuring jug.
▶ Buckets (one empty, one with known quantity of fluid).
▶ ± Stirrup pump.

Procedure

1. Ensure the horse is suitably restrained – ± nose twitch/sedation.
2. Ideally stand on the horse's left side – it is easier to visualise the stomach tube passing down the oesophagus as it courses down the left side of the neck.
3. Estimate the length of the tube required to reach the horse's larynx (Fig. 19.2) and to reach the stomach ± mark with permanent marker pen.
4. Lubricate the tip of the stomach tube, e.g. KY jelly, obstetric lubricant, and ensure the stomach tube is curved with the tip towards the ground.
5. Use your index finger to guide the tube into the ventral meatus using the natural curve of the stomach tube (Fig. 19.3) – this is very important to prevent the tube being passed into the middle meatus, which will result in damage to ethmoturbinates and consequent epistaxis.
6. The tube should pass smoothly along the nasal passages – it must not be forced.
7. Pass the stomach tube to the level of the larynx – some resistance will be felt and the horse may swallow.
8. Flex the horse's neck at this stage – this helps to assist passage of the tube into the oesophagus ± rotate the tube 180° to elevate the end of it.
9. Use a small amount of increased pressure or move the stomach tube backwards and forwards a few centimetres to encourage swallowing of the tube.
10. Air can be gently blown down the end of the tube to encourage swallowing and confirm its location in the oesophagus (boluses of air can be seen passing down the oesophagus) – care must be taken to ensure this is done hygienically and this must not be performed in a horse with suspected colitis/salmonellosis (risk of zoonotic infection).
11. Check that the stomach tube is in the oesophagus – tip of the tube can be subtly visualised as it passes down the left jugular groove region (if unsure gently move the tube backwards and forwards), also it should not be possible to suck air back through the tube (the oesophageal wall will collapse around the end of the tube under negative pressure).
12. If the tube passes into the trachea, the horse will usually (but not always, especially if sedated) cough repeatedly or air will be felt moving in and out of the tube in time with the horse's breathing – if this happens, withdraw the tube back into the nasopharynx and repeat the process again.

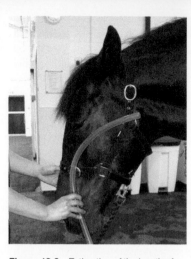

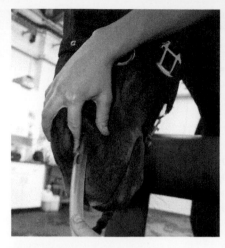

Figure 19.2 Estimation of the length of stomach tube required to reach the horse's larynx.

Figure 19.3 Use of the index finger and the natural curve of the stomach tube to pass the tube into and along the ventral meatus. Take care not to occlude the contra-lateral nasal passage (the horse will resent this).

13. The tube should continue to pass smoothly to the stomach (check the estimated distance on the tube).
14. Mild resistance may be felt as the tip of the tube reaches the cardiac sphincter of the stomach – slightly increased pressure can be used to pass the tube into the stomach (sometimes gently blowing air into the tube can facilitate this).
15. Once the tip of the tube is positioned within the stomach, a bubbling noise will frequently be heard and a slightly sweet smell may be detected.
16. Water can then be administered by gravity flow and the stomach checked for presence of any reflux (this process should be repeated several times and the tube slightly repositioned if reflux is suspected but has not been obtained).
17. To withdraw the tube, empty any fluid from the tube, kink the end and remove smoothly, taking care to avoid aspiration of any fluid/ingesta remaining in the end of the tube (particularly liquid paraffin) into the horse's airways.

Complications

▶ See p. 264.

Normal findings/quantity of fluid to administer

▶ <2 L net fluid retrieved.
▶ The volume to be administered will depend on the horse size and reason for administering oral fluids – as a guide ~ max. 6 L in an adult horse, can be repeated after 1 h.

HANDY TIPS

- Warn the owner of the possibility of epistaxis prior to passing the stomach tube (particularly if the procedure has already been performed recently) and inform the owner that it is common and is usually minor and self-limiting.

- Do not inadvertently occlude the horse's nostrils – this will make it more likely to shake its head and resent the procedure.

- Rarely, horses may have an oesophagus that is positioned on the right side of the neck, making it confusing when trying to visualise the tip of the tube passing down the cervical oesophagus.

- If you are having difficulty passing the tube into the oesophagus despite repeated attempts, try passing the tube up the contralateral nasal passages.

Perform abdominocentesis

Contraindications

▶ Care should be taken (and use of needles avoided) in:
- mares in late gestation (risk of puncturing the uterus)
- horses with marked distension of the large colon/small intestine (risk of laceration of intestine).

Equipment

▶ 19–21G, 50-mm (2") needle.

▶ 19G, 90-mm (3.5") spinal needle individuals with a lot of retroperitoneal fat.

▶ ± Teat cannula and swab.

▶ Clippers and antibacterial scrub.

▶ Sterile gloves.

▶ EDTA and plain blood tubes.

▶ No. 15 scalpel blade and local anaesthetic solution (if using teat cannula).

Procedure

1. Clip a small (10 × 10 cm) area of the ventral abdomen at the most dependent point on the midline (may not be required if fine hair coat).

2. Scrub until the skin site is clean.

3. ± Place a bleb (1–2 ml) of local anaesthetic at the site if using a teat cannula.

4. Put on sterile gloves.

5. Insert needle in the midline/just to the right of midline (Fig. 19.4).

6. If using a teat cannula, use a No. 15 blade to make a small stab incision in the skin, subcutaneous tissues and linea alba and put the cannula through the swab (prevent blood contamination of the sample from the site).

7. Advance the needle/cannula slowly until the peritoneal cavity is entered and peritoneal fluid is obtained (be patient – it can take a few seconds to obtain any fluid).

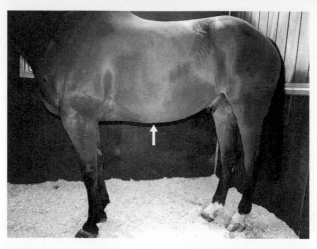

Figure 19.4 Location for performing abdominocentesis on the ventral midline at the most dependent part of the abdomen.

Table 19.2 Assessment of abnormal-looking peritoneal fluid

Colour	Possible diagnosis	Comments
Orange/light red fluid	Ischaemic viscus present ⊡ Possible puncture of small vessel in the abdomen by needle (Fig 19.5a)	Check if consistent with clinical signs; may see 'swirling' of blood into an initially normal-looking sample where puncture of a vessel has occurred
Dark red	Splenic puncture Haemabdomen	Haemabdomen: sample doesn't clot, has a variable PCV (if PCV of sample = systemic PCV, more likely to be splenic puncture), contains no platelets, has evidence of erythrophagocytosis
Green/yellow containing pieces of ingesta	Accidental enterocentesis ⊡	Rarely of consequence to the horse – repeat using a needle at a different site
Brown/red with ingesta	Rupture of a viscus (Fig 19.5b) ⊡	Check horse has clinical signs/ history consistent with this
Turbid (opaque)	Peritonitis (see Fig. 4.4, p. 76) Rarely other causes is chyloabdomen in neonatal foals ⊡	Peritonitis suggestive if: – TP >25 g/L – WBC >5 × 10^9/L

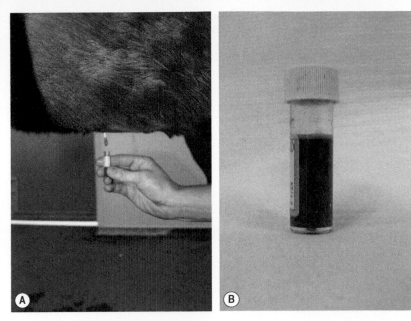

Figure 19.5 (A) Sanguinous peritoneal fluid being obtained. (B) Brown coloured peritoneal fluid containing ingesta that was obtained from a horse in which the stomach had ruptured.

8. If the needle can be seen moving (likely to have penetrated the wall of a viscus), move it back a few mm.
9. If no fluid can be retrieved, consider using a longer needle (there may be a lot of retroperitoneal fat in some horses), or place another needle in a slightly different location.
10. ± Can use abdominal US to identify pockets of peritoneal fluid.
11. Collect retrieved fluid into plain and EDTA tubes.

Normal peritoneal fluid

▶ Yellow, clear fluid.
▶ TP <20–25 g/L.
▶ WBC <5 × 10⁹/L.
▶ Lactate <2.0 mmol/L.

Abnormal peritoneal fluid

See Table 19.2 for assessment of abnormal peritoneal fluid samples.

Perform a rectal examination

Contraindications/increased risk of rectal tears

▶ Foals and small ponies (depending on their size and the size of the examiner's hands).
▶ Horses that are at ↑ risk of rectal tears (where extra care/precautions should be taken):
  ▪ Arab horses
  ▪ small horses
  ▪ young/very nervous horses
  ▪ horses that are unaccustomed to rectal examination
  ▪ male horses – stallions and colts in particular
  ▪ horses with a history of rectal injury
  ▪ horses with colic.

Equipment

▶ Rectal gloves/sleeves.
▶ Obstetric lubricant.
▶ Tail bandage.
▶ ± Sedation/twitch.
▶ ± Butylscopolamine (hyoscine).

Procedure

1. Ensure the horse is suitably restrained and in a suitable location – stocks are ideal if available.
2. ± Sedate the horse (consider particularly in high-risk individuals – see above).
3. ± Administer butylscopolamine (↓ straining).
4. Bandage the tail (minimises the risk of taking hair into the rectum that can cause a laceration).
5. Apply a generous quantity of lubricant to the rectal sleeve.
6. Standing to the side of the horse (if stocks are not used), gently insert a hand into the rectum.
7. Remove any faeces from the rectum.
8. Continue to pass the arm into the rectum – never use any force or push against any peristaltic contractions.
9. Gently sweep across the abdomen, evaluating the structures that can be palpated (Fig. 19.6) – start in the left dorsal region and move in a clockwise direction (Table 19.3).

Assessment of rectal findings

1. Is there any gross distension of any abdominal organs or does the abdomen feel relaxed and relatively empty and does the serosal surface (peritoneum) feel smooth/roughened?
2. If distension of a viscus is evident, what does it feel like and where is it located?
   a. small intestine (feels like inflated inner tubes of bicycle tyres, up to 8 cm in diameter)
   b. large colon (can feel taenial bands/sacculations – firm in impactions/gas filled if colonic obstruction)
   c. small colon (tube-like, approximately 10 cm in diameter)

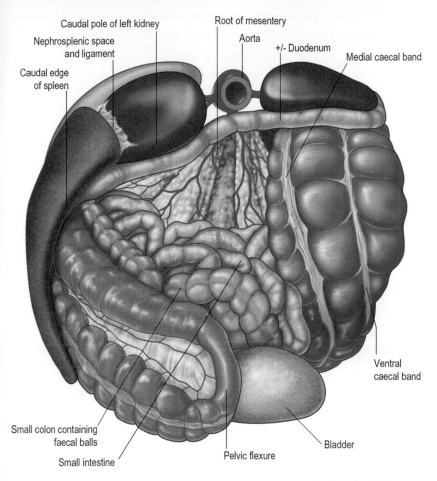

Figure 19.6 Normal cross-section of the caudal abdomen (viewed as standing from the back of the horse) and structures that can be palpated on rectal examination.

d. caecum (always on right side of the abdomen and when distended, can feel a vertical taenial band and cannot palpate between the dorsal caecum and body wall – differentiate from distended large colon)

e. bladder (round and smooth just in front of the pelvis)

f. uterus/ovaries (check for pregnancy/ovarian enlargement)

g. other mass – define size, location, consistency.

Complications

▶ On withdrawal of the examiner's arm from the rectum, check for the presence of any blood on the rectal sleeve in case a rectal tear has occurred (see p. 262).

Table 19.3 Checklist of structures that can normally be palpated during rectal examination

Left dorsal quadrant	Caudal edge of spleen
	Nephrosplenic space*
	Caudal pole of left kidney*
Dorsal	Aorta
	Root of mesentery*
Right dorsal quadrant	Base of caecum*
	Ventral and medial caecal bands*
Ventral/mid abdomen	Bladder
	Ovaries/uterus (females)
	Inguinal rings (male)
Left ventral quadrant	Pelvic flexure and left dorsal colon

*Denotes structures that may be difficult to palpate in larger horses.

Perform synoviocentesis in cases of suspected synovial sepsis

Contraindications

▶ Do not perform if there is evidence of infection/wound/cellulitis at the site due to risk of iatrogenic infection (see p. 272).
▶ Consider alternative approaches to that synovial structure that are distant from the wound.

Equipment

▶ Clippers.
▶ Antibacterial scrub.
▶ Appropriately sized sterile needles and syringes:
  ▪ May need to use a relatively large-bore (18–19G) needle if fluid cannot be retrieved due to fibrin/inflamed synovium blocking the end of the needle (compared to more conventional sizes used for diagnostic analgesia).
▶ Sterile surgical gloves.
▶ EDTA/plain blood tubes.
▶ ± Biphasic culture medium.
▶ ± Sterile saline/LRS.
▶ ± Antimicrobial solutions for intra-articular administration.
▶ ± local anaesthetic solution (can be placed at needle site to facilitate placement).

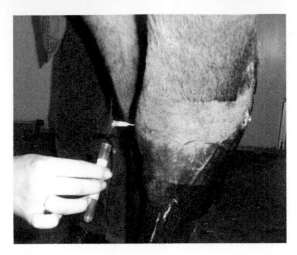

Figure 19.7 Collection of synovial fluid by an assistant from the medial aspect of the tarsocrural joint in a horse that had sustained a wound to the lateral hock region.

Procedure

1. Clip and aseptically prepare the site.
2. ± Infiltrate a small quantity of sterile local anaesthetic subcutaneously at the site.
3. Check the horse is suitably restrained – sedate/twitch if required.
4. Put on sterile gloves and insert a sterile needle at the appropriate site.
5. Retrieve synovial fluid – collect as it drips from the hub of the needle into a collection pot (use an assistant to perform this) or aspirate carefully using a sterile 5-mL syringe (Fig. 19.7).
6. If synovial fluid cannot be obtained and the horse has a wound associated with suspected synovial sepsis, distend the joint/tendon sheath with sterile saline/LRS to confirm or exclude communication between the wound and synovial structure (fluid will either be seen to exit the wound or the structure will become visually distended without exit of fluid).
7. Where sepsis is suspected, administer suitable antimicrobials into the synovial structure, e.g. gentamicin 250 mg or amikacin 125 mg, (adult horse) from new vials prior to removal of the needle (see p. 47).

Evaluation of synovial fluid

▸ Collect into plain and EDTA tubes (be aware that if a small volume is obtained the TP may be falsely ↑).

▸ ± Place some into biphasic culture medium for C&S.

▸ Assess visual appearance and viscosity (see Fig. 3.4, p. 49):

  ▪ normal – yellow, clear and viscous (should form a 'string' between fingers)
  ▪ sepsis – turbid/flocculent yellow/orange/red
  ▪ haemorrhagic – compare with systemic values. If similar, likely haemarthrosis (sepsis less likely).

▸ Measure TP (normal <20 g/L; sepsis often >40 g/L).
▸ Measure WBC (normal <1 × 10⁹/L; variable in cases of sepsis from >5 × 10⁹/L – take TP and cytology into account).
▸ Assess percentage neutrophils (normal <10%; sepsis often >80%).
▸ ± Gram stain to identify bacteria.

Synoviocentesis of selected synovial structures

The following section details approaches to synovial structures that are most commonly affected in cases of traumatic synovial sepsis and which can be performed in the field. See texts for approaches to other synovial structures.

Metacarpophalangeal/metatarsophalangeal (fetlock) joint

▸ Needle: 20G, 25–40 mm (1–1.5").

The landmarks and approaches are shown in Figure 19.8.

Dorsal (A) (Figs 19.8, 19.10)	Usually performed with the limb weight bearing Insert needle medial/lateral to CDET slightly above palpable joint space and pass obliquely into the joint
Proximopalmar/plantar (B) (Fig 19.8)	Usually performed with the limb weight bearing Landmarks: dorsal to SL branch, palmar/plantar to MC/MT3, distal to MC/MT4, proximal to collateral sesamoidean ligament Direct needle slightly distally *blood contamination common
Lateral via collateral sesamoidean ligament (C) (Figs 19.8, 19.9)	Fetlock flexed Landmarks: palpable depression at the end of MC/MT3 cand the dorsal aspect of the proximal sesamoid bone, direct needle 90° to the skin through the collateral sesamoidean ligament
Distopalmar/plantar (D) (Fig. 19.8)	Limb weight bearing Palpable depression between the distodorsal aspect of the sesamoid bone and the proximopalmar/plantar eminence of P1, dorsal to the palmar/plantar digital artery, nerve and vein

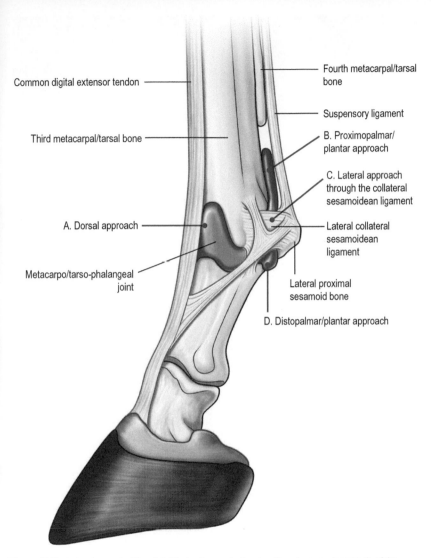

Figure 19.8 Lateral aspect of the distal limb demonstrating locations for synoviocentesis of the metacarpo/tarso-phalangeal (fetlock) joint.

Labels in figure:
- Common digital extensor tendon
- Third metacarpal/tarsal bone
- A. Dorsal approach
- Metacarpo/tarso-phalangeal joint
- Fourth metacarpal/tarsal bone
- Suspensory ligament
- B. Proximopalmar/plantar approach
- C. Lateral approach through the collateral sesamoidean ligament
- Lateral collateral sesamoidean ligament
- Lateral proximal sesamoid bone
- D. Distopalmar/plantar approach

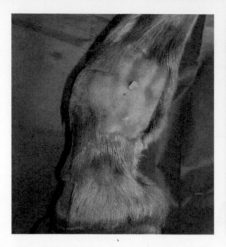

Figure 19.9 Location of needle placement for synoviocentesis of the fetlock joint using a lateral approach through the lateral collateral sesamoidean ligament in a cadaver specimen.

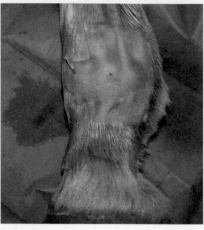

Figure 19.10 Location of needle placement for synoviocentesis of the fetlock joint using a dorsal approach in a cadaver specimen.

Digital flexor tendon sheath

▶ Needle: 20G, 25–40 mm (1–1.5").

Proximal approach (A) (Figs 19.11, 19.12)	Insert the needle ~3 cm proximal to the proximal sesamoid bone along the dorsal edge of the DDFT between the DDFT & SL
	The proximo-lateral out pouching is palpable when the sheath is effused *haemorrhage common with this approach
Mid palmar/ plantar approach (B) (Figs 19.11, 19.12)	Limb flexed or weight bearing
	Palpate for a depression at the base of the proximal sesamoid bone between the palmar/plantar annular ligament and the proximal digital annular ligament, palmar/plantar to the digital neurovascular bundle
	Insert the needle at a 45° upwards angle
Distal palmar/ plantar approach (C) (Figs 19.11, 19.12)	Flexed limb
	Palpate the outpouching of the sheath between proximal and distal digital annular ligaments (easier to palpate the site when the sheath is effused)
	Insert the needle at a shallow angle into the sheath

*See texts for details of alternative palmar/plantar axial sesamoidean approach.

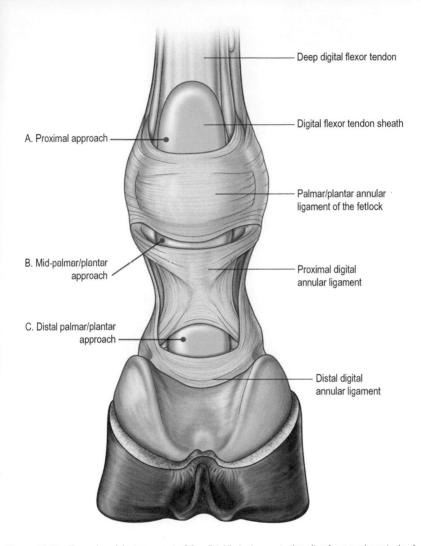

Deep digital flexor tendon

Digital flexor tendon sheath

A. Proximal approach

Palmar/plantar annular ligament of the fetlock

B. Mid-palmar/plantar approach

Proximal digital annular ligament

C. Distal palmar/plantar approach

Distal digital annular ligament

Figure 19.11 The palmar/plantar aspect of the distal limb demonstrating sites for synoviocentesis of the digital flexor tendon sheath (DFTS).

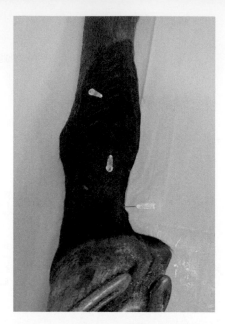

Figure 19.12 Lateral image of the distal limb in a cadaver specimen demonstrating the locations for synoviocentesis of the digital flexor tendon sheath using approaches A, B and C (see text)

Antebrachiocarpal and middle carpal joints

▶ Needle: 20G, 20–40 mm (1–1.5").

A. Dorsal approaches (Figs 19.13, 19.14)	Flexed limb Medial or lateral to the edge of the ECR tendon **Antebrachiocarpal joint** – midway between the distal edge of the radius and the proximal edge of the radiocarpal bone **Middle carpal joint** – midway between the distal edge of the radiocarpal bone and the proximal edge of the 3rd carpal bone
B. Lateral (palmar) approaches (Fig. 19.15)	Limb weight bearing and the needle inserted perpendicular to the limb (easier to palpate when the structures are effused) **Antebrachiocarpal joint** – proximal or distal approaches bordered by the LDE tendon (dorsal) and ulnaris lateralis tendon (palmar). The distal approach is in a shallow recess between the distal lateral radius and the ulnar carpal bone) **Middle carpal joint** – in the shallow depression between the ulnar and 4th carpal bones (~2–2.5 cm below the palpable recess for the antebrachiocarpal joint)

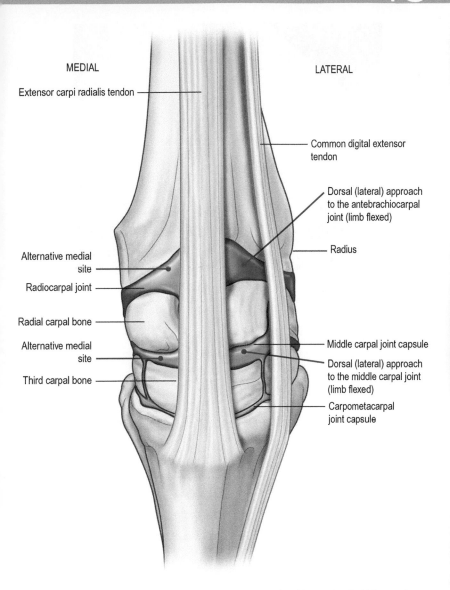

MEDIAL

LATERAL

Extensor carpi radialis tendon

Common digital extensor tendon

Dorsal (lateral) approach to the antebrachiocarpal joint (limb flexed)

Radius

Alternative medial site

Radiocarpal joint

Radial carpal bone

Alternative medial site

Third carpal bone

Middle carpal joint capsule

Dorsal (lateral) approach to the middle carpal joint (limb flexed)

Carpometacarpal joint capsule

Figure 19.13 Dorsal approaches for synovioventesis of the antebrachiocarpal and middle carpal joints.

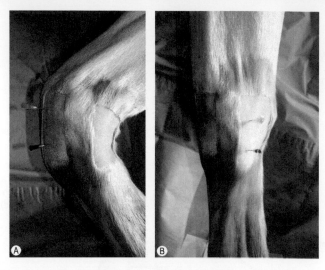

Figure 19.14 Synoviocentesis of antebrachiocarpal and middle carpal joints using a dorsal, (A) or lateral (palmar). (B) approach (lateral aspect of a cadaver limb shown).

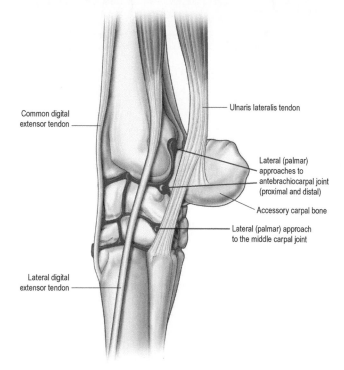

Common digital extensor tendon

Ulnaris lateralis tendon

Lateral (palmar) approaches to antebrachiocarpal joint (proximal and distal)

Accessory carpal bone

Lateral (palmar) approach to the middle carpal joint

Lateral digital extensor tendon

Figure 19.15 Illustration of the carpus demonstrating lateral (palmar) approaches for synoviocentesis of the antebrachiocarpal and middle carpal joints.

Tarsocrural joint

▶ Needle: 20G, 25 mm, (1").

(A) Dorsal approach (Figs 19.16, 19.17)	Approx. 2.5–3.8 cm (1–1.5") distal to the medial malleolus Medial or lateral to the saphenous vein
(B) Plantar approach (Figs 19.16, 19.18)	Medial or lateral approaches – infrequently required The plantar outpouchings of the joint are palpable when the joint is effused

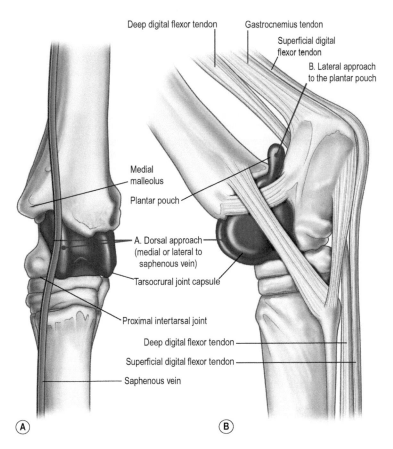

Figure 19.16 (A) Dorsal and (B) lateral views of the hock demonstrating the dorsal and plantar approaches for performing synoviocentesis of the tarsocrural joint.

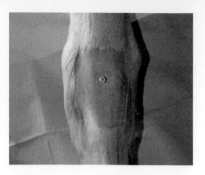

Figure 19.17 Synoviocentesis of the tarsocrural joint using a dorsal approach demonstrated in a cadaver limb.

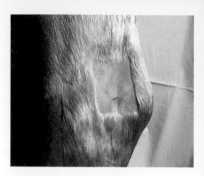

Figure 19.18 Synoviocentesis of the tarsocrural joint using a plantar approach (lateral view of a cadaver limb).

Perform a tracheotomy

Equipment

▸ Equine commercial tracheostomy tube (20-mm internal diameter suitable for most horses, in emergency even 13 mm human commercial tracheostomy tube is fine).

▸ Alternatives: small animal endotracheal tube of suitable diameter, the funnel end of a clean, shortened piece of a stomach tube (do not loose into trachea) or a home-made version using the handle of a clean plastic container, e.g. milk container (Fig. 19.19).

▸ Clippers.

▸ Local anaesthetic solution.

▸ 10-mL syringe and 19–20G, 25–40-mm (1–1.5") needle.

▸ Antibacterial scrub.

▸ Sterile gloves.

▸ Suture kit (in a dire emergency a scalpel blade and handle alone can be used).

▸ Gauze bandage.

▸ Good lighting (head torch useful).

Procedure

(Sections 1–3 may be omitted if the horse has already collapsed.)

1. Clip a 20 × 10 cm area of hair on the midline centred at the junction between the upper and middle thirds of the neck (Fig. 19.19).

2. Palpate the paired sternothyrohyoideus muscles and the trachea.

3. Instil local anaesthetic solution at the site (down to level of tracheal rings) and rescrub.

4. Create a 6–8 cm ventral midline incision at the junction between upper and middle 1/3 of the neck (Fig. 19.20).

5. Incise through the subcutaneous tissues and separate the paired sternothyrohyoideus muscles on the midline – do not dissect the tissues away from the midline (Fig. 19.20).

6. Palpate the two tracheal rings in the centre of the incision.

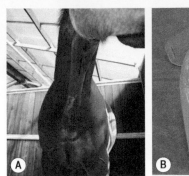
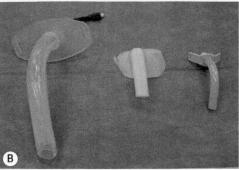

Figure 19.19 (A) Location of tracheotomy incision on the ventral midline of the neck centred at the junction between the upper and middle thirds. (B) Selection of tracheostomy tubes: left, 20-mm equine commercial tube; right, 13-mm human commercial tube; and centre, home- made version using the handle from a plastic container.

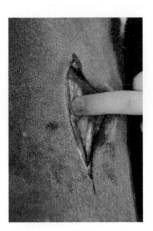

Figure 19.20 Creation of an incision on the ventral midline of the neck to the level of the tracheal rings.

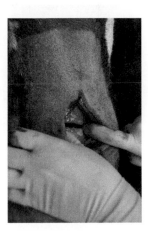

Figure 19.21 An incision is made between two adjacent tracheal rings enabling the tracheal lumen to be penetrated.

7. Make a stab incision between the 2 rings and extend the incision for approximately 1–2 cm each side of the midline (Fig. 19.21).

8. Do not incise more than 1/3 of the tracheal circumference or you may risk injury to the carotid artery/vagus nerve.

9. Insert the tracheostomy tube using a finger to guide it in place – this can be tricky as there is often not much room between the tracheal rings (Fig. 19.22).

10. Check the tube is in place – air can be felt moving in and out of the tube.

11. Secure the tube in place using gauze bandage (thread through a plait on the mane to stop it slipping up/down the neck; Fig. 19.23).

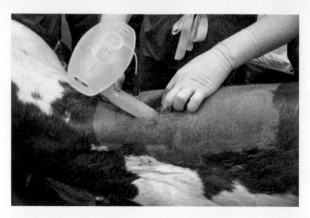

Figure 19.22 A tracheostomy tube is inserted at the site, taking care to ensure the end of the tube is sitting within the tracheal lumen.

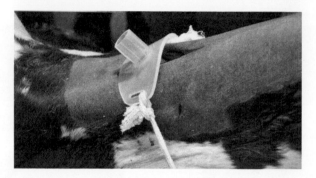

Figure 19.23 Gauze bandage is used to secure the tracheostomy tube in place.

Sedate a fractious/dangerous horse

Horses that are difficult to inject IV

IM sedative mixture

▶ Detomidine alone can be used or can be combined with butorphanol and/or acepromazine in the same syringe for more heavy sedation (NB: this is an unlicenced form of administration):

  ▪ detomidine 0.02 mg/kg

  ▪ butorphanol 0.05 mg/kg

  ▪ acepromazine 0.03 mg/kg.

▶ Inject IM.

  ▪ Leave horse in quiet calm environment but check that it cannot harm itself (e.g. hanging its head over the stable door causing respiratory obstruction/jugular venous occlusion).

  ▪ Peak sedation will take 30 min.

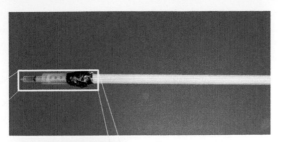

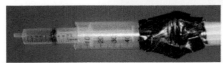

Figure 19.24 Home-made pole syringe prior to placement of the needle.

- Effective in 90% of horses.
- Degree of sedation varies from mild–heavy sedation.
- Can top up with further sedation administered IV.

Horses that are difficult to inject IM

Oral detomidine

▶ A commercially available preparation is available (Domosedan Gel®).

▶ A home-made mixture can be made using the IV preparation – 0.06 mg/kg detomidine PO (unlicenced method of administration):

- absorbed across MM – put into a sugar lump for ponies/small horses or into molasses for larger horses or can administer directly into the mouth
- 60–70% of horses will respond appropriately – may have to repeat or top up sedation in some
- expensive.

Remote injection using a pole syringe

▶ IM sedative mixture (see previous section).

▶ Commercially available pole syringe best (e.g. Wildpharm Ltd, Milverton, UK).

▶ Can make a home-made pole syringe (Fig. 19.24) using:

- 18G, 1.5" (38 mm) needle
- 10-mL syringe (inserted into end of 60-mL syringe barrel once loaded)
- 60-mL syringe with the end cut off
- secured firmly to the end of a pole with heavy-duty tape.

Remote injection

▶ Preloaded high-pressure fluid lines (as used for measurement of arterial pressure in horses) and large-bore needle (19G).

▶ Preload with sedative (IM sedative mixture) followed by saline.

▶ As needle is inserted into horse IM, inject the bolus of drug as the horse moves away.

Impossible to catch/restrain

▸ Darting – contact local zoo/wildlife immobilisation expert.
▸ Oral chloral hydrate (see texts).

Emergency reversal of sedation

▸ Atipamezole (Antisedan®) is not licenced in horses but can be used to reverse sedation in an emergency (e.g. adverse effect of α2 agonist sedative).
▸ Exact dose difficult to suggest – depends on sedation used, duration since given.
▸ As a guide, administer 0.05 mg/kg IM (safer) or slow IV (25 mg for 500-kg horse = 5 mL).

Use sedation infusions

These may be useful where prolonged sedation is required to avoid repeated administration of boluses, which can result in dramatic variation in the degree of sedation (under- to over-dosage).

Equipment

▸ IV catheters and 3-way taps.
▸ 500-mL bags of normal saline.
▸ Small animal giving set.
▸ Sedative agent of choice (detomidine or xylazine used most frequently).

Detomidine infusion

▸ Place an IV catheter.
▸ Sedate the horse with 6 µg/kg detomidine IV (0.006 mg/kg = 3 mg in a 500-kg horse) and wait 5 min before starting the infusion.
▸ Administer butorphanol 0.05–0.1 mg/kg IV.
▸ Add 12 mg detomidine to 500 mL sterile saline/LRS.
▸ For a 500-kg horse start the drip rate at around 4 drops/s (approx. 0.1 µg/kg/min).
▸ When adequately sedated, slow the drip rate to 1–2 drops/s.
▸ Recovery following cessation of infusion = around 15–20 min.

Xylazine infusion

▸ Place IV catheter.
▸ Sedate with 0.5 mg/kg xylazine IV and wait 5 min before starting the infusion.
▸ Administer butorphanol 0.05–0.1 mg/kg IV.
▸ Add 500 mg xylazine to 500 mL sterile saline/LRS.
▸ For a 500-kg horse, start the infusion at 2 drops/s (around 12 µg/kg/min).
▸ Slow the drip rate to 1 drop/s once adequate sedation is achieved.
▸ Recovery following cessation of infusion = around 10–15 min.

Anaesthetise a horse in an emergency

Equipment

▶ Suitable anaesthetic, sedative and analgesic drugs.
▶ IV catheters.
▶ Padded headcollar, soft ropes.
▶ ± Drugs for resuscitation, e.g. adrenaline.
▶ ± Endotracheal tube (ideal).
▶ ± Oxygen and tubing/demand valve (ideal).

Factors to consider beforehand

▶ Consider whether anaesthesia could be avoided, e.g. sedation and nerve blocks, or if euthanasia is a serious alternative.
▶ Ideally have a second veterinary surgeon/nurse with you.
▶ Obtain consent for anaesthesia (have a signed consent form) and discuss the risks associated with anaesthesia (in emergency situations the only alternative may be euthanasia).
▶ Place an IV catheter to ensure secure IV access.
▶ Administer analgesic agents ± antimicrobials as required.
▶ Consider use of local anaesthetic nerve blocks if relevant.

Anaesthetic protocol

Sedation/premedication

▶ ± Acepromazine 0.04 mg/kg IM as a pre-premedicant (needs 30–40 min to achieve effect – unlikely to have time in an emergency).
▶ α2 agonist:
  ▪ xylazine 1.1 mg/kg IV or
  ▪ detomidine 0.01–0.02 mg/kg IV or
  ▪ romifidine 0.06–0.1 mg/kg IV
  ▪ plus butorphanol 0.05–0.2 mg/kg IV.
▶ Wait 5 min.

Induction of anaesthesia

▶ Ketamine 2.2 mg/kg IV ± diazepam 0.05 mg/kg IV.
▶ Alternatively, thiopental 5–8 mg/kg IV ± diazepam 0.05 mg/kg IV.

Maintenance of anaesthesia

▶ Ketamine ± α2 agonist top-ups every 10–12 min (time carefully – don't wait until the horse becomes 'light'):
  ▪ 1/3–1/2 the original premedication and induction doses
  ▪ xylazine premedicant – xylazine and ketamine at 1/3–1/2 original doses every 10–12 min.
  ▪ detomidine premedicant – ketamine top-ups with 1/2 dose detomidine at every third top up (around every 30 min)
  ▪ romifidine premedicant – ketamine top-ups with 1/3–1/2 the original dose of romifidine after 60 min of anaesthesia.
▶ Thiopental 1 mg/kg IV (range 0.5–2.5 mg/kg) as required (total not more than 20 mg/kg).

'Triple drip' combinations

▶ Various combinations used (see texts/website).

Inhalational anaesthesia

▶ See anaesthesia texts for further details.
▶ May not have necessary equipment to hand in emergency situations in the field.

Other considerations

▶ Check position of limbs, padding of head and protection of the eyes.
▶ ± Concurrent administration of IV fluids if the horse is systemically compromised.
▶ Be aware of risks of hypothermia depending on the weather conditions/systemic health of the horse (e.g. if stuck in water for a prolonged period of time).
▶ Ensure the horse is in a safe environment for recovery.

Perform caudal epidural anaesthesia

Equipment

▶ Clippers and tail bandage.
▶ Antibacterial scrub.
▶ Sterile gloves.
▶ Local anaesthetic solution (sterile).
▶ Sterile saline.
▶ Medication of choice (see Table 19.4).
▶ 25G, 16-mm (5/8") needle.
▶ Ideal – spinal needle 19G, 90 mm (3.5").
▶ Can use 18–20G, 40–90 mm (1.5–3.5") needle, depending on size of horse.
▶ 2-mL, 5-mL and 10-mL syringes.

What to inject

▶ Use preservative–free preparations if possible that do not contain adrenaline.
▶ There are a variety of possible drug choices for the injectate – this is largely dependent on personal preference and duration of action (Table 19.4).
▶ Do not inject more than 10 mL in total for a 500-kg horse to avoid the risk of blocking the motor fibres to the hind limbs (risking the horse becoming recumbent).

Technique

1. Bandage the tail, Clip and aseptically prepare the site (Fig. 19.25).
2. Infiltrate 2 mL 2% mepivicaine subcutaneously and along the path that the needle will take (25G, 16-mm (5/8") needle).
3. Check that the horse is standing squarely and is adequately restrained.

Table 19.4 Injectates for caudal epidural anaesthesia*

Drug	Volume	Onset	Duration
Lidocaine 2%	6–8 mL	20 min	1–2 h
Mepivacaine 2%	5 mL	20 min	2 h
Xylazine 0.17 mg/kg	Make up to 10 mL in saline	15 min	2–5 h
Detomidine 0.06 mg/kg	Make up to 10 mL in saline	15 min	2–3 h
Morphine 0.05–0.1 mg/kg + detomidine 0.03 mg/kg	Make up to 10 mL in saline	20 min	17–24 h

*When α2 agonists are used, systemic signs of sedation may be evident.
Modified from Dugdale (2010)

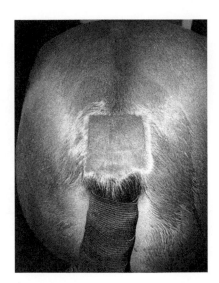

Figure 19.25 Bandaging of the tail and clipping of the site for epidural anaesthesia – the first intercoccygeal space is usually 1–2 cm cranial to the top of the tail hairs.

4. Identify the first intercoccygeal joint by moving the tail up and down and feeling for the most obvious/moveable intervertebral space – it is usually 1–2 cm cranial to the first tail hairs (but can be difficult to palpate in fat individuals); Fig. 19.26.
5. Place the needle perpendicular to the skin with the bevel facing forward.
6. Advance the needle, taking care to stay in a median (midline) plane, perpendicular to the contour of the croup (Fig. 19.27).

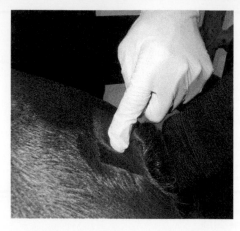

Figure 19.26 Identification of the first intercoccygeal space by placing a finger over the site and moving the tail up and down.

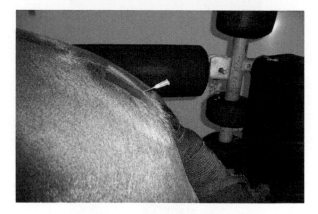

Figure 19.27 Placement of the needle into the intercoccygeal joint space (points 5–9).

7. Withdraw the stylet (if using a spinal needle).
8. Fill the hub of the needle with saline.
9. Advance the needle until one of all of the following occur:
    a. the needle hits bone (dorsal vertebral arch/floor of spinal canal)
    b. there is a change in resistance to advancement of the needle (penetration of interspinous and interarcuate ligament)
    c. saline disappears from the hub (extradural space penetrated)
    d. the horse jumps.

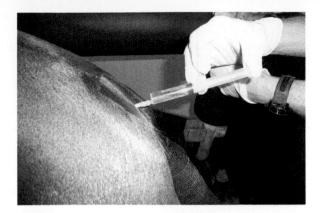

Figure 19.28 Performing test injection (point 10) prior to injecting the local anaesthetic/sedative mixture.

10. Perform a test injection first – with a 5-mL syringe filled with 3 mL saline + 2 mL air, it should be possible to inject the saline without compressing the air bubble (Fig. 19.28).
11. If compression of the air bubble occurs or if blood is seen in the hub, remove the needle and repeat the procedure with a new needle placed at a slightly different angle (making sure it stays on the midline).
12. If the saline can be injected without compression of the air bubble, disconnect the syringe and slowly inject the local anaesthetic/sedative mixture.
13. Assess success by degree of tail/anal sphincter relaxation and response to pin-prick/pinch skin in perineal region (take care to avoid being kicked if the block has not worked!).
14. Be careful if re-performing the block if the first one does not appear to have worked (this could result in HL paralysis if the first one was correctly positioned but the onset of effects were delayed).

Perform local anaesthetic nerve blocks of the head

▶ This section details nerve blocks that are most commonly used in emergency situations – see texts for details of other blocks, e.g. mandibular and retrobulbar nerve blocks.
▶ These are most easily performed with the horse well sedated and the horse's head resting on some form of head support such as a commercial head stand or temporary support, e.g. hay bales covered with a rug.

Equipment

▶ Appropriate sizes of needles and syringes (see relevant nerve block).
▶ ± Clippers.
▶ Antibacterial skin scrub.
▶ Sterile gloves.
▶ Local anaesthetic agent (see Table 19.5).

Choice of nerve block

▶ Where temporary immobilisation of the eyelids is required, an auriculopalpebral nerve block should be placed.
▶ For desensitisation of relevant areas, see Table 19.6.
▶ Figure 19.29 demonstrates the locations of key nerves and foraminae.

Table 19.5 Local anaesthetic agents that can be used for nerve blocks

Agent	Onset	Duration of action
Lidocaine (lignocaine)	5–10 min	1 h (without adrenaline)
Mepivacaine	10–15 min	2 h
Bupivacaine	15–20 min	4–8 h+
Prilocaine	10–15 min	1–2 h (without adrenaline)

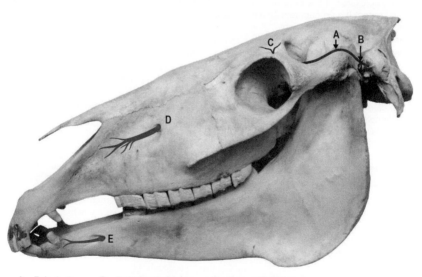

A = Palpebral nerve **B** = Auriculopalpebral nerve **C** = Supraorbital foramen
D = Infraorbital foramen **E** = Mental foramen

Figure 19.29 Cadaver skull demonstrating landmarks A–E.

Table 19.6 Choice of nerve block to perform when desensitising parts of the head

Where desensitisation is required	Local anaesthetic block(s)
Upper eyelid	Supraorbital (middle 2/3)
	Lacrimal (lateral canthus and eyelid)
	Infratrochlear (medial canthus)
Lower eyelid	Zygomatic (most of lower eyelid)
Nostrils	Infraorbital
Upper lip	Infraorbital
Lower lip	Mental
Rostral mandible	Mental (inject into canal)
Rostral maxilla	Infraorbital (inject into canal)

Auriculopalpebral nerve block

Structures desensitised	None – this is a *motor nerve block only* and enables the eyelids to be opened more easily for examination and treatment of the eye
Site of block (Figs 19.29, 19.30)	Where the palpebral nerve crosses the dorsal margin of the zygomatic arch halfway between the eye and ear (A) *or*
	In the triangular depression where a line along the dorsal border of the zygomatic arch transects a vertical line drawn along the caudal border of the vertical ramus of the mandible (B)
Needle	22–25G, 25 mm (1")
Volume of anaesthetic solution	2–5 mL

Supraorbital/frontal nerve block

Structures desensitised	Middle 2/3 upper eyelid
	Skin on the forehead
Site of block (Figs 19.29 and 19.31)	Supraorbital foramen (C)
	Lies halfway between medial and lateral canthi 1–2 cm dorsal to the dorsal rim of the orbit
	Palpate the foramen, insert tip of needle into foramen, check no blood in needle and inject
Needle	23–25G, 16 mm (5/8")
Volume of anaesthetic solution	2–3 mL

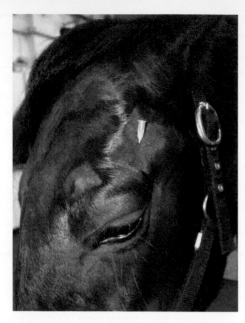

Figure 19.30 Site of needle placement for performing an auriculopalpebral (AP) nerve block.

Infraorbital nerve block

Structures desensitised	Upper lip
	Nostril
	Skin on face rostral to infraorbital foramen
Site of block (Figs 19.29, 19.32)	Infraorbital foramen (D)
	Lift the thin strap-like muscle (levator nasolabialis superioris) and palpate the rim of the foramen
	Insert needle and inject LA where the nerve exits the foramen
	± Can inject up into the canal to desensitise the incisors and canine teeth (need to insert needle approx. 1" into the canal – horse can react violently)
Needle	23–25G, 25–40mm (1–1.5")
Volume of anaesthetic solution	Around 5 mL

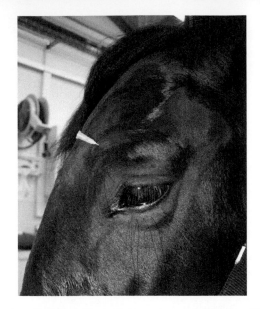

Figure 19.31   Site of needle placement for performing a supraorbital (SO) nerve block.

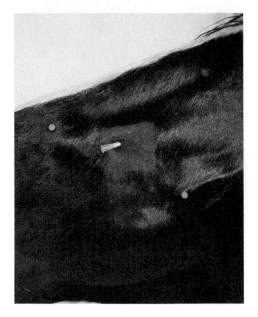

Figure 19.32   Location of needle placement to perform an infraorbital nerve block (the horse's nose is to the left of the picture). The site is halfway along and slightly caudal to a line joining the nasoincisive notch (upper orange dot) and rostral end of the facial crest (lower orange dot).

Mental nerve block

Structures desensitised	Lower lip rostral to mental foramen
Site of block (Figs 19.29, 19.33)	Mental foramen (E) Located in the middle of the interdental space below a strap-like muscle (depressor labii inferioris) Reflect the muscle dorsally Palpate the foramen and insert the needle so the tip is near the site where the nerve exits Can insert needle 1–2" into the foramen if desensitisation of the incisors, canines, premolars and associated bone/oral mucosa is required (horse can react violently)
Needle	20–22G, 25–50 mm (1–2")
Volume of anaesthetic solution	5 mL

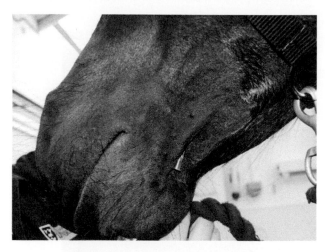

Figure 19.33 Location of needle placement to perform a mental nerve block.

Structures desensitised	Medial canthus and adjacent skin 3rd eyelid and lacrimal duct region
Site of block (Figs 19.34 and 19.35)	Notch in orbital rim just dorsal to the medial canthus (F)
Needle	25G, 16 mm (5/8")
Volume of anaesthetic solution	1–2 mL

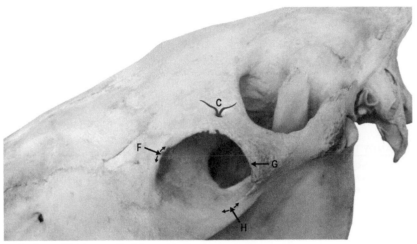

C = Supraorbital foramen (frontal nerve block)
F = Infratrochlear nerve block **G** = Lacrimal nerve block **H** = Zygomatic nerve block

Figure 19.34 Cadaver skull demonstrating landmarks F–H.

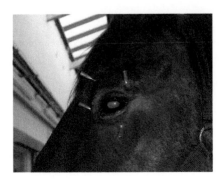

Figure 19.35 Placement of needles for anaesthesia of the entire periocular region.

Lacrimal nerve block

Structures desensitised	Lateral canthus Lateral 1/3 upper eyelid
Site of block (Figs 19.34, 19.35)	Insert needle just medial to the lateral canthus and just beneath the dorsal orbital rim (G)
Needle	25G, 16 mm (5/8")
Volume of anaesthetic solution	1–2 mL

Zygomatic nerve block

Structures desensitised	Lateral 3/4 of the lower eyelid
Site of block (Figs 19.34, 19.35)	Just medial to the lateral canthus along the lower orbital rim (H)
Needle	25G, 16 mm (5/8")
Volume of anaesthetic solution	1–2 mL

> #### HANDY TIP
> If unsure of the location of the infratrochlear, lacrimal and zygomatic nerves, infiltrate local anaesthetic all the way around the orbital rim (0.5–1 mL of local anaesthetic per 1 cm of skin injected subcutaneously).

Place an IV catheter

Equipment

▸ Clippers.
▸ Antibacterial scrub.
▸ 2 mL mepivacaine (or other local anaesthetic) in syringe.
▸ 25G, 16 mm (5/8") needle.
▸ IV catheter (see next section) and extension set, bung/3-way tap.
▸ Suture material (small lengths 3–4 metric suture material threaded into 20G, 25 mm (1") needles useful).
▸ Sterile gloves (required if long-stay catheter being placed).
▸ No. 15 scalpel blade (for long-stay catheter).
▸ 10–20 ml Heparinised saline (5–10 IU heparin per mL in sterile 0.9% NaCl).

Which catheter to use

▸ Material depends on the duration of time it is required for:
  ▪ <24 h – polytetrafluoroethylene (PTFE) catheters ('short stay')
  ▪ >24 h – polyurethane less thrombogenic – 'long stay' catheters.

▸ Size:
  ▪ adult horses – 12G, 8 cm (short stay, 3.1") 14G 13 cm (long stay, 5.25")
  ▪ small pony – 14G, 8 cm (short stay, 3.1")–13 cm (long stay, 5.25").

Where to place

▸ Jugular vein – most commonly used, easy to perform in adult horses.
▸ If the jugular vein cannot be accessed or is thrombosed, alternative sites include:
  ▪ cephalic vein –risk of being kicked/hit in face (easier in neonatal foals)
  ▪ lateral thoracic vein – more tricky to place a catheter, easier in lean horses (± can use US to assist placement).

How to place

1. Clip and aseptically prepare a site over the mid/upper third of the jugular vein (or over other vein if appropriate).
2. Place a subcutaneous bleb (1–2 mL) of local anaesthetic at the site, continue aseptic preparation of the skin ± put on sterile gloves as appropriate.
3. Decide if the catheter is being placed up or down the vein – generally:
   a. uphill – short stay, e.g. anaesthesia/temporary IV access
   b. downhill – long stay, e.g. longer-term fluid therapy/IV medication.
4. ± Make a small incision in the skin (long-stay polyurethane catheters).
5. Use one hand to raise the vein.
6. Insert the catheter at 45° to the skin using the other hand.
7. Advance both the catheter and stylette into the vein until venous blood is obtained (if a high-pressure stream of bright red blood is obtained, most likely from the carotid artery – redirect).
8. Advance a further 5 mm, then flatten the angle of the catheter (in line with the vein).
9. Advance the catheter and stylette a further 5 cm and check for flow of blood.
10. Continue to advance the catheter without the stylette until the catheter hub is sitting against the skin and check the catheter is still in the vein.
11. Attach the catheter bung/3-way tap (or connector if a long-stay catheter is being placed – keep the vein raised until this is connected to prevent aspiration of air).
12. Ensure this is well secured.
13. Secure the wings of the catheter with sutures and make sure the catheter is sitting snugly against the skin (should not see catheter material protruding).
14. Flush the catheter with 10–20 mL heparinised saline.

▸ Ensure the horse cannot catch the catheter on anything – in neonatal foals, the site should be bandaged carefully.
▸ Catheters should only be removed by a vet/nurse or a competent person who has been shown what to do (see Broken catheters, p. 273).

What not to do

▸ Do not catheterise the lower third of the jugular vein – there is more risk of accidental catheterisation of the carotid artery due to the proximity of the vein and artery at this site (suspect if a haematoma develops around the catheter).
▸ Never push the stylette back into the catheter during catheter placement – risk of shearing off the end of the catheter.

Complications

Complications include catheter breakage (p. 273), air embolism (p. 273) and haemorrhage (see below). See texts for complications associated with long-term use, e.g. thrombophlebitis.

Administer IV fluids in the field

This section details how to perform emergency administration of IV fluids in a non-clinic setting. See texts for details of longer-term fluid therapy and hospital-based intensive care.

Equipment

▸ As for IV catheter.
▸ Large animal fluid giving set and high-flow extension set.
▸ Hook/other device (e.g. baler twine/rope) to secure fluid bags.
▸ IV fluids (see relevant sections).

Administering fluids

1. Place IV catheter (see previous section).
2. Connect the fluids and giving set and run through to remove any air – do not overfill the chamber.
3. Thread through a plait on the mane (to prevent tension on the catheter site).
4. Connect the giving set to the IV catheter and ensure it is secured well (Fig. 19.36).

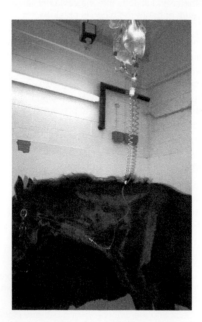

Figure 19.36 Large animal intravenous giving and extension sets being used to administer intravenous fluids in a stable.

5. Monitor for any complications:
   a. catheter blocked/kinked
   b. giving set twisted and blocked
   c. catheter pulled out
   d. giving set disconnected from the catheter – risk of exsanguination (uphill-facing catheter) or air embolus (downhill-facing catheter).

Work out how much and what types of fluid to administer

1. Estimate current fluid deficit (this is a rough estimate):
   - fluid deficit (L) = body weight × estimated % dehydration.

Degree of dehydration	Clinical signs	Volume replacement required in 500-kg horse
5–7%	Semi-dry oral MM, ↓ skin tent, CRT 3 s	25–35 L
8–10%	Dry oral MM, ↓ skin tent, CRT >3 s, ↑ HR	40–50 L
>10%	Skin tent remains raised, v dry MM, weak, cold extremities, recumbent	>50 L

2. Work out the horse's maintenance requirements:
   - around 60 mL/kg/d.

300 kg	400 kg	500 kg	600 kg
18 L/d	24 L/d	30 L/d	36 L/d

3. Estimate ongoing losses (this can be difficult):
   - severe diarrhoea – may be as much as daily maintenance requirement again (or more).
4. Work out what fluids to give (see relevant sections):
   - crystalloids (LRS, Hartmann's) – suitable for most emergency situations
   - hypertonic saline (2–4 mL/kg as a bolus) – administer initially in horses with evidence of moderate dehydration (>8% dehydration) and must be followed up by administration of crystalloids.
   - synthetic colloids can be used in severely hyporolaemic horses (see texts/relevant sections)
   - plasma/blood if required (see relevant sections).
5. Replace the initial fluid deficit within 4–8 h and continue fluid therapy to replace maintenance fluid requirements + ongoing losses:
6. Monitor hydration and other systemic parameters:
   - can monitor PCV/TP to keep within normal limits – more complicated if horse is anaemic or hypoproteinaemic
   - urination is a good general guide in horses with normal renal function:
     » no urination – ↑ fluid rates
     » excessive urination – ↓ fluid rates.
7. Try to get onto oral fluids and feed as soon as possible.

Perform a blood/plasma transfusion

Equipment/materials

▸ Commercial blood collection kit/commercial plasma.
▸ Blood giving set (with filter).
▸ IV catheter, suture and 3-way tap.
▸ Medication for transfusion reaction available (see p. 379).

Obtain blood/plasma

Donor horse

▸ Healthy, large, young gelding (free from infectious disease, e.g. EIA).
▸ PCV >35%, TP >60 g/L.
▸ Ideally a universal donor – Qa and Aa −ve (in reality this is often impractical to achieve).
▸ Decide how much blood is needed by the recipient (see calculation p. 379).
▸ A maximum of 15–18 mL/kg can be taken from the donor horse (Fig. 19.37):
  ▪ 7.5–9 L can be taken from a 500-kg horse at 3–4-week intervals.

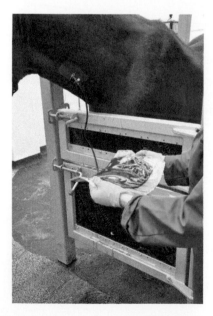

Figure 19.37 Blood being obtained from donor horse; the collection bag should be gently agitated to ensure even mixing of blood and the anticoagulant.

▶ Collect blood into the collection bag containing an anticoagulant.

▶ Administer as whole blood or plasma can be removed (see below).

▶ Blood storage = up to 4 weeks if refrigerated (check manufacturers instructions).

In neonatal isoerythrolysis – the dam is the donor of choice (maternally derived antibodies from colostrum will not attack transfused maternal RBCs). Allow blood to sediment, remove plasma and wash the RBCs 3–5× in normal saline before administering (see p. 243).

Plasma

▶ Commercial plasma:
  - hyperimmunised horses/universal donors guaranteed TP >50 g/L, IgG >24 g/L
  - can be stored for 2 years at −25°C.
▶ From collected blood (above) – allow whole blood to sediment by gravity (Fig. 19.38; reasonable after 2 h, best after 24 h) ; then squeeze the bag from the bottom to collect plasma from the top (Fig. 19.39).
▶ Plasma – best if used fresh but if frozen at −20°C clotting factor stability lasts 2 months, globulin at least 1 year.

± Cross-match blood (see texts)

▶ Antibodies take 5–7 d to be produced by the recipient – if a one-off emergency blood/plasma transfusion is being performed, this step can be missed.

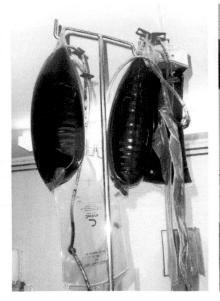

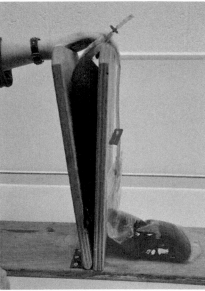

Figure 19.38 RBCs being allowed to sediment prior to collection of plasma.

Figure 19.39 Plasma being removed using a home-made device. A large book will also work well.

How much blood to give

1. Calculate how much blood has been lost (approximate volume may be known if blood has been collected into a container).

$$\begin{array}{c}\text{Estimated amount}\\\text{of blood lost (L)}\end{array} = \frac{\text{normal PCV} - \text{patient PCV}}{\text{normal PCV}} \times 0.08 \times \begin{array}{c}\text{patient body}\\\text{weight(kg)}\end{array}$$

2. Administer 30–40% of the estimated blood volume lost – this is sufficient to maintain life until the bone marrow can respond and is a practical volume that can be obtained from a donor horse (see website also).

How to give

1. Place a 14G IV catheter.
2. Connect plasma/blood to giving set (it must have a filter; Fig. 19.40) and attach to the catheter.
3. Monitor the horse's HR, RR every 2 min for the first 10 min.
4. Start the infusion slowly, e.g. 1 drop/s.
5. If the horse's parameters remain stable, can increase the drip rate progressively and continue until the transfusion is completed (usually takes 30–60 min, depending on the volume being administered).

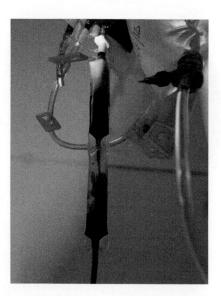

Figure 19.40 Administration of blood via a giving set that contains a filter to remove any particulate matter including blood clots.

6. If any transfusion reactions are seen (see text box -transfusion reactions), stop the infusion immediately (this is infrequent for first-time transfusions).
7. If severe reactions are seen (rare), administer:
   a. furosemide 1 mg/kg IV
   b. dexamethasone 0.05 mg/kg IV or IM
   c. adrenaline 0.01–0.02 mg/kg (1:1000 approx. 1 mL/100 kg) IV, IM or SC
   d. NSAIDs IV
   e. rapid IV administration of sterile fluids (isotonic or hypertonic fluids).

Transfusion reactions

- ↑ RR, ↑ HR , becomes restless/agitated.
- Pyrexia.
- Defecation, urination.
- Colic-like signs.
- Urticaria, pruritus, piloerection.
- ± Haemoglobinuria.
- ± Jaundice.
- ± Dyspnoea (severe).
- ± Dysrhythmias, collapse (severe).

Place a subpalpebral lavage system

Equipment

▶ Specialised ophthalmic catheters – e.g. Mila international (http://www.milainternational.com).
▶ Sedation.
▶ Local anaesthetic (sterile topical ophthalmic preparations and routine preparations).
▶ Sterile gloves (rinse powder off with sterile saline if necessary).
▶ 2% povidone iodine solution.

Technique

1. Sedate the horse (α2 agonist/butorphanol).
2. The catheter can be placed in the upper or lower lid (personal preference).
3. Perform an auriculopalpebral nerve block (see p. 367).
4. Anaesthetise the upper or lower eyelid:
   a. upper lid – supraorbital (frontal) nerve block
   b. lower lid – local infiltration of 1.0–1.5 mL LA at the site (23G, 16-mm (5/8") needle).
5. Anaesthetise the cornea and conjunctiva using topical LA ophthalmic solution.
6. Aseptically prepare the skin of the eyelid with dilute povidone iodine (2%), taking care to avoid getting any into the eye.
7. Check the horse is adequately sedated.
8. Insert a finger at location of intended placement of the catheter between the eyelid and the cornea (Fig. 19.41).

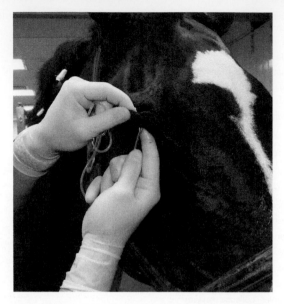

Figure 19.41   Placement of a gloved finger between the cornea and eyelid prior to placing the trochar through the eyelid.

Courtesy Cathy McGowan.

9.   Insert the trochar and catheter tubing through the eyelid and remove the trochar (Fig. 19.42).
10.   Secure the catheter tubing to the head ensuring that the catheter footplate will not migrate out of the conjunctival fornix (Figs 19.43, 19.44).

Maintenance and removal

▸   Infuse 0.2 mL of appropriate medication (see Chapter 6); then inject 1.5 mL air.
▸   The catheter can remain in place for 4 weeks (or more) if looked after properly.
▸   Replace the catheter caps frequently.
▸   Easily removed under sedation:
  ▪   cut the catheter a few cm above the fornix site and remove the catheter attachments to the head
  ▪   the tubing that remains attached to the footplate can be pushed into the fornix and a gloved finger used to retrieve it.

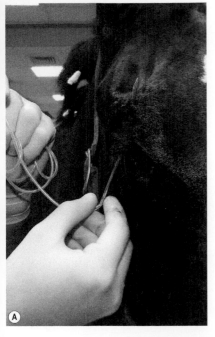
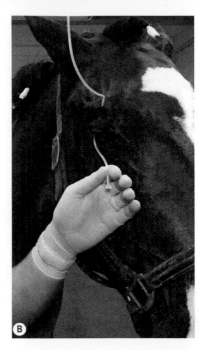

Figure 19.42 (A) Pass the trochar through the eyelid and remove the trochar from the catheter tubing. (B) Pull the catheter tubing through the eyelid to ensure that the footplate sits securely and comfortably in the conjunctival fornix.

Courtesy of Cathy McGowan.

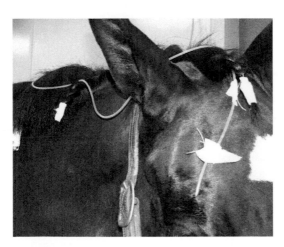

Figure 19.43 Secure the catheter in place to ensure that the footplate does not migrate out of position.

Courtesy of Cathy McGowan.

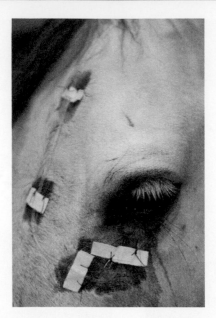

Figure 19.44 Placement of a subpalpebral lavage catheter in the lower eyelid.

Courtesy of Fernando Malalana.

Bandage a limb and foot

Equipment

▸ Soft conforming bandages.
▸ Knitted bandages.
▸ Cotton wool (useful if halved).
▸ Cohesive bandage.
▸ Elastoplast.
▸ ± Primary dressing if wounds present.

Technique

1. Place a primary dressing(s) over any wounds.
2. Apply conforming bandage to the limb, overlapping by half on each turn (same for all layers).
3. Wrap knitted bandage evenly over this layer.
4. Wrap cotton wool down the limb.
5. Wrap knitted bandage evenly and firmly over this layer.
6. ± Repeat a second cotton wool layer (depends on degree of support required/wound exudation).

7. Apply the cohesive bandage firmly but not too tightly.
8. Apply Elastoplast to the top and bottom to prevent migration of material between the bandage and limb.

Foot dressings

▶ A nappy (UK size 4 for most horses) and duct tape are quick, cheap and easy to apply in horses with foot abscesses.
▶ ± Add cotton wool padding if required.

Place a Robert Jones bandage and splints on a limb with a suspected fracture

Equipment

Robert Jones bandage (ranges given for half- and full-limb bandages):

▶ Primary dressing – if required to protect any wound(s).
▶ 15-cm knitted bandages (10–20).
▶ Cotton wool rolls (4–10).
▶ Cohesive bandages (3–7).
▶ Elastoplast (1–2 rolls, more if used instead of cohesive bandages).
▶ Heavy-duty (duct) tape (1–2 rolls).

Splints – whatever you can find (Fig. 19.47):

▶ 5 × 2.5-cm (2 × 1") wooden baton cut to length.
▶ Two broom handles taped together and cut to length.
▶ Fencing rail cut to length.
▶ PVC guttering material (for distal limb – use double, approx. 50-cm long).
▶ ± 12-mm diameter, 3-m-long mild steel rod (certain upper HL fractures).
▶ ± Wooden heel wedge (certain distal limb fractures).

Technique

1. Can be full (to elbow/stifle) or half limb (to carpus/tarsus) depending on the location of the suspected fracture (see Figs 19.45, 19.46).
2. Apply primary dressing and layers as for a normal bandage (see previous section).
3. The layers are repeated until the bandage is 3× the thickness of the limb.
4. Make sure that the layers are not too thick (1.5-cm thickness cotton wool for each).
5. Apply the knitted bandages firmly (↑ pressure with each layer) to ensure suitable compression of the cotton wool layers.
6. Apply additional cotton wool (double-thickness layer) over any areas that narrow on the leg so that a tubular-shaped bandage is created.
7. Finish the bandage with a layer of cohesive bandage and Elastoplast/Elastoplast only.
8. Apply a splint/splints over the bandage if required – the appropriate type will depend on the suspected or known location of the fracture (Figs 19.45, 19.46).
9. Secure the splint firmly in place using large quantities of heavy-duty tape.

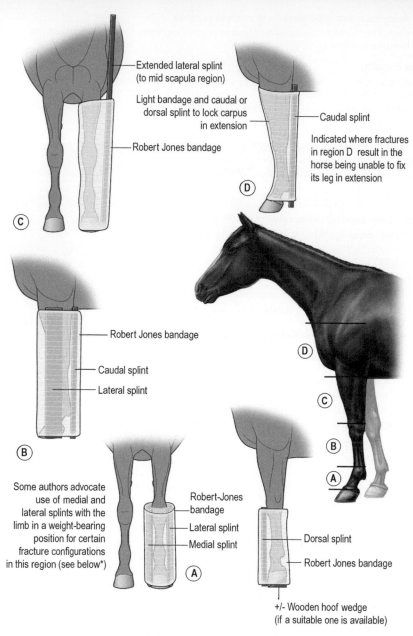

Extended lateral splint
(to mid scapula region)

Light bandage and caudal or
dorsal splint to lock carpus
in extension

Robert Jones bandage

Caudal splint

Indicated where fractures
in region D result in the
horse being unable to fix
its leg in extension

(D)

(C)

Robert Jones bandage

Caudal splint

Lateral splint

(B)

Some authors advocate
use of medial and
lateral splints with the
limb in a weight-bearing
position for certain
fracture configurations
in this region (see below*)

Robert-Jones
bandage

Lateral splint

Medial splint

(A)

(D)

(C)

(B)

(A)

Dorsal splint

Robert Jones bandage

+/- Wooden hoof wedge
(if a suitable one is available)

Figure 19.45 Appropriate bandaging and splinting combinations applied as a first aid measure
depending on the known or suspected location of a forelimb fracture(s) in zones A–D *some surgeons
recommend use of a half limb Robert-Jones bandage together with medial and lateral splints for
suspected P1 or MC/MT3 condylar fractures.

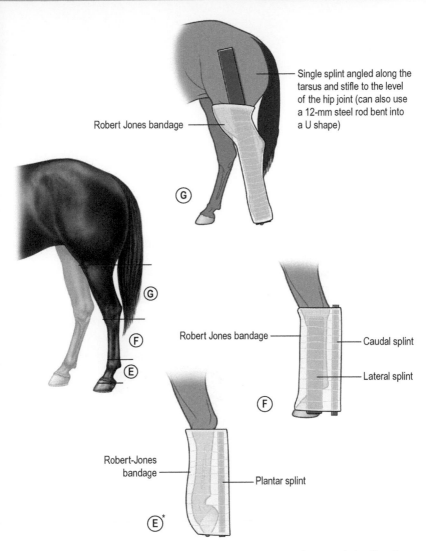

Single splint angled along the tarsus and stifle to the level of the hip joint (can also use a 12-mm steel rod bent into a U shape)

Robert Jones bandage

Ⓖ

Ⓖ

Ⓕ

Ⓔ

Robert Jones bandage — Caudal splint

— Lateral splint

Ⓕ

Robert-Jones bandage

Plantar splint

Ⓔ*

Figure 19.46 Appropriate immobilisation of the hind limb depending on the anatomic location of a suspected fracture (zones E–G). *See comments on splinting of this region in Figure 19.45.

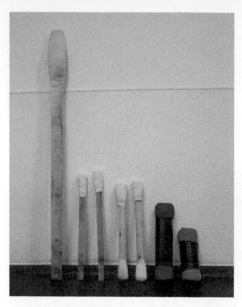

Figure 19.47 Examples of splints that may be required when dealing with a suspected limb fracture.

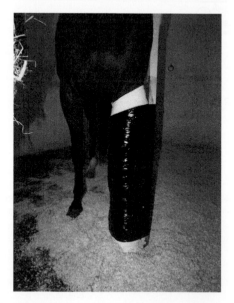

Figure 19.48 Example of full-limb Robert Jones bandage and lateral splint in a horse with a suspected radial fracture.

Isolate a potentially infectious horse

Facilities/equipment

▸ Ideally, the horse should be kept in a separate stable/yard 6–12 m away from other horses that is easy to disinfect (e.g. non-porous walls/floor). See Fig. 19.49.

▸ Footbaths – shallow plastic container filled with disinfectant ± plastic doormat within it.

▸ Disposable gloves.

▸ Foot covers.

▸ Protective overalls.

▸ Barriers.

▸ Stethoscope/thermometer kept outside the stable.

▸ Mucking out and grooming equipment kept with each horse.

▸ Clinical waste bags.

▸ Hand washing facilities.

Ensure that all personnel know the procedures for isolation

▸ Discuss any zoonotic risk (if necessary – see p. 278).

▸ Assign specific people to care for affected horses/deal with them last.

▸ Put on protective clothing before entering the stable, remove and dispose of it appropriately after leaving the stable.

▸ Hand washing (warm water and soap/alcohol gel) following handling of affected horses.

▸ Disinfection of equipment, e.g. stomach tubes.

▸ Stop the area around the stable being used as a passageway.

▸ Limit visitors and stop movement of horses on/off the yard until any disease outbreak has been contained (depending on the suspected pathogen).

Cleaning/disinfection

▸ There are a variety of disinfectants on the market – choose the most appropriate one depending on the pathogen involved and surface (see texts/manufacturer instructions).

Perform euthanasia

Checklist before performing euthanasia

▸ Ensure appropriate appraisal of the horse has been performed – do not be forced into making any rushed decisions about emergency euthanasia (see p. 328).

▸ Obtain a second opinion from another veterinary surgeon if unsure about any decision being taken.

▶ Ensure a consent form has been signed (owner/relevant connections), the insurance company has been contacted (if relevant/possible) and the horse has been correctly identified.

▶ Where the owner is not present, you may have to proceed with only verbal consent (record time, details of conversation).

▶ In the UK, the police have power to authorise euthanasia without the owner's permission.

▶ If there is no owner or police officer present and the horse requires immediate euthanasia, the welfare of the horse must take priority – use clinical judgement (take photos and keep detailed notes of injuries sustained), get an opinion from a second veterinary surgeon (over the telephone if required) and obtain written statements from reliable witnesses.

Performing euthanasia

▶ Check you have the necessary equipment/drugs (Table 19.7)
▶ Check that the site is suitable (unless the horse is stuck/recumbent):
  ▪ consider safety issues
  ▪ out of view of general public/screens used
  ▪ access for removal of the body.
▶ Check that you have a back-up plan if things go wrong (e.g. additional method of euthanasia or additional euthanasia solution).
▶ Ensure the horse's head is properly restrained.
▶ ± Use lunge lines to restrain the horse.
▶ If the horse is fractious/distressed – sedate with α2-agonist/butorphanol first (do not use xylazine if Somulose® is going to be used).
▶ If the IV route is being used, place a 14G catheter (may have to inject off the needle if insufficient time to do this).
▶ Check that assistants have been informed of the procedure, what to expect and not to approach horse during the agonal phase.
▶ Following euthanasia, check the horse is dead:
  ▪ absence of corneal reflex and heart beat (auscultation).

Examine a placenta and investigate a case of abortion/stillbirth

Ideally samples should be submitted to a laboratory that is experienced in dealing with cases of equine abortion. In this case, send the entire foetus, placenta and umbilical cord within two sealed, strong plastic sacs (contact the laboratory first). If this is not possible, examination can be performed on site with submission of samples for further testing. Also ensure that management strategies have been implemented to ↓ risk of abortion occurring in other mares on site (see p. 159), particularly until EHV-1 has been ruled out as a cause.

Examination of the placenta

▶ Weigh the total placental membranes (amnion, chorioallantois and umbilical cord).
▶ Weigh the chorioallantois only.
▶ Inspect the side that is outermost first (usually the allantoic side):
  ▪ spread out into an F-shape
  ▪ check for twinning.

Table 19.7 Options for euthanasia in the horse

Option	Technique	Comments
Quinalbarbitone/ cinchocaine hydrochloride (Somulose®)	Place 14G IV catheter into jugular vein – ideally, do not inject off the needle Inject over 10–15s (speed of injection is important)	Ensure it has not crystallised Do not pre-sedate with xylazine (horses can react violently when solution is injected)
Pentobarbitone (140mg/kg IV)	Inject rapidly Collapse in 35–40s Death 90–150s later	Can collapse violently unless adequately sedated
Free bullet (must have appropriate firearm and licence)	Check no-one is standing in the line of fire Do not cock the hammer until it is brought up to the horse's head Place just below the base of forelock on the midline and aim down the spinal canal (be aware of the position of the horse's head and body). See Figure 19.50	Sedate beforehand (strongly recommended) Cardiac activity may be detected for 15min Use IV agents if unsuccessful
Euthanasia during general anaesthesia	Pentobarbital or concentrated solution of potassium chloride is injected until cardiac arrest occurs	Horse must be under a surgical plane of anaesthesia if potassium chloride is used
Captive bolt	Acceptable if person has suitable experience - brain must be pithed afterwards	
Sedation/GA and aortic transection	Only acceptable if the horse is anaesthetised/heavily sedated Danger to operator Scalpel blade inserted per rectum and used to transect the abdominal aorta	**This must only be used as a last resort where no other option is available** **It is unacceptable to perform this in a conscious or lightly sedated horse**

▶ Assess the allantoic surface (smooth, avillous and pale) (Fig. 19.51):

  ■ assess the allantoic vessels
  ■ piece the blood vessels together and check no portions are missing (particularly the horn tips).

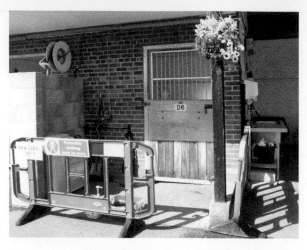

Figure 19.49 Placement of a horse with a possible infectious disease in isolation on a yard.

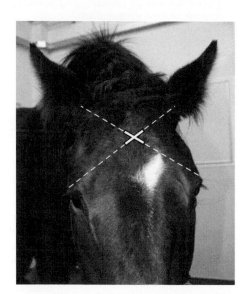

Figure 19.50 Location of bullet entry point at the intersection of lines placed between the middle of the base of the ear and the contralateral lateral canthus of the eye. The gun should be angled (depending on the position of the horse's head and neck) so that the bullet trajectory is down the spinal column.

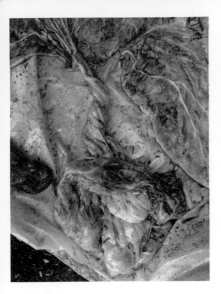

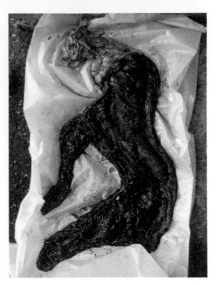

Figure 19.51 Examination of the allantoic surface of the placenta and the umbilical cord.

Figure 19.52 Examination of the chorion of the placenta (dark red, velvet appearance).

▶ Measure the umbilical cord (normal = 36–83 cm, >84 cm high risk for torsion of cord).
▶ Assess the umbilical cord for:
  ▪ oedema
  ▪ focal swellings
  ▪ roughening of the surface/plaques
  ▪ vessel appearance.
▶ Reposition the placenta with the chorion outward (normal = dark red, velvet appearance; Fig. 19.52):
  ▪ assess for abnormal colour/thickness/loss of villous pattern/exudates/tears/shape
    » (tears can be misleading if the mare has stood on it).
▶ Take swabs for microbiology (including at the cervical star).
▶ Take photographs of any lesions identified and record findings.
▶ Place samples of placenta from various sites and place into formalin and viral transport medium (or a sterile container).

Post-mortem examination of foetus/neonate

▶ Weigh.
▶ Place on RHS.
▶ Measure crown–rump length.
▶ Check for congenital defects (umbilical hernia, cleft palate, skeletal deformities).
▶ Record the degree of autolysis and rigor.
▶ Check the umbilicus.

▶ Reflect LF and LH over the back.

▶ Open up the left side of the thorax and abdomen.

▶ Look for excess serosal fluids.

▶ Perform microbiological sampling:

  ▪ use a sterile disposable forceps and scalpel to remove samples of liver, spleen, lung, and thymus into viral transport medium/sterile container for EHV testing

  ▪ take aseptic swabs from the liver, heart, lung and stomach.

▶ Evaluate organs in situ, then remove each.

▶ Check for rib fractures, cardiac bruising, lung aeration.

▶ Check for meconium in stomach/lungs.

▶ Slice organs and, in addition to the samples collected earlier for virology, put pieces (~1 cm diameter) into formalin (spleen, liver, adrenal glands, kidneys, lungs, thymus, heart and thyroid gland).

▶ Check bladder and urachus.

▶ Open limb joints – assess for haemorrhage (especially shoulders and hips).

▶ Remove and split skull if possible – check for haemorrhage and take brain samples if indicated.

▶ Neonate PM – similar approach as for foetus, with the addition of:

  ▪ check for any birth injuries

  ▪ take blood sample for serum IgG

  ▪ herpes virus samples for PCR from tissues as above

  ▪ if neurological signs, take CSF sample from atlanto-occipital site, swab from the meninges and place samples of brain tissue in viral transport medium. Fix the remainder of the brain in an adequate volume of formalin.

  ▪ bacteriology: swab heart blood, liver, lung, kidney, suspected site of infection, e.g. joint, umbilicus, brain

  ▪ take relevant samples for histology.

Perform a field post-mortem

Issues to consider prior to proceeding

▶ Check that the horse does not need to be sent to a specific centre: e.g. as required by insurance company, sport regulatory body, owner request.

▶ If there are potential legal issues, e.g. conflict of interest, this may need to be performed by a different veterinary surgeon/with witnesses present.

▶ Check whether the horse died/was euthanased due to a potentially zoonotic disease – in these situations, PM examination must be performed at a suitable facility with the necessary safety procedures (or in cases such as Hendra virus, may be deemed too risky to perform).

▶ Ideally this is best performed where there are dedicated PM facilities.

▶ PM can be performed on premises – ensure that the following are available:

  ▪ good lighting

  ▪ away from general public viewing/other animals

  ▪ access for disposal of a large carcass

  ▪ containers for disposal of waste

  ▪ water supply

Table 19.8 Equipment required for post-mortem examination

Record keeping	Protective clothing/ disinfection	Dissection, examination and sampling
Clipboard	Waterproof boots	Scalpel blades (Nos. 11 and 22) and handles
Paper (pre-printed checklists very useful)	Overalls	Hacksaw
Pens (including waterproof markers)	Gloves	Bone forceps/rib-cutters
Ruler/tape measure	Plastic apron	Deboning knife
Camera	± Protective eyewear	Forceps
Microchip scanner	Disinfectants for cleaning equipment, clothing and surroundings	Scissors
Scales		Bacteriology swabs (standard and charcoal)
		Blood tubes
		Umbilical tape
		Plastic sealable bags
		Identification tags
		Cutting board(s)
		Leak-proof containers – sample pots, jars and plastic tubs
		Sharps disposal container
		10% formalin

- drainage for disinfection
- human first aid kit/telephone (in case of human injury during the procedure)
- additional personnel to assist with sample collection/taking of photographs
- The necessary equipment is listed in Table 19.8 (above).

Initial procedure

▶ Obtain a full history, including:
  - recent medical history/events leading up to death or euthanasia
  - details of the method and time of euthanasia and carcass storage.
▶ Perform a rigorous, systematic examination.
▶ Keep good records, including the results of any tests.
▶ In welfare and forensic cases, ensure all identifying features are recorded, including:
  - body condition score
  - foot care
  - presence of any external wounds
  - age of any lesions evident
  - evidence of parasitism.

External examination

- ▶ Check for microchip and note coat colour, markings, tattoos/brands/tags.
- ▶ Assess BCS, haircoat and for evidence of external parasites/clip marks/surgical wounds/ catheterisation.
- ▶ Examine for skin lesions/wounds/swellings/depressions/prolapses.
- ▶ Assess state of rigor/hydration/abdominal tympany.
- ▶ Assess external orifices, eyes and conjunctiva.
- ▶ Obtain a jugular blood sample (plain blood tube ± blood culture medium).
- ▶ ± Obtain CSF sample prior to removal of head (sudden death/neurological cases):
  - ▪ flex head until it is 90° to the neck, advance a spinal needle from the rostral edge of the atlas wings, advance towards the nose and aim sagitally.

Internal examination

- ▶ Open carcass:
  - ▪ lateral recumbency (can do in dorsal)
  - ▪ check mammary glands/penis/testicles
  - ▪ make a midline incision, reflect the skin and remove upper FL and HL.
- ▶ Open the abdominal and thoracic cavities:
  - ▪ incise abdominal musculature as a flap
  - ▪ check volume and nature of peritoneal fluid
  - ▪ assess mesenteric and retroperitoneal fat (especially welfare cases)
  - ▪ check the diaphragm and remove attachment
  - ▪ remove the rib cage at its dorsal and ventral extremities.
- ▶ Collect bone marrow from the end of the rib (suction into syringe). Look for gelatinous fat atrophy in welfare cases. If the carcase is not fresh, take a sample of sterum for histology.
- ▶ Examine the GIT:
  - ▪ assess position of organs/tissue compromise
  - ▪ examine large colon and caecum
  - ▪ ligate and cut small colon and oesophagus
  - ▪ detach the mesenteric attachments and remove the GIT
  - ▪ open the stomach and check the entire length of the GIT (± take samples of ingesta)
  - ▪ check the pancreas.
- ▶ Remove liver, kidneys and spleen:
  - ▪ check liver, kidneys, adrenal glands and coeliaco-mesenteric ganglion (craniomedial to left adrenal gland) and spleen
  - ▪ incise into and take any samples (± coeliaco-mesenteric ganglion for EGS confirmation).
- ▶ Open the abdominal aorta.
- ▶ Open the pelvic cavity and remove and examine the urogenital organs:
  - ▪ ± take urine sample.
- ▶ Remove the cardiopulmonary system:
  - ▪ assess thyroid glands
  - ▪ open up the trachea and oesophagus
  - ▪ assess the lungs
  - ▪ open up both sides of the heart and examine the valves/endocardium
  - ▪ assess the coronary fat reserves in welfare cases.

▶ Examine the head and neck:
  ▪ remove skin over head
  ▪ open up the mouth
  ▪ remove the brain
  ▪ examination of the neck in sudden death/neurological/neck trauma cases
  ▪ neck shape, muscle bruising, spinal cord.
▶ Examine the musculoskeletal system:
  ▪ open the limb joints – sepsis/degenerative changes
  ▪ ± take samples from muscles (include diaphragm, intercostal muscles and postural muscles if atypical myopathy suspected).

Where lesion(s) are identified document:

▶ Organ involved and location of lesion.
▶ Size, shape and colour of lesions.
▶ Alterations in surface texture.
▶ Number of lesions/percentage of organ affected.
▶ Contents of lesion, e.g. purulent/haemorrhagic material.
▶ Photographs of lesions/organs useful – label with case number/animal name, cm scale.

Samples to take

▶ Bacteriological swabs – take samples before incising into organs.
▶ Tissue samples from organs of interest/lesions:
  ▪ placed in 10% formalin with ratio of 10:1 formalin:tissue.
▶ Brain – fix whole.
▶ Eye – can inject formalin into the eye to assist preservation.
▶ Fluids for culture – plain blood tubes.
▶ Cytology – EDTA (± a few drops of formalin, especially if contaminated); direct impression smears from lesions.
▶ Faeces for culture/parasitology.
▶ Fresh, unfixed tissues – microbiology/virology or toxicology:
  ▪ place in sealed plastic bags and send on ice.

References and further reading

• Claes, A., Ball, B.A., Brown, J.A., 2008. Evaluation of risk factors, management and outcome associated with rectal tears in horses: 99 cases (1985–2006). J. Am. Vet. Med. Assoc. 233, 1605–1609.

• Dugdale, A., 2010. Veterinary Anaesthesia: Principles to Practice. Wiley Blackwell, Chichester, UK.

• Durham, A.E., 1996. Blood and plasma transfusion in the horse. Equine Vet. Educ. 8, 8–12.

• Hart, K.A., 2011. Pathogenesis, management and prevention of blood transfusion reactions in horses. Equine Vet. Educ. 23, 343–345.

• Jones, R., 1996. Equine euthanasia in the competition situation. In: Dyson, S. (Ed.), British Equine Veterinary Association Manual: A Guide to the Management of Emergencies at Equine Competitions. Equine Veterinary Journal Ltd, Newmarket, UK, pp. 116–121.

• Knottenbelt, D.C., 2006. Equine Formulary (fourth ed.). Elsevier, St. Louis, Missouri.

- **Moyer, W., Schumacher, J., Schumacher, J.,** 2011. In: Equine Joint Injection and Regional Anesthesia. Academic Veterinary Solutions, LLC, Pennsylvania.

- **Senior, M.,** 2008. I need to sedate it but I can't get near. In: Proceedings of the 47th British Equine Veterinary Association Congress 2008. Liverpool, UK, pp. 183–184.

- **Walmsley, J.,** 1999. Emergency management of fractures in horses. In Pract. 21, 122–127.

- **Whitwell, K.,** 2009. Postmortem examination of horses. In Pract. 31, 104–113.

- **Whitwell, K.,** 2009. How to examine a mare's placenta. In: Proceedings of the 48th British Equine Veterinary Association Congress 2009. Brimingham, UK, p. 48.

- **Williams, K.J.,** 2009. Field necropsy of the horse. In: Robinson, N.E., Sprayberry, K.A. (Eds.), Current Therapy in Equine Medicine (sixth ed.). Elsevier, St. Louis, Missouri, pp. 47–52.

Index

Note: Page numbers followed by "*f*", "*t*" and "*b*" refers to figures, tables and boxes respectively.

C

Full into, eyes astream with cold—

With cold?
All right then. With self-knowledge.

Indoors at last, the pages of *Time* are apt
To open, and the illustrated mayor of New York,
Given a glimpse of how and where I work,
To note yet one more house that can be scrapped.

Unwillingly I picture
My walls weathering in the general view.
It is not even as though the new
Buildings did very much for architecture.

Suppose they did. The sickness of our time requires
That these as well be blasted in their prime.
You would think the simple fact of having lasted
Threatened our cities like mysterious fires.

There are certain phrases which to use in a poem
Is like rubbing silver with quicksilver. Bright
But facile, the glamour deadens overnight.
For instance, how 'the sickness of our time'

Enhances, then debases, what I feel.
At my desk I swallow in a glass of water
No longer cordial, scarcely wet, a pill
They had told me not to take until much later.

With the result that back into my imagination
The city glides, like cities seen from the air,
Mere smoke and sparkle to the passenger
Having in mind another destination

Which now is not that honey-slow descent
Of the Champs-Elysées, her hand in his,
But the dull need to make some kind of house
Out of the life lived, out of the love spent.

The whiteness near and far.
The cold, the hush. . . .
A first word stops
The blizzard, steps
Out into fresh
Candor. You ask no more.

Each never taken stride
Leads onward, though
In circles ever
Smaller, smaller.
The vertigo
Upholds you. And now to glide

Across the frozen pond,
Steelshod, to chase
Its dreamless oval
With loop and spiral
Until (your face
Downshining, lidded, drained

Of any need to know
What hid, what called,
Wisdom or error,
Beneath that mirror)
The page you scrawled
Turns. A new day. Fresh snow.

One winter morning as a child
Upon the windowpane's thin frost I drew
Forehead and eyes and mouth the clear and mild
Features of nobody I knew

And then abstracted looking through
This or that wet transparent line
Beyond beheld a winter garden so
Heavy with snow its hedge of pine

And sun so brilliant on the snow
I breathed my pleasure out onto the chill pane
Only to see its angel fade in mist.
I was a child, I did not know

That what I longed for would resist
Neither what cold lines should my finger trace
On colder grounds before I found anew
In yours the features of that face

Whose words whose looks alone undo
Such frosts I lay me down in love in fear
At how they melt become a blossoming pear
Joy outstretched in our bodies' place.

POEM OF SUMMER'S END

The morning of the equinox
Begins with brassy clouds and cocks.
All the inn's shutters clatter wide
Upon Fair Umbria. Twitching at my side
You burrow in sleep like a red fox.

Mostly, these weeks, we toss all night, we touch
By accident. The heat! The food!
Groggily aware of spots that itch
I curse the tiny creatures which
Have flecked our mended sheets with blood.

At noon in a high wind, to bell and song,
Upon the shoulders of the throng,
The gilt bronze image of St. So-and-So
Heaves precipitously along.
Worship has worn away his toe,

Nevertheless the foot, thrust forward, dips
Again, again, into its doom of lips
And tears, a vortex of black shawls,
Garlic, frankincense, Popery, festivals
Held at the moon's eclipse,

As in their trance the faithful pass
On to piazza and café.
We go deliberately the other way
Through the town gates, lie down in grass.
But the wind howls, the sky turns color-of-clay.

The time for making love is done.
A far off, sulphur-pale façade
Gleams and goes out. It is as though by one
Flash of lightning all things made
Had glimpsed their maker's heart, read and obeyed.

Back on our bed of iron and lace
We listen to the loud rain fracture space,
And let at first each other's hair
Be lost in gloom, then lips, then the whole face.
If either speaks the other does not hear.

For a decade love has rained down
On our two hearts, instructing them
In a strange bareness, that of weathered stone.
Thinking how bare our hearts have grown
I do not know if I feel pride or shame.

The time has passed to go and eat.
Has it? I do not know. A beam of light
Reveals you calm but strangely white.
A final drop of rain clicks in the street.
Somewhere a clock strikes. It is not too late

To set out dazed, sit side by side
In the one decent restaurant.
The handsome boy who has already tried
To interest you (and been half gratified)
Helps us to think of what we want.

I do not know—have I ever known?—
Unless concealed in the next town,
In the next image blind with use, a clue,
A worn path, points the long way round back to
The springs we started out from. Sun

Weaker each sunrise reddens that slow maze
So freely entered. Now come days
When lover and beloved know
That love is what they are and where they go.

Each learns to read at length the other's gaze.

AFTER GREECE

Light into the olive entered
And was oil. Rain made the huge pale stones
Shine from within. The moon turned his hair white
Who next stepped from between the columns,
Shielding his eyes. All through
The countryside were old ideas
Found lying open to the elements.
Of the gods' houses only
A minor premise here and there
Would be balancing the heaven of fixed stars
Upon a Doric capital. The rest
Lay spilled, their fluted drums half sunk in cyclamen
Or deep in water's biting clarity
Which just barely upheld me
The next week, when I sailed for home.
But where is home—these walls?
These limbs? The very spaniel underfoot
Races in sleep, toward what?
It is autumn. I did not invite
Those guests, windy and brittle, who drink my liquor.
Returning from a walk I find
The bottles filled with spleen, my room itself
Smeared by reflection onto the far hemlocks.
I some days flee in dream
Back to the exposed porch of the maidens
Only to find my great-great-grandmothers
Erect there, peering
Into a globe of red Bohemian glass.
As it swells and sinks, I call up
Graces, Furies, Fates, removed
To my country's warm, lit halls, with rivets forced

Through drapery, and nothing left to bear.
They seem anxious to know
What holds up heaven nowadays.
I start explaining how in that vast fire
Were other irons—well, Art, Public Spirit,
Ignorance, Economics, Love of Self,
Hatred of Self, a hundred more,
Each burning to be felt, each dedicated
To sparing us the worst; how I distrust them
As I should have done those ladies; how I want
Essentials: salt, wine, olive, the light, the scream—
No! I have scarcely named you,
And look, in a flash you stand full-grown before me,
Row upon row, Essentials,
Dressed like your sister caryatids
Or tombstone angels jealous of their dead,
With undulant coiffures, lips weathered, cracked by grime,
And faultless eyes gone blank beneath the immense
Zinc and gunmetal northern sky . . .
Stay then. Perhaps the system
Calls for spirits. This first glass I down
To the last time
I ate and drank in that old world. May I
Also survive its meanings, and my own.

It is still early, yet
Clear waves of heat,
Eye-watering, dilute
What powers drive
The warped pine to the brink.
You, too, must conquer
Involuntary nausea
Before you look. Far under-
foot are your wept-over
Sunsets, your every year
Deepened perspectives, layer
On monstrous layer of mouse,
Marigold, madder—
All petrifying, not
To be approached without
Propitiatory oohs.
By all means undertake
A descent on gargoyle-faced ass-back
To the degrading yellow
River. This first mistake
Made by your country is also
The most sublime.
Now let its convulsions
Mimic your heart's
And you will guess the source.
Be strong then. Find no fault
With the white-wigged, the quartz-
Pated up there, wrapped
In whipping vestments, neither
Man can corrupt
Nor heaven wholly melt.

They have sat a long time
In one of our highest courts.

Having lately taken up residence
In a suite of chambers
Windless, compact and sunny, ideal
Lodging for the pituitary gland of Euclid
If not for a "single gentleman (references),"
You have grown used to the playful inconveniences,
The floors that slide from under you helter-skelter,
Invisible walls put up in mid-
Stride, leaving you warped for the rest of the day,
A spoon in water; also that pounce
Of wild color from corner to page,
Straightway consuming the latter
Down to your very signature,
After which there is nothing to do but retire,
Licking the burn, into—into—
Look: (Heretofore
One could have said where one was looking,
In or out. But now it almost—) Look:
You dreamed of this:
To fuse in borrowed fires, to drown
In depths that were not there. You meant
To rest your bones in a maroon plush box,
Doze the old vaudeville out, of mind and object,
Little foreseeing their effect on you,
Those dagger-eyed insatiate performers
Who from the first false insight
To the most recent betrayal of outlook,
Crystal, hypnotic atom,
Have held you rapt, the proof, the child
Wanted by neither. Now and then
It is given to see clearly. There

Is what remains ofyou, a body
Unshaven, flung on the sofa. Stains of egg
Harden about the mouth, smoke still
Rises between fingers or from nostrils.
The eyes deflect the stars through years of vacancy.
Your agitation at such moments
Is all too human. You and the stars
Seem both endangered, each
At the other's utter mercy. Yet the gem
Revolves in space, the vision shuttles off.
A toneless waltz glints through the pea-sized funhouse.
The day is breaking someone else's heart.

FOR PROUST

Over and over something would remain
Unbalanced in the painful sum of things.
Past midnight you arose, rang for your things.
You had to go into the world again.

You stop for breath outside the lit hotel,
A thin spoon bitter stimulants will stir.
Jean takes your elbow, Jacques your coat. The stir
Spreads—you are known to all the personnel—

As through packed public rooms you press (impending
Palms, chandeliers, orchestras, more palms,
The fracas and the fragrance) until your palms
Are moist with fear that you will miss the friend

Conjured—but she is waiting: a child still
At first glance, hung with fringes, on the low
Ottoman. In a voice reproachful and low
She says she understands you have been ill.

And you, because your time is running out,
Laugh in denial and begin to phrase
Your questions. There had been a little phrase
She hummed, you could not sleep tonight without

Hearing again. Then, of that day she had sworn
To come, and did not, was evasive later,
Would she not speak the truth two decades later,
From loving-kindness learned if not inborn?

She treats you to a look you cherished, light,
Bold: '*Mon ami*, how did we get along
At all, those years?' But in her hair a long
White lock has made its truce with appetite.

And presently she rises. Though in pain
You let her leave—the loved one always leaves.
What of the little phrase? Its notes, like leaves
In the strong tea you have contrived to drain,

Strangely intensify what you must do.
Back where you came from, up the strait stair, past
All understanding, bearing the whole past,
Your eyes grown wide and dark, eyes of a Jew,

You make for one dim room without contour
And station yourself there, beyond the pale
Of cough or of gardenia, erect, pale.
What happened is becoming literature.

Feverish in time, if you suspend the task,
An old, old woman shuffling in to draw
Curtains, will read a line or two, withdraw.
The world will have put on a thin gold mask.

My mother's lamp once out,
I press a different switch:
A field within the dim
White screen ignites,
Vibrating to the rapt
Mechanical racket
Of a real noon field's
Crickets and gnats.

And to its candid heart
I move with heart ajar,
With eyes that smart less
From pollen or heat
Than from the buried day
Now rising like a moon,
Shining, unwinding
Its taut white sheet.

Two or three bugs that lit
Earlier upon the blank
Sheen, all peaceable
Insensibility, drowse
As she and I cannot
Under the risen flood
Of thirty years ago—
A tree, a house

We had then, a late sun,
A door from which the primal
Figures jerky and blurred
As lightning bugs

From lanterns issue, next
To be taken for stars,
For fates. With knowing smiles
And beaded shrugs

My mother and two aunts
Loom on the screen. Their plucked
Brows pucker, their arms encircle
One another.
Their ashen lips move.
From the love seat's gloom
A quiet chuckle escapes
My white-haired mother

To see in that final light
A man's shadow mount
Her dress. And now she is
Advancing, sister-
less, but followed by
A fair child, or fury—
Myself at four, in tears.
I raise my fist,

Strike, she kneels down. The man's
Shadow afflicts us both.
Her voice behind me says
It might go slower.
I work dials, the film jams.
Our headstrong old projector
Glares at the scene which promptly
Catches fire.

Puzzled, we watch ourselves
Turn red and black, gone up
In a puff of smoke now coiling
Down fierce beams.
I switch them off. A silence.
Your father, she remarks,
Took those pictures; later
Says pleasant dreams,

Rises and goes. Alone
I gradually fade and cool.
Night scatters me with green
Rustlings, thin cries.
Out there between the pines
Have begun shining deeds,
Some low, inconstant (these
Would be fireflies),

Others as in high wind
Aflicker, staying lit.
There are nights we seem to ride
With cross and crown
Forth under them, through fumes,
Coils, the whole rattling epic—
Only to leap clear-eyed
From eiderdown,

Asleep to what we'd seen.
Father already fading—
Who focused your life long
Through little frames,

Whose microscope, now deep
In purple velvet, first
Showed me the skulls of flies,
The fur, the flames

Etching the jaws—father:
Shrunken to our true size.
Each morning, back of us,
Fields wail and shimmer.
To go out is to fall
Under fresh spells, cool web
And stinging song new-hatched
Each day, all summer.

A minute galaxy
About my head will easily
Needle me back. The day's
Inaugural *Damn*
Spoken, I start to run,
Inane, like them, but breathing
In and out the sun
And air I am.

The son and heir! In the dark
It makes me catch my breath
And hear, from upstairs, hers—
That faintest hiss
And slither, as of life
Escaping into space,
Having led its characters
To the abyss

Of night. Immensely still
The heavens glisten. One broad
Path of vague stars is floating
Off, a shed skin
Of all whose fine cold eyes
First told us, locked in ours:
You are the heroes without name
Or origin.

THE LAWN FETE OF HOMUNCULUS ARTIFEX

for Fred and Sandra Segal

Moisten me, press me,
Mold me to tumbler, to tin,
The shallow, the tall, confuse me
With straw and leave me
Where sun is hottest, patted into hills.
Do not forget this bit of mirror:
Half buried in my breast, it will store up
The white blues and the yellow blues of skies
Under which one dreams of living.
There, it is done! Meanwhile
The dishes shall be ceremoniously dotted
With petal of geranium, berries or pebbles,
That there may arise from them
An illusion of food and drink,
A hunger then, a zest for life
Peculiar to those not quite alive,
Who only dream of living, who are not born
In childbed, rather in some hour tense with charms
Glancing off the alembic's giant scrotum
Till sun and moon conjoin, and all is dark
As the wizard's robe, as his drenched brow.
When he could do no more
He fell back spent. Our little party
Got under way as best it could. The twigs
Unclenched, the greedy rosebuds caked with smut.
The ill-knit creatures, now in hues
Of sunstroke, mulberry, white of clown,
Yellow of bile, bruise-blacks-and-blues,
Stumped outward, waving matchstick arms,
Colliding, poking, hurt, in tears

(For the wound became an eye)
Toward the exciting, hostile greens
And the spread cloths of Art.
Already openly in love
With what he saw, one of us disregarded
Common background or future union
Through dissolution in the first real rain
Enough to cry, addressing who
Or what he could not say, "Invest me
With nuance, place on me
Your conical hat of stars,
Hand me the hazel wand
That was my hand—
It stirs! It bends!
When I am base again, and my name mud,
You'll have this likeness of me with a dozen
Of my three billion closest friends."

THE WORLD AND THE CHILD

Letting his wisdom be the whole of love,
The father tiptoes out, backwards. A gleam
Falls on the child awake and wearied of,

Then, as the door clicks shut, is snuffed. The glove-
Gray afterglow appalls him. It would seem
That letting wisdom be the whole of love

Were pastime even for the bitter grove
Outside, whose owl's white hoot of disesteem
Falls on the child awake and wearied of.

He lies awake in pain, he does not move,
He will not scream. Any who heard him scream
Would let their wisdom be the whole of love.

People have filled the room he lies above.
Their talk, mild variation, chilling theme,
Falls on the child. Awake and wearied of

Mere pain, mere wisdom also, he would have
All the world waking from its winter dream,
Letting its wisdom be. The whole of love
Falls on the child awake and wearied of.

CHILDLESSNESS

The weather of this winter night, my dream-wife
Ranting and raining, wakes me. Her cloak blown back
To show the lining's dull lead foil
Sweeps along asphalt. Houses
Look blindly on; one glimmers through a blind.
Outside, I hear her tricklings
Arraign my little plot:
Had it or not agreed
To transplantation for the common good
Of certain rare growths yielding guaranteed
Gold pollen, gender of suns, large, hardy,
Enviable blooms? But in my garden
Nothing is planted. Neither
Is that glimmering window mine.
I lie and think about the rain,
How it has been drawn up from the impure ocean,
From gardens lightly, deliberately tainted;
How it falls back, time after time,
Through poisons visible at sunset
When the enchantress, masked as friend, unfurls
Entire bolts of voluminous pistachio,
Saffron, and rose.
These, as I fall back to sleep,
And other slow colors clothe me, glide
To rest, then burst along my limbs like buds,
Like bombs from the navigator's vantage,
Waking me, lulling me. Later I am shown
The erased metropolis reassembled
On sampans, freighted each
With toddlers, holy dolls, dead ancestors.
One tiny monkey puzzles over fruit.

The vision rises and falls, the garland
Gently takes root
In the sea's coma. Hours go by
Before I can stand to own
A sky stained red, a world
Clad only in rags, threadbare,
Dabbling the highway's ice with blood.
A world. The cloak thrown down for it to wear
In token of past servitude
Has fallen onto the shoulders of my parents
Whom it is eating to the bone.

GETTING THROUGH

I wrote the postcard to you and went out
Through melting snow to mail it. Old Miss Tree
Buttonholed me at the corner with something about
Today being our last chance. Indeed? Well, well,
Not hers and mine, I trusted gallantly,
Disengaging her knuckle from my lapel.

First thing on entering the Post Office,
I made out through my pigeonhole's dim pane
An envelope from you. Cheered up by this,
Card between teeth, I twirled the dials; they whirred
But the lock held. One, two, three times. In vain.
At the stamp window I called for Mr. Bird,

Our friendly Postmaster. Not a soul replied.
Bags of mail lay in heaps, lashed shut, the late
Snowlight upon them. When at last I tried
To avail myself of the emergency stamp machine,
A cancelled 20 franc imperforate
From Madagascar slid out, mocking, green.

Nerves, I thought, wishing more than ever now
You had not gone away, considering mailing
My card unstamped, presuming that somehow. . . .
What's this! Your envelope lies at my feet,
Ripped open, empty, my name running, paling
From snow tracked in by me. Outside, Main Street

Is empty—no: a Telephone Company truck.
Why, I can phone! The mere sound of my voice
Will melt you, help decide you to come back.

But as I hurry home a water drop
Stops me, then little rainbow husks of ice—
From the telephone pole. There at the shivering top

Two men in rubber boots are cutting wires
Which heavily dangle from a further pole.
(Oh, May Day ribbons! Child our town attires
As Queen in tablecloth and paper crown,
Lurching down Main Street blindly as a mole!)
When the last wire is severed I lurch down

The street myself, my blankness exquisite.
Beyond a juniper hedge sits Mrs. Stone,
Mute on her dazzling lawn. Bracing to sit
In such fresh snow, I brightly call. Her hard
Gaze holds me like amber. I drop my own,
And find I cannot now read the postcard

Still in my grasp, unspotted and uncrushed.
My black inkstrokes hover intensely still
Against the light—starlings gunshot has flushed
That hover one split second, so, then veer
Away for good. The trees weep, as trees will.
Everything is cryptic, crystal-queer.

The stationery store's brow drips, ablaze
Where the pink sun has struck it with the hand
Of one remembering after days and days—
Remembering what? I am a fool, a fool!
I hear with joy, helpless to understand
Cries of snow-crimson children leaving school.

FIVE OLD FAVORITES

1. *A Dream of Old Vienna*

The mother sits, the whites of her eyes tinted
By a gas lamp of red Bohemian glass.
Her one gray lock could be a rosy fireworks.
She hums the galop from Lehár's Requiem Mass.

Deepening a blood-red handkerchief the father
Has drawn over his face, the warm beams wreathe
Its foldings into otherworldly features
Now and then stirred lightly from beneath.

The child, because of his extreme pallor,
Acquires a normal look as the lamp glows,
For which the mother is and is not grateful,
Torn between conflicting libidos.

To wed the son when he has slain the father,
Or thrust the brat *at once* into the damp . . . ?
Such are the throbbing issues that enliven
Many a cozy evening round the lamp.

2. *The Midnight Snack*

When I was little and he was riled
It never entered my father's head
Not to flare up, roar and turn red.
Mother kept cool and smiled.

Now every night I tiptoe straight
Through my darkened kitchen for
The refrigerator door—
It opens, the inviolate!

Illumined as in dreams I take
A glass of milk, a piece of cake,
Then stealthily retire,

Mindful of how the gas stove's black-
Browed pilot eye's blue fire
Burns into my turned back.

3. *Sundown and Starlight*

He licks the tallest tree, and takes a bite.
His day's excess has left him flushed and limp. Then, too,
It is time she changed for the evening. Hadn't she better
Be thinking what to wear? Nothing seems quite

To match her mood. Women! She must consider
One dress after another of pale or fiery hue.
At the hour's end, as foreseen, her favorite dark blue
Comes fold by fold out of its chest of cedar.

His jaws have closed on the tree's base.
Moments like this, he turns into a compulsive eater.
Men! Let him burn all night. She has other things to do
Than care for him. She opens her jewel case.

4. *Event without Particulars*

Something will be hanging from the ceiling—
A dagger fern in chains? Shroud of a chandelier?
One feebly blinking bulb? Be that as it may,
Something you notice right away.

*Something will decorate the wall—*a calendar?
A looking-glass? A scorched place? One never can say.
*And something lie on the table—*a teacup or book
You may care to read if you dare to look.

Then comes the opening of the door.
*Somebody enters—*young, face deep in a nosegay,
Or with a drink, or a crutch and milk-blind eyes.
In any case *you will rise*

And go to her over whatever is underfoot
To make you feel at home, since you have come to stay—
Black and white marble might be used for some;
For others, roses of linoleum.

5. *The Dandelion Sermon*

In the heat of a sentence I stopped. You waited
Complacently, but the mind
Had been breathed upon at last.
Innumerable feathery particles rose in less than wind

Out over the nude waters where both suns
Fierily, the reflected and the seen,
Strove to be one, then perhaps were, within
A white haze not at once or ever with ease construed.

I may be oversusceptible to news
But what I see in the papers leaves me numb.
The bomb. The ultimatum. Wires hum—
Adult impersonators giving interviews,

As if that helped. What would? I've thought of it.
With all due ceremony—flags unfurled,
Choirs, priests—the leaders of a sobered world
Should meet, kneel down, and, joining hands, submit

To execution: say in Rome or Nice—
Towns whose economy depends on crowds.
Ah, but those boys, their heads aren't in the clouds.
They would find reasons not to die for peace.

Damn them. I'd give *my* life. Each day I meet
Men like me, young, indignant. We're not cranks.
Will some of them step up? That's plenty. Thanks.
Now let's move before we get cold feet.

Music we'll need, and short, clear speeches given
Days of maximum coverage in the press.
We'll emphasize disinterestedness,
Drive the point home that someone could be driven

To do this. Where to go? Why not Japan,
Land of the honorable suicide.
And will the world change heart? Until we've tried,
No one can say it will not. No one can.

THE RECONNAISSANCE

Up from the ranks a body volunteers
For the difficult assignment, hears
That it may not come back, smartly replies
Far better I than you, Sir. Tears
Spring to the General's eyes.

The body now dons a disguise
That turns it thin and sallow. It is gowned
In white, and given to memorize
Things to be heard by none but a renowned
Leader of the Underground.

Fevers. Vigils. Not till the sixth moon's
Dead shimmer gloats upon the last
River struggled across, is the pigeon released
Whose return to Headquarters invariably means
Mission Accomplished.

The General stiffens. He began
As a young officer learning strategy,
Also the languages of flower and fan.
In those days would he have made so free
With the life of any man?

Dully he lifts a gloved fist to his face.
The tears however do not fall.
Too few are left and he will need them all
Now word has come of an unassailable place
Far from the sirens' call.

When I was four or so
I used to read aloud
To you—I mean, recite
Stories both of us knew
By heart, the book held close
To even then nearsighted
Eyes. It was morning. You,
Still in your nightgown
Over cold tea, would nod
Approval. Once I caught
A gay note in your quiet:
The book was upside down.

Now all is upside down.
I sit while you babble.
I watch your sightless face
Jerked swiftly here and there,
Set in a puzzled frown.
Your face! It is no more yours
Than its reflected double
Bobbing on scummed water.
Other days, the long pure
Sobs break from a choked source
Nobody here would dare
Fathom, even if able.

With you no longer able,
I tried to keep apart,
At first, or to set right
The stories you would tell.
The European trip,
The fire of 1908—

I could reel them off in sleep,
Given a phrase to start;
Chimneys of kerosene
Lamps only you could clean
Because your hands were small . . .
I have them all by heart

But cannot now find heart
To hinder them from growing
Together, wrong, absurd.
Do as you must, poor stranger.
There is no surer craft
To take you where you are going
—A story I have heard
And shall over and over
Till you are indeed gone.
Last night the mockingbird
Wept and laughed, wept and laughed,
Telling it to the moon.

Your entire honeymoon,
A ride in a rowboat
On the St. Johns River,
Took up an afternoon.
And by that time, of course,
The water hyacinth
Had come here from Japan,
A mauve and rootless guest
Thirsty for life, afloat
With you on the broad span
It would in sixty years
So vividly congest.

ANNIE HILL'S GRAVE

Amen. The casket like a spaceship bears her
In streamlined, airtight comfort underground.
Necropolis is a nice place to visit;
One would not want to live there all year round.

So think the children of its dead, emerging
From shadow by the small deep gates of clay,
Exclaiming softly, joyful if bewildered,
To see each other rouged, heads bald or gray.

Some have not met, though constant to the City,
For decades. Now their slowly sunnier
Counterclockwise movement, linked and loving,
Slackens the whirlpool that has swallowed her.

Alone, she grips, against confusion, pictures
Of us the living, and of the tall youth
She wed but has not seen for thirty summers.
Used to the dark, he lies in the next booth,

Part of that whole, poor, overpopulated
Land of our dreams, that 'instant' space
—To have again, just add stars, wind, and water—
Shrinkingly broached. And, as the brief snail-trace

Of her withdrawal dries upon our faces
The silence drums into her upturned face.

ANGEL

Above my desk, whirring and self-important
(Though not much larger than a hummingbird)
In finely woven robes, school of Van Eyck,
Hovers an evidently angelic visitor.
He points one index finger out the window
At winter snatching to its heart,
To crystal vacancy, the misty
Exhalations of houses and of people running home
From the cold sun pounding on the sea;
While with the other hand
He indicates the piano
Where the Sarabande No. 1 lies open
At a passage I shall never master
But which has already, and effortlessly, mastered me.
He drops his jaw as if to say, or sing,
'Between the world God made
And this music of Satie,
Each glimpsed through veils, but whole,
Radiant and willed,
Demanding praise, demanding surrender,
How can you sit there with your notebook?
What do you think you are doing?'
However he says nothing—wisely: I could mention
Flaws in God's world, or Satie's; and for that matter
How did he come by *his* taste for Satie?
Half to tease him, I turn back to my page,
Its phrases thus far clotted, unconnected.
The tiny angel shakes his head.
There is no smile on his round, hairless face.
He does not want even these few lines written.

TO A BUTTERFLY

Already in midsummer
I miss your feet and fur.
Poor simple creature that you were,
What have you become!

Your slender person curled
About an apple twig
Rebounding to the winds' clear jig
Gave up the world

In favor of obscene
Gray matter, rode that ark
Until (as at the chance remark
Of Father Sheen)

Shining awake to slough
Your old life. And soon four
Dapper stained glass windows bore
You up—ENOUGH.

Goodness, how tired one grows
Just looking through a prism:
Allegory, symbolism.
I've tried, Lord knows,

To keep from seeing double,
Blushed for whenever I did,
Prayed like a boy my cheek be hid
By manly stubble.

43

I caught you in a net
And first pierced your disguise
How many years ago? Time flies,
I am not yet

Proof against rigmarole.
Those frail wings, those antennae!
The day you hover without any
Tincture of soul,

Red monarch, swallowtail,
Will be the day my own
Wiles gather dust. Each will have flown
The other's jail.

THE PARROT FISH

The shadow of the little fishing launch
Discreetly, inch by inch,
Crept after us on its belly over
The reef's uneven floor.

The motor gasped out drowsy vapor.
Seconds went by before
Anyone thought to interpret
The jingling of Inez's bracelet.

Chalk-violet, olive, all veils and sequins, a
Priestess out of the next Old Testament extravaganza,
With round gold eyes and minuscule buck-teeth,
Up flaunted into death

The parrot fish. And for a full hour beat
Irregular, passionate
Tattoos from its casket lined with zinc.
Finally we understood, I think.

Ashore, the warm waves licked our feet.
One or two heavy chords the heat
Struck, set the white beach vibrating.
And throwing back its head the sea began to sing.

When our son died
We cured his little frame,
Scoured, pickled, overlaid head to toe
The ultimate forged antique
With augmentingly non-literal translations
Into gold, of the boy, into alabaster,
His face's full moon setting
Beneath an earth chewed bare by beetles,
And all at length, with tutors and possessions
Packed into a gold—into *four* gold
Garages at the heart
Of four three-sided glassy slopes
Upheaved through layers of blue and yellow gas.
The gods our cousins were reduced
To looking on, bird-eyed or jackal-eyed,
His guests who had been theirs.
My sister and I stood
As we stand now, in red
Granite, chins high, fists drugged
Upon symbols of rank. We must
Apparently have felt
Shock of a sort. We are shown taking
A rigid backward step
Into this world of giant papyrus-sheaves,
Sunwashed, pitted with inventory.
It was 'the dawn of history.'
Do not judge us unkindly, friend
Whose heart still beats and bleeds.
States noway known till we induced them
Propel one bride and groom, your autumn night,
Into the living area

Of a first apartment. Openarmed,
Goat-footed chairs the worm has drilled,
A quarter year been traded to possess,
In the bronze glow of missiles become lamps
Receive the pair. His cup
Poured, sweetened, her small voice goes on:
Each day should be *composed*,
Should have 'shape' and 'texture'—living was an art!...
He nods, on fire. Back of her fair young face
Is hung her other, her unchanging face
Launched free of earth between sun-whitened waves.
Her slaves, his senses, rend their clothing.
Eyes she will never look through look through him
To chill themselves in a transparence
On whose far side, all night
Enthralled, press wings, press tiny wings.
Illumined therefore unbudging, we rule here.
Exerting no pressure. Only
When stones he gave her, that will cost one year,
Glitter, glittering back.
Too late the ritual of blinds.
Both now, as all before them, have seen us—grown
Taller than buildings, masked in magnets,
Traffic of stars, the myriad needles plunged
Green into that arterial heaven
Our loss, which is your gain.

THE SMILE

It was going to rain.
Beneath his scalp
The silver ached. He got
With no one's help
To his feet. A cane
Steadied him up the stair.

It was warm there
On the sleeping porch.
His jacket hung
Over a chair would not
Let go his form.
He placed his round gold watch,

Unwound, among
Dimes, quarters, lunatic change . . .
He woke in bed,
Missing his spectacles.
He felt the strange
Palms laid on his forehead.

Then he heard other palms
Rattling in wind.
More time passed. He had dreams.
In one, rain fell
And fell, and when
The sun rose near at hand

Stood his life gleaming full.
The bubble-beaded
Tumbler magnified

A false and grinning friend
No longer needed.
He turned his face and died.

SWIMMING BY NIGHT

A light going out in the forehead
Of the house by the ocean,
Into warm black its feints of diamond fade.
Without clothes, without caution

Plunging past gravity—
Wait! Where before
Had been floating nothing, is a gradual body
Half remembered, astral with phosphor,

Yours, risen from its tomb
In your own mind,
Haunting nimbleness, glimmerings a random
Spell had kindled. So that, new-limned

By this weak lamp
The evening's alcohol will feed
Until the genie chilling bids you limp
Heavily over stones to bed,

You wear your master's robe
One last time, the far break
Of waves, their length and sparkle, the spinning globe
You wear, and the star running down his cheek.

A TENANCY

Something in the light of this March afternoon
Recalls that first and dazzling one
Of 1946. I sat elated
In my old clothes, in the first of several
Furnished rooms, head cocked for the kind of sound
That is recognized only when heard.
A fresh snowfall muffled the road, unplowed
To leave blanker and brighter
The bright, blank page turned overnight.

A yellow pencil in midair
Kept sketching unfamiliar numerals,
The 9 and 6 forming a stereoscope
Through which to seize the Real
Old-Fashioned Winter of my landlord's phrase,
Through which the ponderous *idées reçues*
Of oak, velour, crochet, also the mantel's
Baby figures, value told me
In some detail at the outset, might be plumbed
For signs I should not know until I saw them.

But the objects, innocent
(As we all once were) of annual depreciation,
The more I looked grew shallower,
Pined under a luminous plaid robe
Thrown over us by the twin mullions, sashes,
And unequal oblong panes
Of windows and storm windows. These,
Washed in a rage, then left to dry unpolished,
Projected onto the inmost wall
Ghosts of the storm, like pebbles under water.

And indeed, from within, ripples
Of heat had begun visibly bearing up and away
The bouquets and wreathes of a quarter century.
Let them go, what did I want with them?
It was time to change that wallpaper!
Brittle, sallow in the new radiance,
Time to set the last wreath floating out
Above the dead, to sweep up flowers. The dance
Had ended, it was light; the men looked tired
And awkward in their uniforms.
I sat, head thrown back, and with the dried stains
Of light on my own cheeks, proposed
This bargain with—say with the source of light:
That given a few years more
(Seven or ten or, what seemed vast, fifteen)
To spend in love, in a country not at war,
I would give in return
All I had. All? A little sun
Rose in my throat. The lease was drawn.

I did not even feel the time expire.

I feel it though, today, in this new room,
Mine, with my things and thoughts, a view
Of housetops, treetops, the walls bare.
A changing light is deepening, is changing
To a gilt ballroom chair a chair
Bound to break under someone before long.
I let the light change also me.
The body that lived through that day
And the sufficient love and relative peace

Of those short years, is now not mine.
Would it be called a soul?
It knows, at any rate,
That when the light dies and the bell rings
Its leaner veteran will rise to face
Partners not recognized
Until drunk young again and gowned in changing
Flushes; and strains will rise,
The bone-tipped baton beating, rapid, faint,
From the street below, from my depressions—

From the doorbell which rings.
One foot asleep, I hop
To let my three friends in. They stamp
Themselves free of the spring's
Last snow—or so we hope.

One has brought violets in a pot;
The second, wine; the best,
His open, empty hand. Now in the room
The sun is shining like a lamp.
I put the flowers where I need them most

And then, not asking why they come,
Invite the visitors to sit.
If I am host at last
It is of little more than my own past.
May others be at home in it.

JAMES MERRILL

James Merrill was born in New York in 1926. He
lives in Stonington, Connecticut, but spends part of
the year traveling. He is the author of two earlier
books of poems, *First Poems* (1951), and *The Country of
a Thousand Years of Peace* (1959); a novel, *The Seraglio*
(1957); and two plays, *The Immortal Husband* (given
an off-Broadway production in 1955 and published
the following year in *Playbook*) and, in one act,
The Bait, published in *Artists' Theatre* (1960).